TOPICS IN PREVALENT DISEASES: A MINORITY'S PERSPECTIVE

TOPICS IN PREVALENT DISEASES: A MINORITY'S PERSPECTIVE

NORBERTO C. CHAVEZ-TAPIA
AND MISAEL URIBE
EDITORS

Nova Biomedical Books
New York

For permission to use material from this book please contact us:
Telephone 631-231-7269; Fax 631-231-8175
Web Site: http://www.novapublishers.com

Library of Congress Cataloging-in-Publication Data

Topics in prevalent diseases : a minority's perspective / [edited by] Norberto C. Chavez-Tapia and Misael Uribe.
p.; cm.
Includes bibliographical references and index.
ISBN 978-1-60456-959-9 (hardcover)
1. Minorities--Medical care. 2. Minorities--Diseases. I. Chavez-Tapia, Norberto C. II. Uribe, Misael.
[DNLM: 1. Minority Health. 2. Healthcare Disparities. WA 300.1 T674 2008]
RA563.M56T67 2008
362.1089--dc22

2008032766

Published by Nova Science Publishers, Inc. ; New York

Contents

Preface		**vii**
Chapter 1	Introduction *Norberto C. Chavez-Tapia and Misael Uribe*	**1**
Chapter 2	Prostate Cancer in Minorities *Takashi Kobayashi, Osamu Ogawa and Toshiyuki Kamoto*	**5**
Chapter 3	Colorectal Cancer in Minorities *Sandra Garcia Osogobio and Félix Ignacio Téllez Ávila*	**31**
Chapter 4	Acquired Immune Deficiency Syndrome in Minorities *Karina F. Zihlmann and Jorge Casseb*	**47**
Chapter 5	Ischemic Heart Disease in Minorities *Fernando Lanas and Pamela Serón*	**63**
Chapter 6	Stroke in Minorities *Fahmi Yousef Khan*	**85**
Chapter 7	Ethnicity and the Metabolic Syndrome *Roopa Mehta and Carlos A. Aguilar-Salinas*	**95**
Chapter 8	Prevalence of Diabetes: An International Perspective *Hamid R Baradaran and Mohammad E. Khamseh*	**113**
Chapter 9	Hypercholesterolemia in Minorities *Carlos J. Rodriguez and Juan C. Brenes*	**125**
Chapter 10	Involuntary Exposure to Environmental Tobacco Smoke in Vulnerable Groups *Tonatiuh Barrientos-Gutiérrez and David Gimeno Ruiz de Porras*	**137**
Chapter 11	Tuberculosis in Minorities *Ahmet Emin Erbaycu*	**163**
Chapter 12	Parasitic Diseases of Infants *B.R. Mirdha and Nishat Ahmad*	**177**

Chapter 13 Gastrointestinal Viral Infections in Children **225**
Gabriel Ignacio Parra, Karin Bok and José Paulo Gagliardi Leite

Chapter 14 Asthma among Rural Bangladeshi Children: Prevalence and Risk Factors **253**
K. Zaman, Haruko Takeuchi and Shams El Arifeen

Chapter 15 Maternal Mortality in Minorities **259**
Abha Aggarwal, Arvind Pandey, Rohini Sehgal and Suneeta Mittal

Chapter 16 Depression in Minorities **279**
Asae Oura and Mitsuru Mori

Chapter 17 Osteoporosis in Minorities **287**
Marta Pentek, Ildiko Kaposi, Laszlo Gulacsi and Gyula Poor

Chapter 18 Road Traffic Crashes and Injury Prevention among Racial/Ethnic Minorities in the United States **303**
Paul D. Juarez

Index **333**

Preface

This book is a new, exciting editorial project designed to provide high-quality information about the most important worldwide diseases affecting minorities groups. Information on this topic is commonly diffuse and not always highlighted. Consequently, preventive, diagnostic, and treatment issues could differ from classical (most cited) information. This is a classical text for those practitioners or researchers who have interest about medical troubles in the most numerous groups of patients (all minorities). In this book you will find scientific data regarding the most imperative diseases worldwide derived from miniority groups. Taking into consideration the information in this book you may be able to analyze with a critical and constructive view the standard of care in prevalent diseases. Additionally, this could be a great opportunity for researchers to identify limitations in the available information and in the future help to solve these restrictions.

In: Topics in Prevalent Diseases
Editors: N. C. Chavez-Tapia and M. Uribe
ISBN 978-1-60456-959-9

Chapter 1

Introduction

Norberto C. Chavez-Tapia and Misael Uribe
Department of Gastroenterology, Instituto Nacional de Ciencias Medicas y Nutrición Salvador Zubirán, Mexico City, México

There is no universally accepted definition of "minorities", and the word is interpreted differently in different societies. The United Nations (UN) has failed to reach consensus in a definition of what constitutes a minority, beyond what is implied in the title of the UN Declaration on the Rights of Persons belonging to National or Ethnic, Religious and Linguistic Minorities. Attempting a more precise statement has been fraught with difficulties, as the motivation for a tighter definition has been often to deny certain rights to specific groups of people. The Minority Rights Group International defines "minorities" as those subjects belonging to a non-dominant ethnic, religious or linguistic community, who may not necessarily be numerical minorities [1].

Usually minorities experience several inequalities and, although some of them are diminishing, opportunities for improvement can still be found. In the health field, several measures for improvement can be identified, such as preventive services, treatment of acute illness, management of chronic disease and disability, timeliness, and patient centeredness [2]. As demonstrated by extensive research and confirmed by previous National Healthcare Disparities Reports, racial and ethnic minorities, as well as people from low socioeconomic statuses, are disproportionately represented in scientific studies and trials [3].

Obviously, to reach significant improvement on health issues, it is necessary to expand the research topics to these groups, thus, generating information useful to improve the quality of life of these persons.

The participation of racial/ethnic minorities and other underrepresented groups in clinical trials is a critical link between scientific innovation and improvements in healthcare delivery and health. Since 1993, the National Institutes of Health requires that all sponsored research, including cancer-related trials, ensure the inclusion of women and members of minority groups. Between 1993 and 2002, the budget of the National Cancer Institute (NCI) doubled, and clinical trial accrual increased. Nevertheless, only 2.5% of cancer patients are enrolled into trials, being African-American men, Latinos/Hispanics, Asian and Pacific Islanders, American Indians/Alaska Natives, adolescents, elder adults, individuals who reside in rural areas, and individuals of low socioeconomic status underrepresented among participants. Most publications reporting the results from cancer clinical trials do not describe participants' race or ethnicity. Lack of diversity in randomized study populations reduces opportunities for discovering effects that may be particularly relevant to underrepresented populations, and contributes to inequitable distribution of benefits and risks of trial participation. Age, gender, race, socioeconomic status, comorbidities, and disease severity are still common ground for misrepresentation of important population groups in clinical trials [5].

Previous research has found racial disparities in the delivery of quality health care. Many explanations for these differences have been offered, including the possibility that providers' attitudes about individuals of certain racial or ethnic backgrounds are associated with differences in care. Such stereotyping may result from the complex decisions faced by healthcare providers, which can have negative consequences. Very little, however, is known about how stereotypes are incorporated into clinical decision-making. Clinicians' practices regarding substance use may be a useful venue to examine the processes that give rise to racially disparate treatment. Illicit drug use is stigmatizing and is often linked to racial minorities, even though epidemiologic evidence does not suggest that rates of substance use among minority women are higher than those of White women [6].

Participation of minorities in public affairs, such as research, is essential to their sense of identity, being crucial to the development of a sense of belonging to a wider community. Also, participation is a fundamental way to assure minorities' well-being protection, building channels of communication with the society at large, allowing a better collective decision-making and implementation of public policies [7].

In this book we present a general overview about existing gaps in world-wide health care, discussing the most important causes of death and disease from an international perspective. This effort is not exhaustive and only represents a small piece of this complex puzzle. However, the contribution of each author is in accordance with the responsibility to divulge and promote information related to minorities' health.

References

[1] MRG. State of the World's Minorities 2008. In: Matheson I, ed.: Minority Rights Group International 2008.

[2] Key Themes and Highlights from the National Healthcare Disparities Report. Rockville: Agency for Healthcare Research and Quality 2007.

[3] National Healthcare Disparities Report. Rockville: Agency for Healthcare Research and Quality 2006.

[4] Du W, Gadgeel SM, Simon MS. Predictors of enrollment in lung cancer clinical trials. *Cancer* 2006;106:420-5.

[5] Mosenifar Z. Population issues in clinical trials. *Proceedings of the American Thoracic Society* 2007;4:185-7; discussion 7-8.

[6] Kirk JK, Graves DE, Bell RA, *et al.* Racial and ethnic disparities in self-monitoring of blood glucose among US adults: a qualitative review. *Ethnicity & disease* 2007;17:135-42.

[7] MRG. Public Participation and Minorities. In: Ghai Y, ed.: Minority Rights Group International 2003.

In: Topics in Prevalent Diseases
Editors: N. C. Chavez-Tapia and M. Uribe
ISBN 978-1-60456-959-9

Chapter 2

Prostate Cancer in Minorities

Takashi Kobayashi, Osamu Ogawa and Toshiyuki Kamoto
Department of Urology, Kyoto University Graduate School of Medicine
54 Shogoinkawahara-cho, Sakyo-ku, Kyoto 606-8507, Japan

Introduction

Prostate cancer (CaP) is a disease of older men. Although autopsy series have revealed small CaP in up to 29% of men aged 30–40 years [1], clinical manifestations of the disease are generally observed in men aged >50 years. The main tumor is located in the peripheral zone of the prostate gland in 85% of non-palpable CaP cases, and the high frequency of CaP located in the peripheral zone allows some cancers to be detected by digital rectal examination (DRE). Before the advent of the serum tumor marker prostate-specific antigen (PSA) in the late 1980s to early 1990s, a number of CaPs were diagnosed by clinical manifestation, for example, abnormal DRE findings or bone metastasis. Currently, in the PSA era, a large majority of CaPs are detected by abnormal PSA and the incidence of locoregional disease has increased, whereas the incidence of metastatic disease has decreased.[2] Most CaPs are diagnosed by fine needle biopsy by a transrectal or transperineal approach, under transrectal ultrasonography imaging, while some other CaPs are detected incidentally by histopathological examination, after transurethral prostatectomy for the treatment of benign prostatic hypertrophy. Although PSA is a very useful tumor marker, which reflects the extent of disease in most cases, its diagnostic sensitivity and specificity for CaP are not satisfactorily high if the conventional cutoff value of >4.0 ng/ml is used. The incidence of detectable CaP in men with PSA levels of 2.0–4.0 ng/ml is reported to be 23.6–26.9%.[3, 4] Lowering the cutoff of PSA may allow detection of more CaPs, although it may increase the detection of clinically indolent cancers that have no influence on life expectancy. A number of studies have been conducted to determine truly effective methods for the detection of clinically significant CaP.

Definitive diagnosis of CaP is usually made by pathological examination of biopsy specimens. Most CaPs are classified as adenocarcinoma, and diagnosis of prostate adenocarcinoma requires both cellular atypia and abnormal architecture of prostatic acini or ducts. Lesions with architecturally normal prostatic acini or ducts, lined by cytologically atypical cells, are defined as prostatic intraepithelial neoplasia (PIN), and high-grade PIN is considered as a precursor of prostate adenocarcinoma. The most frequently used histological grading of prostate adenocarcinoma is the Gleason grading system, which is based on the glandular pattern of the tumor, as identified at relatively low magnification, without considering cytological features.[5] Gleason scores of 1 (the most differentiated) to 5 (the least differentiated) are assigned to the two most prevalent architectural patterns. Gleason sum is the sum of the two Gleason scores and ranges from 2 to 10, and generally, a Gleason sum of ≥ 7 indicates more aggressive disease. Disease stage is defined by the American Joint Committee for Cancer Staging and End Results Reporting tumor-node-metastasis (TNM) criteria.[6] Gleason grade and serum PSA level are useful for the prediction of TNM disease stage, and TNM criteria are helpful for estimating disease prognosis and consequent decision-making for reasonable treatment options.

Treatment for CaP comprises radical surgery, radiotherapy, cryotherapy, androgen-deprivation therapy (ADT) and chemotherapy. The first three are primarily definitive therapies, which are indicated for localized CaP, with curative intent. In radical surgery for CaP, the whole prostate gland is removed concomitantly with both seminal vesicles. Radical prostatectomy (RP) is classified into retropubic (RRP), laparoscopic (LRP) and perineal (PRP) prostatectomy, according to surgical approach. Radiotherapy includes external beam radiation (EBR), and brachytherapy with intracorporeal seeding of irradiating agents. In some cases, RP and EBR are selected as salvage treatment for relapsed disease after other definitive local therapies. Although ADT and chemotherapy are systemic, the former is sometimes selected for patients with localized CaP. The current standard first-line treatment option for metastatic CaP is ADT, and chemotherapy is one of the limited treatment options for hormone-refractory prostate cancer (HRPC).

Generally, survival rates of localized CaP treated appropriately are very good, irrespective of treatment options selected and some investigators have reported 5–10-year relapse-free survival of >90%.[7, 8] Therefore, the question of treatment-induced disturbance of quality of life (QOL) should be discussed in selecting treatment strategy for localized CaP. All therapeutic modalities can cause some treatment-induced morbidity, including urinary dysfunction, erectile dysfunction, rectal injury, general loss of muscle strength and osteoporosis. Compared to the life expectancy of patients with localized CaP, survival rates of metastatic CaP are poor. The most frequent primary metastatic sites of CaP are regional lymph nodes and bones. In these cases, surgery and radiotherapy are no longer effective, although some cases need them as a palliative treatment to control local symptoms; transurethral resection or irradiation of the prostate for bladder outlet obstruction, and bone irradiation for metastatic pain. Even in such metastatic diseases, tumor growth is initially androgen dependent and ADT results in regression of androgen-dependent tumors, as reported by Huggins over 30 years ago.[9] However, many men eventually fail this therapy and die of HRPC. At present, there are limited effective therapies for HRPC.[10]

As described above, there remains much about prostate cancer to be elucidated at the clinical and basic levels, and detailed discussion on each issue is beyond the scope of this article. Whatever we discuss regarding CaP, we must remember that there are some racial/ethnic and regional differences in the nature of this disease.[11] These differences involve epidemiology, biological features, diagnosis and treatment, and socioeconomic factors, and this article focuses on discussion and exploration of these issues.

Epidemiology

Worldwide, CaP is the fourth most common male malignant neoplasm. The incidence of CaP varies more than 100-fold across the regions and among the various racial/ethnic populations. Based on data from the Surveillance Epidemiology and End Results (SEER) program, a nationwide population-based cancer registry system, the overall incidence of CaP in the United States between 2000 and 2004 was 168.0 per 100,000 persons (Table 1)[12], and it is the most commonly diagnosed cancer in men in that country. The same is true in men in Canada, Australia, Israel and South America.[13] In Europe, CaP is one of the five most commonly diagnosed cancers, whereas it is the sixth to tenth most common cancer in Asia. In Japanese men, CaP is the sixth most commonly diagnosed cancer, and its incidence between 1998 and 2000 was 21.7 per 100,000 persons (Table 1). This incidence is considerably less than that in North and South America and Europe, but higher than in other Asian countries, where CaP incidence is the lowest in the world. Rates of CaP in African countries were thought to be much the same as those in Asia. However, it seemed to be affected by access to and quality of health care, accuracy of cancer registries, and dissemination of PSA screening. As reliable data are accumulated, it has been shown that CaP is one of the most common cancer among men in Uganda [14] and Nigeria.[15, 16]

In the United States, African American men have the highest incidence, followed by Caucasian, Hispanic, Asian/Pacific Islander and American Indian/Alaskan Native people (Table 1). The difference among racial/ethnic groups living in the same country indicates that genetic background has some influence on the incidence of CaP. On the other hand, there are some indications that environment plays an important role in modulating CaP risk around the world.

Table 1. Incidence and mortality rates of prostate cancer by race

Race/Ethnicity	Age-adjusted incidence rates (per 100,000)	Age-adjusted death rates (per 100,000)	Mortality (%)
United States [12]			
Overall	168.0	27.9	16.6
White	161.4	25.6	15.9
Black	255.5	62.3	24.4
Asian/Pacific Islander	96.5	11.3	11.7
American Indian/Alaska Native	68.2	21.5	31.5
Hispanic	140.8	21.2	15.1
Japan [22]			
Japanese	21.7	8.5	39.1

One of the most prominent susceptibility factors is a Western lifestyle, especially a diet that includes a high intake of fat, meat and dairy products. Japanese and Chinese men in the United States have a higher risk for development of CaP than their relatives in Japan and China. [17, 18] The incidence of CaP in Uganda and Zimbabwe is still lower compared to that in African American men in the United States,[19] although it has been revealed to be more common than previously expected. The recent rapid increase in CaP incidence in Japan is supposed to be caused by westernization of lifestyles.[20] The evidence collectively indicates that both genetic and environmental background play an important role in determining CaP predisposition. When we consider the highest CaP incidence of 255.5 per 100,000 African American men in the United States, it appears most likely that the black race and westernized lifestyle have the strongest impact on CaP risk.

CaP mortality also varies widely between countries and racial/ethnic populations. It is highest in North American and North European countries, and is approximately as high as 20 per 100,000 persons, [21] and the second leading cause of cancer death. It is as low as <5 per 100,000 in Asian countries, except Japan, where the age-adjusted death rate was 8.5 per 100,000 in 1999, and CaP is the seventh leading cause of cancer death. [22] In the United States, age-adjusted CaP-related mortality is 2.4 times higher for African Americans than for Caucasians (Table 1). This difference in mortality rate is still observed when adjusted with disease incidence (Table 1). Recent research based on health care insurance data has demonstrated a 1.8-year shorter survival for African Americans with localized CaP treated with RP, 0.7 years shorter after radiotherapy, and 1 year in those choosing active surveillance, even after adjustment for other covariates, including education and income levels.[23] (See also "Treatment" section)

These findings strongly suggest that genetic structure and function play an important role in modulating biological features of CaP, as well as its carcinogenesis. In addition, there is evidence that diet and lifestyle are also responsible for CaP mortality. Ornish and colleagues [24] have randomized known early non-aggressive CaP patients into two groups: an experimental group who changed their lifestyle to a vegan diet and moderate aerobic exercise, and a control group without any intervention. In the 12 months after diagnosis, serum PSA decreased by 4% in the experimental group, whereas it increased by 6% in the control group. In addition, growth of androgen-dependent human prostate cancer LNCaP cells was inhibited almost eight times more by serum from the experimental than from the control group. Ngo and colleagues have demonstrated, using a mouse xenograft model, that a high-fat Western diet resulted in a shorter time to hormone resistance and shorter survival.[25] With regard to high fat intake, there have been some reports that higher incidence of obesity in African Americans is associated with CaP incidence and aggressiveness.[26-29] It should be noted, however, that there is no definitive evidence for a direct association between obesity and CaP incidence and progression.[30]

Results of these studies have suggested that Japanese lifestyle inhibits progression of CaP. In this regard, an autopsy series has shown that the incidence of latent CaP is not so different between Japanese men in Japan and the United States.[31, 32] Another study has clarified that the prevalence of microscopic or latent prostate tumors is similar in most populations, [33] although clinical prostate cancer incidence and death rate are markedly different in diverse geographic regions and among various racial/ethnic groups. These findings collectively indicate that some environmental factors affect at least progression of CaP to clinically significant disease after CaP carcinogenesis.

Genetics and Biology

Epidemiological data clearly show the difference in incidence and mortality of CaP between countries and racial/ethnic groups around the world. There is cumulative evidence that may explain these differences genetically and biologically. Determining genetic variants that indisputably affect CaP risk and explain racial/ethnic disparities has been challenging. Although a number of regions have been linked to CaP, few have been consistently replicated across different studies and populations. [34, 35] Recent genome-wide linkage studies have detected overlapping signals for CaP on chromosome 8q24, and have found that relatively common variants are strongly associated with CaP risk. [36, 37] In addition, more recent studies have found three neighboring regions within a 600-kb segment of 8q24 that independently harbor variants associated with CaP risk, [38-40] and importantly, the risk alleles are more common among African Americans.[39, 40] Although the individual associations of the 8q24 variants with CaP are relatively modest (odds ratio <2.0), a combination of multiple variants shows considerably larger associations. The results of these studies are important in that racial/ethnic variance in CaP incidence may be explained by the specific genetic variances.

The chromosomal region of 8q24 is considered to be associated with CaP risk. [41] It is one of the most commonly amplified regions [42] and well known to contain copy number variants [43, 44] in prostate tumors. The biological mechanisms underlying these findings that the multiple variants independently contribute to CaP risks remain unclear. None of the variants seems to be functional and is located within or near known genes. Although it is well known that 8q24 contains a proto-oncogene *MYC*, which is considered to be associated with CaP carcinogenesis, [45] some of the associated variants do not seem to affect *MYC* expression. [38] In addition to their epidemiological significance, there are several implications derived from these findings, which contribute to public health and clinical management of CaP. Pre-diagnostic risk assessment based on associated variants is of benefit to CaP mass screening. Precise understanding of the biological mechanisms would enable us to prevent and treat CaP by modulating these mechanisms. Therefore, substantial efforts will need to be focused on this issue, and important evidence will be rapidly accumulated, and consequently, the genetic basis for the racial/ethnic variance may be clarified.

Many researchers have attempted to explain racial/ethnic and geographical differences in CaP incidence and mortality in relation to androgens and associated molecules. It has been reported that serum total and free testosterone levels are higher in African Americans than in whites, [46] whereas another study has demonstrated no significant differences in androgens and sex hormone-binding globulins between African Americans and whites.[47] The longitudinal Physicians' Health Study has demonstrated a positive correlation between plasma testosterone levels and CaP risk.[48] However, other longitudinal and case-control studies have found no association of CaP risk with androgens and sex hormone-biding proteins.[47, 49-52]

5α-reductase is the enzyme that converts testosterone to dihydrotestosterone (DHT), which has a greater ligand activity on the androgen receptor. The difference in 5α-reductase activity that affects DHT-to-testosterone ratio may also explain the higher CaP incidence in African Americans and whites than in Japanese subjects. [47, 53] A variety of polymorphisms have been detected in *SRD5A2*, a 5α-reductase-coding gene, and have been reported to be associated with racial differences in CaP risk.[54] A polymorphism in the *CYP3A4* gene, which codes for a cytochrome enzyme involved oxidative degradation of testosterone, has also been reported to be associated with CaP risk.[55] A trinucleotide (CAG) repeat polymorphism in exon 1 of androgen receptor gene is thought to modify its transcriptional activity; the shorter the repeat, the higher the transcriptional activity. Numerous studies have identified that a shortened CAG repeat length is associated with increased incidence as well as development of advanced, hormone-refractory disease.[56, 57] Sartor and colleagues have reported that CAG repeat length in African Americans is significantly shorter than that in whites.[58]

Insulin-like growth factor-I (IGF-1) stimulates cell proliferation, decreases apoptosis, and has been implicated in cancer development.[59, 60] Some investigators have reported that higher plasma levels of IGF-1 are associated with an increased risk of CaP, in longitudinal [61, 62] and case-control [63, 64] studies. IGF-binding protein 3 (IGFBP-3) is a carrier protein that modulates the effect of IGF-1 by preventing binding of the hormones to IGF or insulin receptors, through high-affinity coupling [59, 60] Lower plasma levels of IGFBP-3 have been reported to be associated with an increased risk of colorectal cancer, [65, 66] although some studies have shown no direct association between IGFBP-3 and CaP. [61, 62, 67] There have been a number of studies on racial/ethnic differences in plasma concentration of IGF-1 and IGFBP-3. Some have shown that IGF-1 levels are rather lower in African Americans than in whites, [68, 69]and others have found no significant difference between the two ethnicities. [67, 70] Plasma IGFBP-3 levels have been reported to be lower in African Americans than in whites.[67-70]

Although some investigators have claimed the importance of IGF-1/IGFBP-3 ratio as an indicator of IGF-1 bioavailability, results have been inconsistent. McGreevy and colleagues have reported a higher IGF-1-to-IGFBP-3 ratio in African Americans than in whites, [68] whereas no significant difference was observed in the study by Platz and colleagues.[69] It has been reported that plasma levels of IGF and associated parameters can be influenced by some nutritional factors. According to another recent cross-sectional study by McGreevy and colleagues, intake of total, saturated and non-saturated fats is positively associated with the IGF-1-to-IGFBP-3 molar ratio in whites but not in African Americans.[71] Intake of calcium and dairy products is positively associated with IGF-1 levels and increased vegetable intake is positively associated with IGFBP-3 levels in African Americans but not in whites. The results indicate that the impact of nutrients on IGF and IGFBP levels is different in African Americans and whites.

Besides the plasma concentrations, genetic variation in IGF-1 and IGFBP-3 has been studied to elucidate possible explanations for racial/ethnic difference in biological features of CaP. There is a cytosine-adenine $(CA)_{19}$ repeat polymorphism located upstream of the gene's transcription start site, which is associated with lower plasma concentration [72, 73] and consequent possible decrease in CaP risk. Schildkraut and colleagues have found that carrying homozygous $(CA)_{19}$ alleles is inversely associated with CaP risk in African Americans (OR, 0.2; 95% CI, 0.0–0.8). [74] A similar association has been found in white men (OR, 0.4; 95% CI, 0.1–1.6). Importantly, the prevalence of the homozygous IGF-1 $(CA)_{19}$ genotype is significantly lower in African American than in white controls. Another case-control study by Chen and colleagues has shown inconsistent results, in that there was no significant association between the number of CA repeats in IGF-1 genotype and plasma levels of IGF-1 or CaP risk. [75] A similar significantly lower prevalence of the homozygous IGF-1 $(CA)_{19}$ genotype in African American compared to white controls was reported in this study. This polymorphism has also been shown to affect the prognosis of CaP. According to a case-control study on Japanese men, the longer allele (over 18 [CA] repeats) was significantly associated with worse prognosis of metastatic CaP. [76] With regard to other polymorphism in IGF-1 gene, a recent report on 2320 patients and 2290 control subjects from the Multiethnic Cohort Study has shown that certain single nucleotide polymorphisms (SNPs) and haplotypes, characterized by genotyping 64 SNPs that span 156 kb around the IGF-1 gene, are associated with CaP risk. [77]

The A allele of the IGFBP-3 –202A/C promoter region polymorphism has been reported to be associated with higher plasma levels of IGFBP-3. [78, 79] However, some investigators have reported that no significant association is found between genotype and CaP risk in either African Americans or whites. Although similar negative results about IGFBP-3 –202 A/C polymorphisms and susceptibility to CaP have been reported for a Japanese population, the presence of the C allele was significantly associated with higher grade and more advanced stage of the disease. [80] Interestingly, C allele frequency for Japanese controls reported in this study was 30%, [80] which seems much lower than that for African Americans (46–50%) or whites (55–59%) reported in Western case–control studies.[78, 79]

It seems very complicated to interpret and apply the accumulated knowledge for the prevention of CaP in multiethnic populations. Collectively, although variation in plasma levels and genetic polymorphisms of IGF-1 may play a role in the risk of CaP, they do not seem to account for the racial difference in CaP incidence. The same holds true for IGFBP-3, while its genetic variation may contribute to the racial difference in biological aggressiveness of CaP.

There are some genes whose genetic polymorphisms have been reported to be associated with CaP risk. Polymorphisms of the vitamin D receptor (VDR) gene, which may play an inhibitory role in the development and progression of CaP, has been found to be associated with CaP risk in African Americans but not in whites.[81, 82] Another study has suggested that VDR polymorphism was associated with CaP risk in a Japanese population.[83] Since these three reports have investigated different polymorphisms within the VDR gene, comprehensive analysis for a multiethnic cohort is warranted. E-cadherin (CDH-1) gene may play a role in tumor initiation and progression, and the A allele in the –160 C/A polymorphism has been reported to be associated with CaP in whites but not in African Americans.[84] In a Japanese population, a similar association of the A allele with increased CaP risk has been reported,[85] whereas no significant association was found in another study in a Japanese population.[86] Since the prevalence of the A/A genotype is similar between ethnic groups, the CDH-1 polymorphism does not seem to contribute to racial differences in CaP incidence. However, the prevalence of the A/A genotype is very low (0.0–

3.6%) in every ethnic group, and therefore, large scale studies with substantial statistical power are warranted in the future. There have been numerous reports on the association between CaP risk and genetic polymorphisms in various genes, including XRCC1,[87] APE1,[87] UGT2B17, [88] FHIT,[89] BRCA1 [90] and SOD2.[91] It is interesting that the impact of these polymorphisms on CaP risk differs between ethnic groups; a significant association was only found in whites for the polymorphisms of XRCC1,[87] APE1,[87] UGT2B17[88] and SOD2.[91]

Selenium is a chemical element of the sulfur group and is essential to the functioning of several enzymes, including the antioxidant enzyme glutathione peroxidase. The organic form of selenium is contained in a variety of foods and there is marked geographical variation of selenium in foods, related to local soil content. Geographical studies have shown an inverse relationship between environmental selenium levels and cancer incidence and mortality.[92, 93] As Klein [94] and Moyad [95] have reviewed , both case-control and randomized placebo-controlled trials in humans have also suggested that selenium can decrease the risk for development of CaP. In addition, selenium inhibits tumorigenesis in a variety of experimental models, and a number of potential mechanisms have been proposed for its antitumorigenic effects. [94] Therefore, selenium is considered to be one of the potential effective agents for chemoprevention of CaP. Vogt and colleagues have found that serum selenium concentrations in African Americans are 6% lower than those in whites.[96] This significant difference remains after adjustment for known selenium predictors, including a proxy for geographical variation, although it was reduced to about 3%.

In addition to selenium intake, numerous dietary factors seem responsible for the racial/ethnic disparity in CaP incidence and mortality as we have already discussed in "Epidemiology" section. Interestingly, there seem to be some genetic disparities that affect CaP incidence and mortality not only directly as described above, but also indirectly by modulating the sensitivity to environmental risk factors for CaP. Soybean isoflavones (genistein, daidzein and equol) have been suggested to have suppressive effect on prostate cancer.[97] It has been also reported that some individuals are able to degrade daidzein into equol and others are not, and that equol producers are associated with lower CaP risk.[98] A case-control study [99] revealed that rates of equol producer were significantly lower in Japanese (29%) and Korean (30%) CaP patient groups than those in control groups (46 and 59%, respectively). This trend was not observed in US residents (unfortunately unconfirmed race); rate of equol producer was 17 and 14% for patients and controls, respectively. These findings suggest that effect of some chemopreventive agents may vary by race/ethnicity. Therefore, results of chemoprevention trials should be interpret with cautious with regard to race/ethnicity and recruitment of racial/ethnic minority is very important in these trials as described later (see also "Clinical trials" section).

Diagnosis

Currently, the large majority of CaP is detected by PSA elevation, and the use of PSA has resulted in increased diagnosis of early-stage CaP, decreased incidence of metastatic disease, and a decrease in age-adjusted CaP mortality.[2] Similar patterns of incidence, survival and mortality rates have been observed in African Americans and whites, although the improvement in mortality in African Americans is of a smaller magnitude and was observed 2 years later than that in whites.[100] In Japan, decrease in CaP mortality is yet manifested by far, although it may be caused by lower penetrance of PSA screening.

There are also some racial/ethnic differences in the properties of PSA, as well as other clinicopathological features of CaP. In men without detectable CaP, serum PSA levels are affected by the presence of benign enlargement or inflammation of the prostate, or other non-malignant signs, and tend to be higher in those with lower urinary tract symptoms than in those without. In addition, PSA levels increase with age and age-associated patterns of PSA elevation are similar between racial/ethnic groups.[101-103] Even with adjustment of these factors, however, absolute serum PSA levels in African Americans have been reported to be higher than those in whites[101], and levels in Asians are also lower than those in whites.[102] Therefore, it has been reported that cut-off values for PSA for prostate biopsy should be determined in age- and race-specific manners.[101] Indeed, the detection rate of CaP in patients with PSA >4.0ng/ml is higher in African Americans than in whites.[104] In addition, recent studies have shown that CaP can be detected at PSA levels <4.0 ng/ml, [3, 4] and the detection rate at this PSA level is also higher in African Americans than in whites.[105] Thus, African Americans are more likely to have high-grade and advanced CaP than younger whites of the same age and with the same PSA level, and therefore, improvement in CaP detection techniques are warranted for this high-risk ethnic group. However, the diagnostic performance of percent free PSA, one of the strongest tools for enhancing PSA-based CaP detection at low to intermediate PSA levels, is rather worse in African Americans than in whites.[106]

There have been some reports on the racial/ethnic disparity in clinicopathological features at the time of diagnosis of CaP. Most studies of this kind have been undertaken at medical institutes with equal access, in which men of similar economic status are provided a medical service that is essentially free of charge, in order to nullify the impact of economic factors. A report from a tertiary care military medical center by Moul and colleagues [107] has shown that the mean PSA value at the time of CaP diagnosis was 14.0 ng/ml for African Americans compared with 8.3 ng/ml for whites. This difference was observed across all stages, grades and age categories, and was still significant when these factors were simultaneously controlled for. Other investigators have reported similar results that support Moul's findings.[108, 109] Although the differences in PSA levels were initially thought to reflect differences in tumor volume between racial/ethnic groups,[107] later studies that incorporate tumor volume have shown that PSA levels in African American men at diagnosis of CaP are still higher than for white men, after controlling tumor volume.[109, 110]

With regard to disease stage, it has been reported that African American patients had distant metastasis more often than white patients did in the pre-PSA era (1973–1992) [111, 112]. However, a later report from the same equal-access medical institute showed that there was no significant difference in disease stage between African American and white patients in the PSA era (1991–1997).[108] With regard to tumor grade, there seem to be some racial/ethnic differences. Freedland and colleagues have reported that average Gleason scores for 230 African American patients was slightly higher than for 247 white patients (6.2 vs 5.9, $p=0.0025$).[108] Results from the SEER program have supported Freedland's findings, although the stage-specific racial/ethnic differences are not large and have declined over time.113 These findings suggest that racial/ethnic differences in the frequency of advanced or high-grade CaP have resulted from differences in PSA-based screening rates.

Treatment

There is racial/ethnic disparity in the treatment of CaP. According to two studies by Underwood and colleagues based on data from the SEER program,[114, 115] African American men are more likely to receive ADT/expectant management as the primary treatment for locoregional (up to stage D1 disease with regional lymph node involvement) CaP, compared to both Hispanic and white men, whereas another study reported that the likelihood of secondary treatment after failure of primary treatment was not significantly associated with race/ethnicity and socioeconomic factors. [116] In other words, African American patients are less likely to receive definitive therapy as the primary treatment for curable CaP, and the authors suggested that it is one of the non-biological contributory factors for racial/ethnic disparity in CaP mortality. Two questions are raised with regard to the cause and consequence of this racial/ethnic disparity in the choice of CaP treatment; what the reason for the disparity is, and whether the disparity results in worse treatment outcome or higher CaP mortality rate in African American men.

The wide variation in treatment options for locoregional CaP without definitive systematic decision process might influence the racial difference in the decision making of CaP treatment. According to the report by Steginga and colleagues, CaP treatment decisions are influenced by referral physicians' recommendations, the positive and negative experiences of other patients, and pre-existing beliefs that a certain treatment modality is better than another. [117] These miscellaneous factors are likely to be influenced by socioeconomic status and patients' distrust of physician. Since race/ethnicity, socioeconomic position and distrust of health provider seem to be closely intertwined each other (see also "Socioeconomics" and "Clinical trials" sections), it seems very difficult to evaluate these, so as to incorporate them into the analysis, and it should be noted that socioeconomic status was not incorporated in Underwood's reports. In addition, with the advent and popularization of novel, less invasive treatment modalities such as brachytherapy and cryotherapy, treatment decision making for localized CaP has become more complicated. It has been suggested that large-scale efforts to promote evidence-based, high-quality care are needed for this kind of study to elucidate the impact of race/ethnicity on treatment trends and outcomes.

In addition to above-mentioned nonbiological factors, potential racial/ethnic differences in biological feature of CaP could influence on decision making of treatment. It is possible that higher PSA levels in African American men than other racial/ethnic groups with similar disease extent[109, 110] influence treatment decision making. It is also possible that differences in tumor grade between races/ethnicities [108, 113] (see also "Diagnosis" section) influence decision making, although the difference was reported very small. Although above-mentioned Underwood's reports did not incorporate disease stage, there has been a report that there is no significant difference in the rate of lymph node involvement between racial/ethnic groups.[118]

In this regard, Underwood and colleagues have also found that the racial/ethnic differences in treatment trends appear to have lessened over time between 1992 and 1999, when PSA-based screening was rapidly popularized.[114, 115] This lessened disparity in treatment trends among racial/ethnic groups might have resulted from the "shift of disease stage" due to PSA-based screening [119, 120] and consequent decrease in the disease stage differences among racial/ethnic groups. This possibility was supported by another study using the same registry program, which has shown that racial/ethnic differences in the use of aggressive and conservative therapies increase for men aged ≥65 years, who seemed less influenced by population-based CaP screening using PSA. [118]

Moreover, some studies on CaP treatment outcome in equal-access medical care delivery systems have shown no such significant racial/ethnic differences. Eastham and Kattan have reviewed the records of 218 African American and 257 white patients with localized CaP (T1–T2) and found no racial/ethnic differences in pathological stage, surgical margin status and recurrence-free survival.[121] Freedland and colleagues have retrospectively reviewed the records of 125 African American and 148 white patients with CaP undergoing RP and have found no differences in the pathological features of the RP specimens and recurrence rates after RP.[122] Optenberg and colleagues have retrospectively studied survival of patients with CaP registered at the US Department of Defense Tumor Registry and have found that race does not affect survival.[112] Collectively, racial/ethnic difference in primary treatment trends for locoregional CaP seems secondary to racial/ethnic difference in miscellaneous non-biological factors including socioeconomic status, access to healthcare and distrust of health providers.

On the other hand, does the disparity in decision making of CaP treatment between racial/ethnic groups directly cause worse treatment outcome or higher CaP mortality rate in African American men? Different from the consistent results from the equal-access medical institutes, data from the large scale registry program has shown remarkable disparities in treatment outcomes of patients with localized CaP. As mentioned above, Godley's report based on the SEER program database has demonstrated that overall survival was 1.8 years shorter for African Americans than for whites treated by RP, 0.7 years shorter after radiotherapy, and 1.0 year shorter in those choosing active surveillance.[23] Another study based on the same SEER program has shown that the disease-free survival for African Americans with localized CaP was 3.3 years shorter than for their Asian counterparts and 2.5 years shorter than for Hispanics.[123] Meanwhile, other reports have shown that there is no significant difference in disease-free survival between whites and Hispanics undergoing RP,[124] and no significant difference in survival rates between African Americans and whites with advanced (stage C or more) CaP.[125]

As described above, a remarkable racial/ethnic difference in treatment trends in active surveillance has been reported can be a possible explanation for the worse treatment outcome of localized CaP in African American men compared to other racial/ethnic groups. Two studies by Shavers and colleagues have suggested that it is not only because active surveillance was inappropriate and definitive therapy should have selected in some cases, but also because of the quality of management. First they have found in the SEER database that African American and Hispanic men are significantly more likely to receive active surveillance in multivariate analysis incorporating age, co-morbidity, stage, grade and life expectancy.[126] It has also been supposed that educational levels have a significant impact on the likelihood of active surveillance. It should be noted that men are determined to receive active surveillance as initial treatment of CaP if they do not receive surgery, radiotherapy or hormonal treatment within the first 6 months after diagnosis, according to SEER and medical claims data. This was a limitation of the study based on the SEER database, and it is supposed that some of the patients determined to have received active surveillance actually needed definitive treatment, but were lost to follow-up. In this regard they have shown in their second report that 6% of African American and 5% of Hispanic men did not have any medical monitoring visits or procedures during the 60-month follow-up period, compared to only 1% of white men.[127] These men did not seem to be selected for active surveillance as a treatment option for CaP, and this may at least partially explain the difference in the likelihood of active surveillance and poor outcomes of men who had received expectant management.

It is possible that poor quality of patient follow-up accounts for the worse outcome of treatment for localized CaP other than ADT/expectant management. However, there may be other potential contributory factors since Godley and colleagues demonstrated that the poor treatment outcome of localized CaP in African American men was consistent even after adjustment for other clinical, pathological and socioeconomic covariates.[23] It cannot exclude the possible efficacy of further efforts including establishment of better patient-physician relationship with informed consent, reform of healthcare system and effectual educational campaign for the correction of racial/ethnic disparity in treatment outcome of localized CaP.

In addition to disease control, alteration of quality of life (QOL) is a very important measure of treatment outcome, especially for localized CaP in which fairly good survival can be expected. Penedo and colleagues have shed light on this issue by studying racial disparities in QOL outcomes after treatment for localized CaP.[128] Ethnicity is related to QOL, such that African Americans and Hispanics have lower QOL than whites, and this association is partially mediated by sociodemographic, medical and health behavior factors.

Besides approved treatment modalities, the use of complementary and alternative medicine (CAM) has become increasingly common. Some surveys have revealed that approximately one-fifth to one-third of patients reported using at least one of more than 50 types of CAM.[129-132] Initiation of CAM after diagnosis of CaP is associated with being a member of an ethnic minority group and higher level of education, whereas herbal/dietary use before diagnosis is associated with being white.[129] Other reports have also suggested that sociodemographic factors strongly influence the likelihood of using CAM.[130, 131] Since there has been limited evidence for the efficacy of CAM on CaP, it is unclear if differences in the use of CAM can explain racial/ethnic differences in CaP incidence and mortality. If future studies elucidate the impact of CAM on controlling CaP, especially with regard to possible racial/ethnic differences in the efficacy of CAM, it will help to clarify whether use of CAM has any influence on the racial/ethnic difference in CaP incidence and mortality.

Socioeconomics

Socioeconomic factors are very important when discussing racial/ethnic differences in CaP incidence and mortality, because both race/ethnicity and clinical knowledge and behavior regarding CaP seem to be directly associated with socioeconomic background. Chan and colleagues have reported the results of a survey in which men attending outpatient clinics were surveyed for their knowledge about and experience with PSA-based CaP screening.[133] Although African Americans had less knowledge than whites, the difference was due to differences in educational level and experience with PSA screening. According to a recent questionnaire survey by Talcott and colleagues, African American patients with CaP are younger, less often married, and have lower educational level, job status, income and medical access than their white counterparts.[134] Although African American patients are aware of their increased risk of cancer, the importance of treatment, and responsibility for their own health, their worse socioeconomic position seems to result in reduced access and consequent distrust of physicians. These findings suggest that public health efforts are needed to promote informed decision making, particularly in peoples of lower socioeconomic status.

Socioeconomic status has a substantial impact on CaP mortality, particularly in older patients. Du and colleagues have studied SEER–Medicare linked data and have found that low economic status is significantly associated with decreasing survival in all men with locoregional CaP.[135] It has also been noted that socioeconomic status remains significant after adjustment for race/ethnicity, while race/ethnicity is also generally significant after adjustment for socioeconomic differences. Albano and colleagues have studied estimated age-adjusted cancer death rates using race and education details from death certificates and population denominator data from the US Bureau of the Census.[136] They have found that African American men who have completed 12 or fewer years of education have a CaP death rate more than double that of African American men with more schooling (10.5 *vs* 4.8 per 100,000 men; relative risk=2.17; 95% CI=1.82–2.58), although the relative risk associated with race was higher than that associated with educational level within each racial/ethnic group.

These findings collectively suggest that socioeconomic factors are strongly associated with CaP risk. However, whether socioeconomic status and race/ethnicity affect independently CaP risk, or whether the former can be an explanation for the racial/ethnic disparity in CaP risk, is still unclear. Since race/ethnicity and socioeconomic status are closely intertwined, it is difficult to determine the extent to which the reported racial/ethnic healthcare differences are due to differences in socioeconomic status.[137] In addition, it is difficult to estimate the effect of improving socioeconomic status on subsequent risk of cancer death.[138] Moreover, socioeconomic status can affect that of family members. In this respect, it has a sort of inherited tendency, similar to genetic differences. Although it seems too complicated to be clearly understood, continuous efforts should be focused on this issue to establish helpful measures for socioeconomics to improve public health regarding CaP.

Clinical Trials

It is extremely important to enroll members of ethnic minority groups in clinical trials on CaP screening or treatment. This is because there is racial/ethnic disparity in almost everything about CaP, as described above. Therefore, results from clinical trials on white populations cannot be directly applied to other racial/ethnic groups. In addition, well-designed, multiethnic, population-based clinical trials are needed to reveal possible disparities between racial/ethnic groups. Consequently, since 1993 the National Institutes of Health has required that all sponsored clinical trials ensure that women and members of minorities are included in all human research.[139] Nevertheless, recruitment of ethnic minorities into clinical trials has failed to enroll sufficient numbers of participants. Indeed, a study by Murthy and colleagues based on the results of the National Cancer Institute Clinical Trial Cooperative Group Breast, Colorectal, Lung, and Prostate Cancer Clinical Trials has shown significantly lower enrollment among African American and Hispanic compared to white patients.[140] According to another study by Moinpour and colleagues based on the Prostate Cancer Prevention Trial (PCPT) sponsored by the Southwestern Oncology Group (SWOG), African American men comprised only 4% of the total randomized sample compared to the study goal of 8%, despite emphasized minority recruitment, including distribution of recruitment materials, engagement of recruitment consultants, production of a recruitment manual and assignment of recruiters.[141]

There seems to be numerous barriers to recruiting racial/ethnic minorities into cancer clinical trials.[142, 143] Barber and colleagues have found that African American men were half as likely as to choose community-based CaP mass screening programs, and a private health care setting is more important to them than white men.[144] Advani and colleagues have demonstrated that African American patients with malignant disease have significantly less willingness to participate in clinical trials than do their white counterparts.[145] Robinson and colleagues have reported that low socioeconomic status African Americans expressed less willingness to participate in CaP clinical trials than did men of middle socioeconomic status.[146] They have also noted that barriers to participation in CaP clinical trials include concerns about drug toxicity, medical experimentation and distrust of the medical profession.

Although difficulty with the recruitment of ethnic minorities has been recognized for quite some time, and a variety of efforts have been focused on the recruitment of minorities, there is limited evidence for effective strategies to recruit racial/ethnic minority populations.[147] As a matter of fact, a definition of "success" in recruitment of minority populations has only just published.[148] Barber and colleagues have reported the efficacy of watching an educational video to improve knowledge of CaP.[144] They have also noted that radio reached the largest number of African Americans, while newspapers reached most white men.

In the African American Hereditary Prostate Cancer (AAHPC) study organized by Howard University, Washington DC, USA, a historical African American institution, six Collaborative Recruitment Centers were responsible for the identification and enrollment of 100 African American families with hereditary CaP. Their recruitment strategies included mass media campaigns, physician referrals, community health affairs/CaP screenings, support groups, tumor registries, as well as visits to churches, barber shops, and universities. It has been reported that the most productive recruitment mechanisms were physician referrals and tumor registries, which yielded 81% of recruited families.[149] The AAMEN project was designed to recruit African American men aged 55–74 years in a prostate, lung and colorectal cancer screening trial, and to randomize subjects to a control group or to one of three increasingly intensive intervention arms, which used different combinations of mail, phone and in person, church-based recruitment. As a result, a significantly greater enrollment yield was seen in the most intensive, church-based intervention arm.[150] A literature review has suggested that several medical-provider-related factors substantially influence recruitment of minorities into clinical trials.[151] These results have indicated that face-to-face contact is the most important factor in the interventions that yield high enrollment rates, especially for elderly African Americans.

The Selenium and Vitamin E Cancer Prevention Trial (SELECT) is a US national primary prevention trial for CaP, and the recruitment goal was 24% ethnic minorities, with 20% black, 3% Hispanic and 1% Asian participants. It has been reported that, of the 35,534 participants enrolled, 21% were from minorities, with 15% black, 5% Hispanic and 1% Asian, which achieved the largest ever recruitment of minority participants into a cancer prevention trial.[152] The recruitment strategies were to: (i) consider minority recruitment during site selection; (ii) expand the eligibility criteria by lowering the age criterion for black men and including men with controlled co-morbid illnesses; (iii) develop a national infrastructure; (iv) give additional funds to sites with the potential to increase black enrollment; and (v) provide resources to maximize free media opportunities to promote SELECT.

The success of SELECT has some important implications; cancer-related clinical trials should have clear measurement approaches for recruiting minority populations, with the recruitment goals specified a priori.[148] With regard to measurement approaches, effective use of the mass media is increasingly important. The influence of some kind of medium differs among racial/ethnic or socioeconomic populations, as reported by Barber and colleagues.[144] The recent explosive popularization of the internet is noteworthy and may make some changes in strategies for minority recruitment. In this regard, the California Men's Health Study (CMHS), based online (or on paper), has been initiated.[153] So far, 84,170 participants have been recruited, with approximately 40% from minority populations. A wide variety and range of body mass index, sexual habits, education, and income were observed. The investigators expect that a wide variety of epidemiological, health services, and outcomes research utilizing a rich array of electronic, biological and clinical resources is possible within this multiethnic cohort.

Summary

In this chapter, racial/ethnic differences in CaP incidence and mortality have been discussed. Although the reasons for the racial/ethnic differences seem too complicated to explain accurately, recent advances in genetics may have an important clue for more precise understandings of racial/ethnic disparities in CaP risk. In the population-based screening or clinical diagnosis of CaP, the use of race/ethnicity-specific cut off of PSA may strengthen the diagnostic ability of PSA. Then, racial/ethnic disparity in the disease stage at diagnosis may be removed, and a fair comparison, without bias, of disease extent will be possible. To obtain more objective and supportive information, well-designed clinical trials with proper and balanced recruitment of race/ethnic populations are warranted.

However, there seem to be too many socioeconomic, educational, behavioral, occupational and environmental factors known to be associated with CaP risk. Moreover, it is possible that there remain other unknown factors. Since some of these factors affect and reflect each other and even CaP mortality, it seems almost impossible to control all of these underlying factors completely.

Elucidating the reason for the health disparities, including those concerning CaP, is only an intermediate objective. Our primary goal is to prevent morbidity and mortality from CaP in all populations regardless of race/ethnicity, education level and socioeconomic status. Comprehensive understanding of the CaP-related health disparities will be achieved by an adequate combination of molecular genetics and descriptive and analytical epidemiology. Our continuous efforts for better understanding of the disease and proper interventional measures to conquer the problems may eventually lead to improved public health.

References

[1] Sakr WA, Grignon DJ, Crissman JD, Heilbrun LK, Cassin BJ, Pontes JJ, et al. High grade prostatic intraepithelial neoplasia (HGPIN) and prostatic adenocarcinoma between the ages of 20-69: an autopsy study of 249 cases. *In Vivo* 1994;8(3):439-43.

[2] Newcomer LM, Stanford JL, Blumenstein BA, Brawer MK. Temporal trends in rates of prostate cancer: declining incidence of advanced stage disease, 1974 to 1994. *J. Urol.* 1997;158(4):1427-30.

[3] Thompson IM, Pauler DK, Goodman PJ, Tangen CM, Lucia MS, Parnes HL, et al. Prevalence of prostate cancer among men with a prostate-specific antigen level < or =4.0 ng per milliliter. *N. Engl. J. Med.* 2004;350(22):2239-46.

[4] Kobayashi T, Nishizawa K, Ogura K, Mitsumori K, Ide Y. Detection of prostate cancer in men with prostate-specific antigen levels of 2.0 to 4.0 ng/mL equivalent to that in men with 4.1 to 10.0 ng/mL in a Japanese population. *Urology* 2004;63(4):727-31.

[5] Gleason DF, Mellinger GT. Prediction of prognosis for prostatic adenocarcinoma by combined histological grading and clinical staging. *J. Urol.* 1974;111(1):58-64.

[6] Flemming ID, Cooper JS, Hemson DE, et al., editors. American Joint Committee on Cancer Staging Manual. 5th ed. Philadelphia: JP Lippincott; 1997. p. 219-222.

[7] Hull GW, Rabbani F, Abbas F, Wheeler TM, Kattan MW, Scardino PT. Cancer control with radical prostatectomy alone in 1,000 consecutive patients. *J. Urol.* 2002; 167 (2 Pt 1):528-34.

[8] D'Amico AV, Schultz D, Loffredo M, Dugal R, Hurwitz M, Kaplan I, et al. Biochemical outcome following external beam radiation therapy with or without androgen suppression therapy for clinically localized prostate cancer. *JAMA* 2000; 284 (10):1280-3.

[9] Huggins C. Endocrine-induced regression of cancers. *Cancer Res.* 1967; 27 (11): 1925-30.

[10] Petrylak DP, Tangen CM, Hussain MH, Lara PN, Jr., Jones JA, Taplin ME, et al. Docetaxel and estramustine compared with mitoxantrone and prednisone for advanced refractory prostate cancer. *N. Engl. J. Med.* 2004;351(15):1513-20.

[11] French DB, Jones LA. Minority issues in prostate disease. *Med. Clin. North Am.* 2005; 89 (4):805-16.

[12] Surveillance Epidemiology and End Results. SEER Cancer Statistics Review. Available at: http://seer.cancer.gov/statfacts/html/prost.html. Accessed November 7, 2007

[13] International Agency for Research on Cancer. Cancer incidence on five continents: World Health Organization; 2005.

[14] Wabinga HR, Parkin DM, Wabwire-Mangen F, Nambooze S. Trends in cancer incidence in Kyadondo County, Uganda, 1960-1997. Br J Cancer 2000;82(9):1585-92.

[15] Osegbe DN. Prostate cancer in Nigerians: facts and nonfacts. *J. Urol.* 1997; 157 (4):1340-3.

[16] Ogunbiyi JO, Shittu OB. Increased incidence of prostate cancer in Nigerians. *J. Natl. Med. Assoc.* 1999;91(3):159-64.

[17] Shimizu H, Ross RK, Bernstein L, Yatani R, Henderson BE, Mack TM. Cancers of the prostate and breast among Japanese and white immigrants in Los Angeles County. *Br. J. Cancer* 1991;63(6):963-6.

[18] Muir CS, Nectoux J, Staszewski J. The epidemiology of prostatic cancer. Geographical distribution and time-trends. *Acta Oncol.* 1991; 30 (2):133-40.

[19] Gronberg H. Prostate cancer epidemiology. *Lancet* 2003; 361(9360):859-64.

[20] Landis SH, Murray T, Bolden S, Wingo PA. Cancer statistics, 1999. CA *Cancer J. Clin.* 1999; 49 (1):8-31, 1.

[21] Quinn M, Babb P. Patterns and trends in prostate cancer incidence, survival, prevalence and mortality. Part I: international comparisons. *BJU Int.* 2002;90(2):162-73.

[22] The Editorial Board of the Cancer Statistics in Japan. Cancer Statistics in Japan 2005: Foundation for Promotion of Cancer Research; 2005.

[23] Godley PA, Schenck AP, Amamoo MA, Schoenbach VJ, Peacock S, Manning M, et al. Racial differences in mortality among Medicare recipients after treatment for localized prostate cancer. *J. Natl. Cancer Inst.* 2003;95(22):1702-10.

[24] Ornish D, Weidner G, Fair WR, Marlin R, Pettengill EB, Raisin CJ, et al. Intensive lifestyle changes may affect the progression of prostate cancer. *J. Urol.* 2005;174 (3): 1065-9; discussion 1069-70.

[25] Ngo TH, Barnard RJ, Anton T, Tran C, Elashoff D, Heber D, et al. Effect of isocaloric low-fat diet on prostate cancer xenograft progression to androgen independence. *Cancer Res.* 2004;64 (4):1252-4.

[26] Amling CL, Kane CJ, Riffenburgh RH, Ward JF, Roberts JL, Lance RS, et al. Relationship between obesity and race in predicting adverse pathologic variables in patients undergoing radical prostatectomy. *Urology* 2001;58 (5):723-8.

[27] Amling CL, Riffenburgh RH, Sun L, Moul JW, Lance RS, Kusuda L, et al. Pathologic variables and recurrence rates as related to obesity and race in men with prostate cancer undergoing radical prostatectomy. *J. Clin. Oncol.* 2004;22(3):439-45.

[28] Freedland SJ, Aronson WJ, Kane CJ, Presti JC, Jr., Amling CL, Elashoff D, et al. Impact of obesity on biochemical control after radical prostatectomy for clinically localized prostate cancer: a report by the Shared Equal Access Regional Cancer Hospital database study group. *J. Clin. Oncol.* 2004;22(3):446-53.

[29] Freedland SJ, Terris MK, Presti JC, Jr., Amling CL, Kane CJ, Trock B, et al. Obesity and biochemical outcome following radical prostatectomy for organ confined disease with negative surgical margins. *J. Urol.* 2004;172(2):520-4.

[30] Freedland SJ. Obesity and prostate cancer: importance of race and stage of disease. *J. Urol.* 2007;178(5):1842-3.

[31] Shimizu H, Ross RK, Bernstein L. Possible underestimation of the incidence rate of prostate cancer in Japan. *Jpn. J. Cancer Res.* 1991;82(5):483-5.

[32] Shiraishi T, Watanabe M, Matsuura H, Kusano I, Yatani R, Stemmermann GN. The frequency of latent prostatic carcinoma in young males: the Japanese experience. *In Vivo* 1994;8(3):445-7.

[33] Breslow N, Chan CW, Dhom G, Drury RA, Franks LM, Gellei B, et al. Latent carcinoma of prostate at autopsy in seven areas. The International Agency for Research on Cancer, Lyons, France. *Int. J. Cancer* 1977;20(5):680-8.

[34] Ostrander EA, Stanford JL. Genetics of prostate cancer: too many loci, too few genes. *Am. J. Hum. Genet* 2000; 67 (6):1367-75.

[35] Schaid DJ. The complex genetic epidemiology of prostate cancer. *Hum. Mol. Genet.* 2004; 13 Spec No 1:R103-21.

[36] Amundadottir LT, Sulem P, Gudmundsson J, Helgason A, Baker A, Agnarsson BA, et al. A common variant associated with prostate cancer in European and African populations. *Nat. Genet* 2006;38(6):652-8.

[37] Freedman ML, Haiman CA, Patterson N, McDonald GJ, Tandon A, Waliszewska A, et al. Admixture mapping identifies 8q24 as a prostate cancer risk locus in African-American men. *Proc. Natl. Acad. Sci. USA* 2006;103(38):14068-73.

[38] Gudmundsson J, Sulem P, Manolescu A, Amundadottir LT, Gudbjartsson D, Helgason A, et al. Genome-wide association study identifies a second prostate cancer susceptibility variant at 8q24. *Nat. Genet.* 2007;39(5):631-7.

[39] Haiman CA, Patterson N, Freedman ML, Myers SR, Pike MC, Waliszewska A, et al. Multiple regions within 8q24 independently affect risk for prostate cancer. *Nat. Genet.* 2007; 39(5):638-44.

[40] Yeager M, Orr N, Hayes RB, Jacobs KB, Kraft P, Wacholder S, et al. Genome-wide association study of prostate cancer identifies a second risk locus at 8q24. *Nat. Genet.* 2007; 39(5):645-9.

[41] Nelson WG, De Marzo AM, Isaacs WB. Prostate cancer. *N. Engl. J. Med.* 2003; 349 (4):366-81.

[42] Wong KK, deLeeuw RJ, Dosanjh NS, Kimm LR, Cheng Z, Horsman DE, et al. A comprehensive analysis of common copy-number variations in the human genome. *Am. J. Hum. Genet.* 2007;80(1):91-104.

[43] Cher ML, Bova GS, Moore DH, Small EJ, Carroll PR, Pin SS, et al. Genetic alterations in untreated metastases and androgen-independent prostate cancer detected by comparative genomic hybridization and allelotyping. *Cancer Res.* 1996; 56 (13):3091-102.

[44] Elo JP, Visakorpi T. Molecular genetics of prostate cancer. *Ann. Med.* 2001;33(2):130-41.

[45] Gil J, Kerai P, Lleonart M, Bernard D, Cigudosa JC, Peters G, et al. Immortalization of primary human prostate epithelial cells by c-Myc. *Cancer Res.* 2005;65(6):2179-85.

[46] 46. Ross R, Bernstein L, Judd H, Hanisch R, Pike M, Henderson B. Serum testosterone levels in healthy young black and white men. *J. Natl. Cancer Inst.* 1986; 76 (1):45-8.

[47] Wu AH, Whittemore AS, Kolonel LN, John EM, Gallagher RP, West DW, et al. Serum androgens and sex hormone-binding globulins in relation to lifestyle factors in older African-American, white, and Asian men in the United States and Canada. *Cancer Epidemiol. Biomarkers Prev.* 1995;4(7):735-41.

[48] Gann PH, Hennekens CH, Ma J, Longcope C, Stampfer MJ. Prospective study of sex hormone levels and risk of prostate cancer. *J. Natl. Cancer Inst.* 1996;88(16):1118-26.

[49] Eaton NE, Reeves GK, Appleby PN, Key TJ. Endogenous sex hormones and prostate cancer: a quantitative review of prospective studies. *Br. J. Cancer* 1999;80(7):930-4.

[50] Heikkila R, Aho K, Heliovaara M, Hakama M, Marniemi J, Reunanen A, et al. Serum testosterone and sex hormone-binding globulin concentrations and the risk of prostate carcinoma: a longitudinal study. *Cancer* 1999;86(2):312-5.

[51] Chen C, Weiss NS, Stanczyk FZ, Lewis SK, DiTommaso D, Etzioni R, et al. Endogenous sex hormones and prostate cancer risk: a case-control study nested within the Carotene and Retinol Efficacy Trial. *Cancer Epidemiol. Biomarkers Prev.* 2003;12 (12): 1410-6.

[52] Kaaks R, Lukanova A, Rinaldi S, Biessy C, Soderberg S, Olsson T, et al. Interrelationships between plasma testosterone, SHBG, IGF-I, insulin and leptin in prostate cancer cases and controls. *Eur. J. Cancer Prev.* 2003;12(4):309-15.

[53] Ross RK, Bernstein L, Lobo RA, Shimizu H, Stanczyk FZ, Pike MC, et al. 5-alpha-reductase activity and risk of prostate cancer among Japanese and US white and black males. *Lancet* 1992;339(8798):887-9.

[54] Hsing AW, Chen C, Chokkalingam AP, Gao YT, Dightman DA, Nguyen HT, et al. Polymorphic markers in the SRD5A2 gene and prostate cancer risk: a population-based case-control study. *Cancer Epidemiol. Biomarkers Prev.* 2001;10(10):1077-82.

[55] Bangsi D, Zhou J, Sun Y, Patel NP, Darga LL, Heilbrun LK, et al. Impact of a genetic variant in CYP3A4 on risk and clinical presentation of prostate cancer among white and African-American men. *Urol. Oncol.* 2006;24(1):21-7.

[56] Balic I, Graham ST, Troyer DA, Higgins BA, Pollock BH, Johnson-Pais TL, et al. Androgen receptor length polymorphism associated with prostate cancer risk in Hispanic men. *J. Urol.* 2002;168(5):2245-8.

[57] Taplin ME, Rajeshkumar B, Halabi S, Werner CP, Woda BA, Picus J, et al. Androgen receptor mutations in androgen-independent prostate cancer: Cancer and Leukemia Group B Study 9663. *J. Clin. Oncol.* 2003;21(14):2673-8.

[58] Sartor O, Zheng Q, Eastham JA. Androgen receptor gene CAG repeat length varies in a race-specific fashion in men without prostate cancer. *Urology* 1999;53(2):378-80.

[59] Stewart CE, Rotwein P. Growth, differentiation, and survival: multiple physiological functions for insulin-like growth factors. *Physiol. Rev.* 1996;76(4):1005-26.

[60] Monzavi R, Cohen P. IGFs and IGFBPs: role in health and disease. *Best Pract. Res. Clin. Endocrinol. Metab.* 2002;16(3):433-47.

[61] Chan JM, Stampfer MJ, Giovannucci E, Gann PH, Ma J, Wilkinson P, et al. Plasma insulin-like growth factor-I and prostate cancer risk: a prospective study. *Science* 1998;279(5350):563-6.

[62] Harman SM, Metter EJ, Blackman MR, Landis PK, Carter HB. Serum levels of insulin-like growth factor I (IGF-I), IGF-II, IGF-binding protein-3, and prostate-specific antigen as predictors of clinical prostate cancer. *J. Clin. Endocrinol. Metab.* 2000;85 (11): 4258-65.

[63] Mantzoros CS, Tzonou A, Signorello LB, Stampfer M, Trichopoulos D, Adami HO. Insulin-like growth factor 1 in relation to prostate cancer and benign prostatic hyperplasia. *Br. J. Cancer* 1997;76(9):1115-8.

[64] Wolk A, Mantzoros CS, Andersson SO, Bergstrom R, Signorello LB, Lagiou P, et al. Insulin-like growth factor 1 and prostate cancer risk: a population-based, case-control study. *J. Natl. Cancer Inst.* 1998;90(12):911-5.

[65] Ma J, Pollak MN, Giovannucci E, Chan JM, Tao Y, Hennekens CH, et al. Prospective study of colorectal cancer risk in men and plasma levels of insulin-like growth factor (IGF)-I and IGF-binding protein-3. *J. Natl. Cancer Inst.* 1999;91(7):620-5.

[66] Giovannucci E, Pollak MN, Platz EA, Willett WC, Stampfer MJ, Majeed N, et al. A prospective study of plasma insulin-like growth factor-1 and binding protein-3 and risk of colorectal neoplasia in women. *Cancer Epidemiol. Biomarkers Prev.* 2000;9(4):345-9.

[67] DeLellis K, Rinaldi S, Kaaks RJ, Kolonel LN, Henderson B, Le Marchand L. Dietary and lifestyle correlates of plasma insulin-like growth factor-I (IGF-I) and IGF binding protein-3 (IGFBP-3): the multiethnic cohort. *Cancer Epidemiol. Biomarkers Prev.* 2004; 13 (9):1444-51.

[68] McGreevy K, Hoel B, Lipsitz S, Bissada N, Hoel D. Racial and anthropometric differences in plasma levels of insulin-like growth factor I and insulin-like growth factor binding protein-3. *Urology* 2005;66(3):587-92.

[69] Platz EA, Pollak MN, Rimm EB, Majeed N, Tao Y, Willett WC, et al. Racial variation in insulin-like growth factor-1 and binding protein-3 concentrations in middle-aged men. *Cancer Epidemiol. Biomarkers Prev.* 1999;8(12):1107-10.

[70] Winter DL, Hanlon AL, Raysor SL, Watkins-Bruner D, Pinover WH, Hanks GE, et al. Plasma levels of IGF-1, IGF-2, and IGFBP-3 in white and African-American men at increased risk of prostate cancer. *Urology* 2001;58(4):614-8.

[71] McGreevy KM, Hoel BD, Lipsitz SR, Hoel DG. Impact of nutrients on insulin-like growth factor-I, insulin-like growth factor binding protein-3 and their ratio in African American and white males. *Public Health Nutr.* 2007;10(1):97-105.

[72] Allen NE, Davey GK, Key TJ, Zhang S, Narod SA. Serum insulin-like growth factor I (IGF-I) concentration in men is not associated with the cytosine-adenosine repeat

polymorphism of the IGF-I gene. Cancer Epidemiol Biomarkers Prev 2002;11(3):319-20.

[73] Rietveld I, Janssen JA, Hofman A, Pols HA, van Duijn CM, Lamberts SW. A polymorphism in the IGF-I gene influences the age-related decline in circulating total IGF-I levels. *Eur. J. Endocrinol.* 2003;148(2):171-5.

[74] Schildkraut JM, Demark-Wahnefried W, Wenham RM, Grubber J, Jeffreys AS, Grambow SC, et al. IGF1 (CA)19 repeat and IGFBP3 -202 A/C genotypes and the risk of prostate cancer in Black and White men. *Cancer Epidemiol. Biomarkers Prev.* 2005; 14 (2):403-8.

[75] Chen C, Freeman R, Voigt LF, Fitzpatrick A, Plymate SR, Weiss NS. Prostate cancer risk in relation to selected genetic polymorphisms in insulin-like growth factor-I, insulin-like growth factor binding protein-3, and insulin-like growth factor-I receptor. *Cancer Epidemiol. Biomarkers Prev.* 2006;15(12):2461-6.

[76] Tsuchiya N, Wang L, Suzuki H, Segawa T, Fukuda H, Narita S, et al. Impact of IGF-I and CYP19 gene polymorphisms on the survival of patients with metastatic prostate cancer. *J. Clin. Oncol.* 2006;24(13):1982-9.

[77] Cheng I, Stram DO, Penney KL, Pike M, Le Marchand L, Kolonel LN, et al. Common genetic variation in IGF1 and prostate cancer risk in the Multiethnic Cohort. *J. Natl. Cancer Inst.* 2006;98(2):123-34.

[78] Deal C, Ma J, Wilkin F, Paquette J, Rozen F, Ge B, et al. Novel promoter polymorphism in insulin-like growth factor-binding protein-3: correlation with serum levels and interaction with known regulators. *J. Clin. Endocrinol. Metab.* 2001; 86 (3): 1274-80.

[79] Schernhammer ES, Hankinson SE, Hunter DJ, Blouin MJ, Pollak MN. Polymorphic variation at the -202 locus in IGFBP3: Influence on serum levels of insulin-like growth factors, interaction with plasma retinol and vitamin D and breast cancer risk. *Int. J. Cancer* 2003;107(1):60-4.

[80] Wang L, Habuchi T, Tsuchiya N, Mitsumori K, Ohyama C, Sato K, et al. Insulin-like growth factor-binding protein-3 gene -202 A/C polymorphism is correlated with advanced disease status in prostate cancer. *Cancer Res.* 2003;63(15):4407-11.

[81] Oakley-Girvan I, Feldman D, Eccleshall TR, Gallagher RP, Wu AH, Kolonel LN, et al. Risk of early-onset prostate cancer in relation to germ line polymorphisms of the vitamin D receptor. *Cancer Epidemiol. Biomarkers Prev.* 2004;13(8):1325-30.

[82] Kidd LC, Paltoo DN, Wang S, Chen W, Akereyeni F, Isaacs W, et al. Sequence variation within the 5' regulatory regions of the vitamin D binding protein and receptor genes and prostate cancer risk. *Prostate* 2005;64(3):272-82.

[83] Habuchi T, Suzuki T, Sasaki R, Wang L, Sato K, Satoh S, et al. Association of vitamin D receptor gene polymorphism with prostate cancer and benign prostatic hyperplasia in a Japanese population. *Cancer Res.* 2000; 60(2):305-8.

[84] Bonilla C, Mason T, Long L, Ahaghotu C, Chen W, Zhao A, et al. E-cadherin polymorphisms and haplotypes influence risk for prostate cancer. *Prostate* 2006; 66 (5):546-56.

[85] Kamoto T, Isogawa Y, Shimizu Y, Minamiguchi S, Kinoshita H, Kakehi Y, et al. Association of a genetic polymorphism of the E-cadherin gene with prostate cancer in a Japanese population. *Jpn. J. Clin. Oncol.* 2005; 35 (3):158-61.

[86] Tsukino H, Kuroda Y, Imai H, Nakao H, Qiu D, Komiya Y, et al. Lack of evidence for the association of E-cadherin gene polymorphism with increased risk or progression of prostate cancer. *Urol. Int.* 2004;72(3):203-7.

[87] Chen L, Ambrosone CB, Lee J, Sellers TA, Pow-Sang J, Park JY. Association between polymorphisms in the DNA repair genes XRCC1 and APE1, and the risk of prostate cancer in white and black Americans. *J. Urol.* 2006;175(1):108-12; discussion 112.

[88] Park J, Chen L, Ratnashinge L, Sellers TA, Tanner JP, Lee JH, et al. Deletion polymorphism of UDP-glucuronosyltransferase 2B17 and risk of prostate cancer in African American and Caucasian men. *Cancer Epidemiol. Biomarkers Prev.* 2006; 15 (8): 1473-8.

[89] Levin AM, Ray AM, Zuhlke KA, Douglas JA, Cooney KA. Association between germline variation in the FHIT gene and prostate cancer in Caucasians and African Americans. *Cancer Epidemiol. Biomarkers Prev.* 2007;16(6):1294-7.

[90] Douglas JA, Levin AM, Zuhlke KA, Ray AM, Johnson GR, Lange EM, et al. Common variation in the BRCA1 gene and prostate cancer risk. *Cancer Epidemiol. Biomarkers Prev.* 2007; 16 (7):1510-6.

[91] Kang D, Lee KM, Park SK, Berndt SI, Peters U, Reding D, et al. Functional variant of manganese superoxide dismutase (SOD2 V16A) polymorphism is associated with prostate cancer risk in the prostate, lung, colorectal, and ovarian cancer study. *Cancer Epidemiol. Biomarkers Prev.* 2007;16(8):1581-6.

[92] Shamberger RJ, Willis CE. Selenium distribution and human cancer mortality. *CRC Crit. Rev. Clin. Lab. Sci.* 1971;2(2):211-21.

[93] .Clark LC, Cantor KP, Allaway WH. Selenium in forage crops and cancer mortality in U.S. counties. *Arch Environ Health* 1991;46(1):37-42.

[94] .Klein EA. Selenium: epidemiology and basic science. *J. Urol.* 2004;171(2 Pt 2):S50-3; discussion S53.

[95] .Moyad MA. Selenium and vitamin E supplements for prostate cancer: evidence or embellishment? *Urology* 2002;59(4 Suppl 1):9-19.

[96] .Vogt TM, Ziegler RG, Patterson BH, Graubard BI. Racial differences in serum selenium concentration: analysis of US population data from the Third National Health and Nutrition Examination Survey. *Am. J. Epidemiol.* 2007;166(3):280-8.

[97] .Severson RK, Nomura AM, Grove JS, Stemmermann GN. A prospective study of demographics, diet, and prostate cancer among men of Japanese ancestry in Hawaii. *Cancer Res.* 1989;49(7):1857-60.

[98] Akaza H, Miyanaga N, Takashima N, Naito S, Hirao Y, Tsukamoto T, et al. Is daidzein non-metabolizer a high risk for prostate cancer? A case-controlled study of serum soybean isoflavone concentration. *Jpn. J. Clin. Oncol.* 2002;32(8):296-300.

[99] Akaza H, Miyanaga N, Takashima N, Naito S, Hirao Y, Tsukamoto T, et al. Comparisons of percent equol producers between prostate cancer patients and controls: case-controlled studies of isoflavones in Japanese, Korean and American residents. *Jpn. J. Clin. Oncol.* 2004;34(2):86-9.

[100] Chu KC, Tarone RE, Freeman HP. Trends in prostate cancer mortality among black men and white men in the United States. *Cancer* 2003;97(6):1507-16.

[101] Morgan TO, Jacobsen SJ, McCarthy WF, Jacobson DJ, McLeod DG, Moul JW. Age-specific reference ranges for prostate-specific antigen in black men. *N. Engl. J. Med.* 1996; 335 (5):304-10.

[102] Oesterling JE, Kumamoto Y, Tsukamoto T, Girman CJ, Guess HA, Masumori N, et al. Serum prostate-specific antigen in a community-based population of healthy Japanese men: lower values than for similarly aged white men. *Br. J. Urol.* 1995;75(3):347-53.

[103] Kobayashi T, Kinoshita H, Nishizawa K, Mitsumori K, Ogawa O, Kamoto T. Age-associated increase of prostate-specific antigen in a high level of men visiting urological clinics. *Int. J. Urol.* 2005; 12 (8):733-8.

[104] Fowler JE, Jr., Bigler SA, Farabaugh PB. Prospective study of cancer detection in black and white men with normal digital rectal examination but prostate specific antigen equal or greater than 4.0 ng/mL. *Cancer* 2002;94(6):1661-7.

[105] Smith DS, Carvalhal GF, Mager DE, Bullock AD, Catalona WJ. Use of lower prostate specific antigen cutoffs for prostate cancer screening in black and white men. *J. Urol.* 1998; 160(5):1734-8.

[106] Fowler JE, Jr., Sanders J, Bigler SA, Rigdon J, Kilambi NK, Land SA. Percent free prostate specific antigen and cancer detection in black and white men with total prostate specific antigen 2.5 to 9.9 ng./ml. *J. Urol.* 2000;163(5):1467-70.

[107] Moul JW, Sesterhenn IA, Connelly RR, Douglas T, Srivastava S, Mostofi FK, et al. Prostate-specific antigen values at the time of prostate cancer diagnosis in African-American men. *JAMA* 1995;274(16):1277-81.

[108] Freedland SJ, Sutter ME, Naitoh J, Dorey F, Csathy GS, Aronson WJ. Clinical characteristics in black and white men with prostate cancer in an equal access medical center. *Urology* 2000;55(3):387-90.

[109] Pettaway CA, Troncoso P, Ramirez EI, Johnston DA, Steelhammer L, Babaian RJ. Prostate specific antigen and pathological features of prostate cancer in black and white patients: a comparative study based on radical prostatectomy specimens. *J. Urol.* 1998;160(2):437-42.

[110] Moul JW, Connelly RR, Mooneyhan RM, Zhang W, Sesterhenn IA, Mostofi FK, et al. Racial differences in tumor volume and prostate specific antigen among radical prostatectomy patients. *J. Urol.* 1999;162(2):394-7.

[111] Powell IJ, Schwartz K, Hussain M. Removal of the financial barrier to health care: does it impact on prostate cancer at presentation and survival? A comparative study between black and white men in a Veterans Affairs system. *Urology* 1995;46(6):825-30.

[112] Optenberg SA, Thompson IM, Friedrichs P, Wojcik B, Stein CR, Kramer B. Race, treatment, and long-term survival from prostate cancer in an equal-access medical care delivery system. *JAMA* 1995;274(20):1599-605.

[113] Polednak AP. Black-white differences in tumor grade (aggressiveness) at diagnosis of prostate cancer, 1992-1998. *Ethn. Dis.* 2002;12(4):536-40.

[114] Underwood W, 3rd, Jackson J, Wei JT, Dunn R, Baker E, Demonner S, et al. Racial treatment trends in localized/regional prostate carcinoma: 1992-1999. *Cancer* 2005; 103 (3): 538-45.

[115] Underwood W, De Monner S, Ubel P, Fagerlin A, Sanda MG, Wei JT. Racial/ethnic disparities in the treatment of localized/regional prostate cancer. *J. Urol.* 2004; 171 (4): 1504-7.

[116] Krupski TL, Saigal CS, Hanley J, Schonlau M, Litwin MS. Patterns of care for men with prostate cancer after failure of primary treatment. *Cancer* 2006;107(2):258-65.

[117] Steginga SK, Occhipinti S, Gardiner RA, Yaxley J, Heathcote P. Making decisions about treatment for localized prostate cancer. *BJU Int.* 2002; 89(3):255-60.

[118] Zeliadt SB, Potosky AL, Etzioni R, Ramsey SD, Penson DF. Racial disparity in primary and adjuvant treatment for nonmetastatic prostate cancer: SEER-Medicare trends 1991 to 1999. *Urology* 2004; 64(6):1171-6.

[119] Ung JO, Richie JP, Chen MH, Renshaw AA, D'Amico AV. Evolution of the presentation and pathologic and biochemical outcomes after radical prostatectomy for patients with clinically localized prostate cancer diagnosed during the PSA era. *Urology* 2002;60(3):458-63.

[120] Galper SL, Chen MH, Catalona WJ, Roehl KA, Richie JP, D'Amico AV. Evidence to support a continued stage migration and decrease in prostate cancer specific mortality. *J. Urol.* 2006;175(3 Pt 1):907-12.

[121] Eastham JA, Kattan MW. Disease recurrence in black and white men undergoing radical prostatectomy for clinical stage T1-T2 prostate cancer. *J. Urol.* 2000; 163 (1): 143-5.

[122] Freedland SJ, Jalkut M, Dorey F, Sutter ME, Aronson WJ. Race is not an independent predictor of biochemical recurrence after radical prostatectomy in an equal access medical center. *Urology* 2000;56(1):87-91.

[123] Cohen JH, Schoenbach VJ, Kaufman JS, Talcott JA, Schenck AP, Peacock S, et al. Racial differences in clinical progression among Medicare recipients after treatment for localized prostate cancer (United States). *Cancer Causes Control* 2006;17(6):803-11.

[124] Lam JS, Sclar JD, Desai M, Mansukhani MM, Benson MC, Goluboff ET. Is Hispanic race an important predictor of treatment failure following radical prostatectomy for prostate cancer? *J. Urol.* 2004;172(5 Pt 1):1856-9.

[125] Polednak AP. Black-white differences in survival from late-stage prostate cancer. *Ethn. Dis.* 2003;13(2):220-5.

[126] Shavers VL, Brown ML, Potosky AL, Klabunde CN, Davis WW, Moul JW, et al. Race/ethnicity and the receipt of watchful waiting for the initial management of prostate cancer. *J. Gen. Intern. Med.* 2004;19(2):146-55.

[127] Shavers VL, Brown M, Klabunde CN, Potosky AL, Davis W, Moul J, et al. Race/ethnicity and the intensity of medical monitoring under 'watchful waiting' for prostate cancer. *Med. Care* 2004;42(3):239-50.

[128] Penedo FJ, Dahn JR, Shen BJ, Schneiderman N, Antoni MH. Ethnicity and determinants of quality of life after prostate cancer treatment. *Urology* 2006; 67 (5): 1022-7.

[129] Diefenbach MA, Hamrick N, Uzzo R, Pollack A, Horwitz E, Greenberg R, et al. Clinical, demographic and psychosocial correlates of complementary and alternative medicine use by men diagnosed with localized prostate cancer. *J. Urol.* 2003; 170 (1): 166-9.

[130] Boon H, Westlake K, Stewart M, Gray R, Fleshner N, Gavin A, et al. Use of complementary/alternative medicine by men diagnosed with prostate cancer: prevalence and characteristics. *Urology* 2003;62(5):849-53.

[131] Chan JM, Elkin EP, Silva SJ, Broering JM, Latini DM, Carroll PR. Total and specific complementary and alternative medicine use in a large cohort of men with prostate cancer. *Urology* 2005;66(6):1223-8.

[132] Yoshimura K, Ichioka K, Terada N, Terai A, Arai Y. Use of complementary and alternative medicine by patients with localized prostate carcinoma: study at a single institute in Japan. *Int. J. Clin. Oncol.* 2003;8(1):26-30.

[133] Chan EC, Vernon SW, O'Donnell FT, Ahn C, Greisinger A, Aga DW. Informed consent for cancer screening with prostate-specific antigen: how well are men getting the message? Am J Public Health 2003;93(5):779-85.

[134] Talcott JA, Spain P, Clark JA, Carpenter WR, Do YK, Hamilton RJ, et al. Hidden barriers between knowledge and behavior: the North Carolina prostate cancer screening and treatment experience. *Cancer* 2007;109(8):1599-606.

[135] Du XL, Fang S, Coker AL, Sanderson M, Aragaki C, Cormier JN, et al. Racial disparity and socioeconomic status in association with survival in older men with local/regional stage prostate carcinoma: findings from a large community-based cohort. *Cancer* 2006;106(6):1276-85.

[136] Albano JD, Ward E, Jemal A, Anderson R, Cokkinides VE, Murray T, et al. Cancer mortality in the United States by education level and race. *J. Natl. Cancer Inst.* 2007;99(18):1384-94.

[137] Fiscella K, Franks P, Gold MR, Clancy CM. Inequality in quality: addressing socioeconomic, racial, and ethnic disparities in health care. *JAMA* 2000;283(19):2579-84.

[138] Wacholder S. Untangling differences in cancer mortality rates: a closer look at race and education. *J. Natl. Cancer Inst.* 2007;99(18):1356-7.

[139] National Institutes of Health. Monitoring adherence to the NIH policy on the inclusion of women and minoritiesas subjects in clinical research; 2003.

[140] Murthy VH, Krumholz HM, Gross CP. Participation in cancer clinical trials: race-, sex-, and age-based disparities. *JAMA* 2004;291(22):2720-6.

[141] Moinpour CM, Atkinson JO, Thomas SM, Underwood SM, Harvey C, Parzuchowski J, et al. Minority recruitment in the prostate cancer prevention trial. *Ann. Epidemiol.* 2000; 10(8 Suppl):S85-91.

[142] Talone P. Establishing trust after Tuskegee. *Int. J. Radiat. Oncol. Biol. Phys.* 1998; 40 (1):3-4.

[143] Ford JG, Howerton MW, Lai GY, Gary TL, Bolen S, Gibbons MC, et al. Barriers to recruiting underrepresented populations to cancer clinical trials: A systematic review. *Cancer* 2007.

[144] Barber KR, Shaw R, Folts M, Taylor DK, Ryan A, Hughes M, et al. Differences between African American and Caucasian men participating in a community-based prostate cancer screening program. *J. Community Health* 1998;23(6):441-51.

[145] Advani AS, Atkeson B, Brown CL, Peterson BL, Fish L, Johnson JL, et al. Barriers to the participation of African-American patients with cancer in clinical trials: a pilot study. *Cancer* 2003;97(6):1499-506.

[146] Robinson SB, Ashley M, Haynes MA. Attitude of African-Americans regarding prostate cancer clinical trials. *J. Community Health* 1996;21(2):77-87.

[147] Lai GY, Gary TL, Tilburt J, Bolen S, Baffi C, Wilson RF, et al. Effectiveness of strategies to recruit underrepresented populations into cancer clinical trials. *Clin. Trials* 2006; 3 (2):133-41.

[148] Bolen S, Tilburt J, Baffi C, Gary TL, Powe N, Howerton M, et al. Defining "success" in recruitment of underrepresented populations to cancer clinical trials: moving toward a more consistent approach. *Cancer* 2006;106(6):1197-204.

[149] Royal C, Baffoe-Bonnie A, Kittles R, Powell I, Bennett J, Hoke G, et al. Recruitment experience in the first phase of the African American Hereditary Prostate Cancer (AAHPC) study. *Ann. Epidemiol.* 2000;10(8 Suppl):S68-77.

[150] Ford ME, Havstad SL, Davis SD. A randomized trial of recruitment methods for older African American men in the Prostate, Lung, Colorectal and Ovarian (PLCO) Cancer Screening Trial. *Clin. Trials* 2004;1(4):343-51.

[151] Howerton MW, Gibbons MC, Baffi CR, Gary TL, Lai GY, Bolen S, et al. Provider roles in the recruitment of underrepresented populations to cancer clinical trials. *Cancer* 2007; 109(3):465-76.

[152] Cook ED, Moody-Thomas S, Anderson KB, Campbell R, Hamilton SJ, Harrington JM, et al. Minority recruitment to the Selenium and Vitamin E Cancer Prevention Trial (SELECT). *Clin. Trials* 2005; 2 (5):436-42.

[153] Enger SM, Van den Eeden SK, Sternfeld B, Loo RK, Quesenberry CP, Jr., Rowell S, et al. California Men's Health Study (CMHS): a multiethnic cohort in a managed care setting. *BMC Public Health* 2006;6:172.

In: Topics in Prevalent Diseases
Editors: N. C. Chavez-Tapia and M. Uribe
ISBN 978-1-60456-959-9

Chapter 3

Colorectal Cancer in Minorities

***Sandra Garcia Osogobio*[1] *and Félix Ignacio Téllez Ávila*[2]**
[1] Department of Surgery, McMaster University, St. Joseph's Healthcare, Hamilton, Ontario, Canada
[2] Department of Gastroenterology and Endoscopy, Instituto Nacional de Ciencias Médicas y Nutrición Salvador Zubirán, México City, Mexico

Epidemiology

In countries with a westernized lifestyle about half of all deaths are caused by circulatory disease and a quarter by cancer. Cancer is an important problem in both public health and political terms worldwide, irrespective of a country's development.

Colorectal cancer (CRC) is the fourth commonest form of cancer occurring worldwide. It affects men and women almost equally, with about 401 000 new cases in men annually and 381 000 in women. The number of new cases of colorectal cancer worldwide has been increasing rapidly since 1975. Worldwide, colorectal cancer represents 9.4% of all incident cancer in men and 10.1% in women. Colorectal cancer, however, is not equally common throughout the world. If the westernised countries (North America; those in northern, southern, and western Europe; Australia; and New Zealand) are combined, colorectal cancer represents 12.6% of all incident cancer in men and 14.1% in women. Elsewhere colorectal cancer represents 7.7% and 7.9% of all incident cases in men and women respectively.

Data about Latin American Countries are scarce. In Mexico, cancer in general is a major public health problem. It is the second cause of mortality after cardiovascular diseases, with a rate around 51.6 per 100,000 inhabitants, amounting for 46,423 deaths in 1994.

Throughout Mexico, 2,361 new cases of colorectal cancer and a total of 1,809 deaths were reported in 1993. This accounts for 4 percent of all cancer deaths in the country, with a specific mortality rate for colorectal cancer of 2.48 per 100,000 inhabitants. A recent study shows an increase in colon cancer frequency over the past 25 years. Rates of advanced disease diagnosed are high in Mexico (metastatic disease in 25% and 15% at Instituto

Nacional de Nutricion and Centro Medico de Occidente, respectively) and percentage of patients with curative disease amenable for surgical treatment is low (67%-76%).

Data from the Surveillance, Epidemiology, and End Results (SEER) program indicate that the overall incidence of and mortality from colorectal cancer have been decreasing in the United States, unfortunately, mortality rates in Mexico have been increasing in the last 15 years.

Genetics

The development of colorectal cancer involves a progression from normal mucosa through adenoma to carcinoma. A genetic model of colorectal carcinogenesis has been proposed that describes a sequence of key mutations driving the process of colorectal carcinogenesis. This process may involve the accumulation of mutations in both, tumor suppressor genes and proto-oncogenes, as well as epigenetic phenomena such as DNA hypermethylation or hypomethylation. The onset of genomic instability increases the mutation rate and accelerates this progression. Inactivation of the adenomatous polyposis coli (APC) gene on chromosome 5q is thought to be one of the earliest mutations in sporadic cancers and is seen as a germline mutation in patients with familial polyposis. Mutations in other tumor suppressor genes play an important role in this pathway as well, including mutations in DCC, SMAD2, and SMAD4 on chromosome 18q and p53 on chromosome 17p; these events are thought to occur at a later stage of tumor progression. Mutations in the K-ras oncogene occur at an intermediate stage.

Microsatellite instability (MSI) is an alternative pathway to genomic instability and subsequent colorectal carcinogenesis. This phenomenon arises from defects in mismatch repair genes, which cause significantly increased mutation rates in comparison with those in normal cells. MSI in hereditary nonpolyposis colorectal cancer (HNPCC)is most commonly attributable to germline mutations in the hMLH1 and hMSH2 genes. MSI in sporadic colorectal cancer is most frequently associated with hypermethylation of the promoter region of the hMLH1 gene, which leads to inactivation of the gene and loss of expression of the hMLH1 protein.

Risk Factors

A number of risks factors for CRC have been described, including a family history of cancer or adenomatous polyps, familial colorectal cancer syndromes, inflammatory bowel disease, and dietary and lifestyle factors.

The vast majority of colorectal cancers worldwide are sporadic. No more than 5% of colorectal cancers are associated with known genetic syndromes.

The relative risk of colorectal cancer in those with an affected first-degree relative is 2.25, it rises to 4.25 if more than one relative is involved and to 3.87 if colorectal cancer was diagnosed before the age of 45.

Table 1. Amsterdam II Criteria

1. Three or more relatives with HNPCC-related cancers (colon, uterine, stomach, ovarian, small bowel, and urinary tract), one of whom should be a first-degree relative of the other two
2. At least two successive generations should be affected
3. In one of the relatives, colorectal carcinoma should have been diagnosed when the patient was younger than 50 years of age.

Table 2. Screening for colorectal cancer and polyps

Risk Category	Screening Method
Average risk*	FOBT annually Flexible sigmoidoscopy every 5 yr FOBT annually + flexible sigmoidoscopy every 5 yr Air contrast barium enema every 5–10 yr Colonoscopy every 10 yr
Personal History	Colonoscopy every 3-5 yr
Family History	Colonoscopy at 40 yr or 10 yr before diagnosis of the youngest affected family member; if normal repeat every 10 yr
IBD	Colonoscopy every 1-2 yr, after 8 yr or 15 yr with pancolitis or left-sided colitis, respectively
HNPCC	Colonoscopy every 1-2 yr at age of 20-25 yr or 10 yr earlier than the youngest case of CRC
FAP	Sigmoidoscopy or colonoscopy annually

* Choose one of the following

The National Polyp Study found that the relative risk of colorectal cancer was 1.78 in first-degree relatives of patients with adenomatous polyps.

The most common of the genetic syndromes known to be associated with colorectal cancer is HNPCC, which accounts for the majority of patients with familial colorectal cancer. HNPCC can be diagnosed clinically on the basis of what are known as the Amsterdam II Criteria (Table 1). The lifetime risk of CRC in HNPCC patients is approximately 80%.

Familial adenomatous polyposis (FAP) accounts for the remainder of patients with familial colorectal syndromes. It has a nearly 100% risk of CRC by the age of 40 if prophylactic colectomy is not performed.

The lifetime risk of colorectal cancer for patients with ulcerative colitis is 3.7%, which increases to 5.4% for patients with pancolitis and rises further with greater duration of disease. Crohn´s disease may be associated with a similarly increased risk of colorectal cancer.

Lifestyle and dietary factors have been put forward as potential causes of increased colorectal cancer risk. Lower levels of physical activity and increased body mass index are associated with an increased risk of colorectal cancer in man and women. The western style diet, which is high in calories and fat and low fiber, is associated with high rates of colorectal cancer. There is some evidence that increased dietary intake of calcium may confer some protection against the development of colorectal cancer and adenomatous polyps.

Screening

The recognition that virtually all colorectal cancers arise from a discrete and accessible precursor lesion raises the prospect that cancer can essentially be prevented with appropriate screening. The "dwell time" between the initiation of a polyp and development of an invasive cancer has been estimated to be as long as 10 years. This provides an ideal opportunity to intervene and alter the natural history of the disease. Proof of this principle was provided by the National Polyp Study, which established that colonoscopic polypectomy can dramatically reduce the incidence of colorectal cancer. First of all, it is essential to stratify patients into risk groups for CRC: average, moderate and high risk patients (Table 2).

Average Risk

Average risk patients are those greater than 50 years old who do not have any of the risk factors listed before. The vast majority of the population (70%) will fall into the average risk group.

Recommendations

1. Annually, two samples from each of three consecutive stools should be examined without rehydration using a guaiac-impregnated slide. Patients are to avoid ASA/NSAIDS, foods high in vitamin C, and red meat for three days before the examination. Any positive test should be followed up with colonoscopy.
2. Flexible sigmoidoscopy every five years.

It has been hypothesized that the combination of flexible sigmoidoscopy and FOBT would increase the overall detection rate of CRC. While this approach has not been rigorously tested, the sensitivity of this combined screening strategy was estimated by analyzing patients who had undergone both a full colonoscopy and FOBT.

3. Double Contrast Barium Enema (DCBE) every 5-10 years. As such, DCBE is considerably less sensitive than colonoscopy. The sensitivity of DCBE for polyps > 1 cm is 48% and for CRC 82.9%. Nevertheless, this does represent another modality for visualization of the entire colon, particularly in those cases in which the cecum cannot be intubated or there are contraindications to colonoscopy.
4. Colonoscopy every ten years. It has been convincingly demonstrated that colonoscopic polypectomy results in a decreased incidence of CRC, which is again likely to translate to a decrease in mortality from CRC.

Moderate Risk

Moderate risk individuals include those with 1) a personal history of adenomatous polyps or CRC, 2) a family history of adenomatous polyps or CRC, or 3) chronic inflammatory bowel disease.

Recommendations

1. Patients with an advanced adenoma (>1 cm, villous histology, high-grade dysplasia, or cancer) or ≥3 adenomas should have a follow-up colonoscopy in three years. Patients with 1 or 2 small (≤1 cm) tubular adenomas should have a follow-up colonoscopy in five years.
2. Patients with CRC should have a complete colonoscopy at the time of diagnosis to rule out synchronous lesions. Follow-up colonoscopy should be performed at three years and if normal, again at five years.
3. Patients with one 1st degree relative with CRC or adenomatous polyps diagnosed at <60 years old or two 1st degree relatives with CRC diagnosed at any age should start screening colonoscopy at 40 years old or 10 years before the earliest diagnosis in the family. This should be repeated every five years.
4. Patients with one 1st degree relative with CRC or adenomatous polyps diagnosed at >60 years old or two 2nd degree relatives with CRC should begin screening at 40 years old. If normal, examinations should be repeated every 10 years.
5. In patients with Inflammatory Bowel Disease surveillance colonoscopy is recommended every 1 to 2 years after 8 years of disease in patients with pancolitis and after 15 years in those with left-sided disease. Four-quadrant biopsies should be taken every 10 cm throughout the colon. Additional biopsies should be taken of any suspicious lesions.

High Risk

Patients at high risk include those with a hereditary colon cancer syndrome. Approximately 5% of all colorectal cancers occur in association with a hereditary colon cancer syndrome. Three of the most common and best understood are the Hereditary Nonpolyposis Colorectal Cancer (HNPCC), Familial Adenomatous Polyposis (FAP), and MYH-Associated Polyposis (MAP) syndromes.

Recommendations

1. Patients with FAP need an annual sigmoidoscopy starting at 10-12 years old. In attenuated FAP, full colonoscopy should be performed annually starting at age 25 years.

2. Patients with HNPCC need colonoscopy every 1-2 years starting at age 20-25 years or 10 years earlier than the youngest case of CRC diagnosis in the family. Annual colonoscopy after age 40 years.

Clinical Evaluation

Unfortunately, colon cancer in Mexico is diagnosed in advanced stages. Some patients present with occult GI bleeding and anemia. The duration of symptoms, however, is not necessarily associated with the stage of tumor. The most common symptoms of colorectal cancer are bleeding per rectum, abdominal or back pain, and changes in bowel habits or stool caliber. Other symptoms are fatigue, anorexia, weight loss, nausea, and vomiting. Some patients present with acute bowel obstruction o perforation.

Careful digital assessment of the rectal tumor may yield valuable information. Important parameters that should be recorded during the physical examination of a rectal tumor are: location, morphology, number of quadrants involved, degree of fixation, mobility, extra rectal growths and direct continuity. A clinical staging system based on tumor mobility has been established. In this clinical staging system, tumor mobility is correlated with the level of tumor penetration in the different layers of the rectal wall (Table 3). It has been clearly showed that useful information can be obtained from digital examination of rectal tumors.

Staging, Diagnosis and Prognosis

Traditionally, staging of colorectal cancer has been based on modifications of the Dukes classification, which was initially developed for rectal cancer. This classification has undergone multiple modifications, of which the most widely used is the modified Astler-Coller system. Currently, the TNM classification, developed by the American Joint Committee on Cancer (AJCC) and the International Union against Cancer (UICC), is the preferred staging system (Table 4). This system takes into account the depth of penetration into the bowel wall (T), the presence and number of involved mesenteric nodes (N), and the presence of distant metastases (M).

Table 3. Clinical staging system*

Clinical stage	Mobility	Pathologic correlation (level of invasion)
CS1	Freely mobile	Submucosa
CS2	Mobile with rectal wall	
CS3	Tethered mobility	Muscularis propria
CS4	Fixed/tethered fixation	
		Perirectal fat
		Adjacent tissues

* The accuracy is directly proportional to the experience of the examiner.

Table 4. Staging system of CRC

Dukes Classification
A: Tumor does not grow beyond muscularis propria
B: Tumor grows beyond muscularis propria
C: Lymph node metastasis/es with the tumor
D: Distant metastasis/es
Astler Coller Classification
A: Tumor limited to mucosa; carcinoma in situ
B1: Tumor grows through muscularis mucosae but not through muscularis propria
B2: Tumor grows beyond muscularis propria
C1: Stage B1 with regional lymph node metastases
C2: Stage B2 with regional lymph node metastases
D: Distant metastases.
TNM Classification
TX: Primary tumor cannot be assessed
T0: No evidence of primary tumor
Tis: Carcinoma in situ: intraepithelial or invasion of the lamina propria
T1: Tumor invades submucosa
T2: Tumor invades muscularis propria
T3: Tumor invades through the muscularis propria into the subserosa, or into nonperitonealized pericolic or perirectal tissues
T4: Tumor directly invades other organs or structures, and/or perforates visceral peritoneum
NX: Regional nodes cannot be assessed
N0: No regional lymph node metastasis
N1: Metastasis in 1 to 3 regional lymph nodes
N2: Metastasis in 4 or more regional lymph nodes
MX: Distant metastasis cannot be assessed
M0: No distant metastasis
M1: Distant metastasis
AJCC Stage
Stage 0 Tis N0 M0
Stage I T1 N0 M0 T2 N0 M0
Stage IIA T3 N0 M0
Stage IIB T4 N0 M0
Stage IIIA T1 N1 M0 T2 N1 M0
Stage IIIB T3 N1 M0 T4 N1 M0
Stage IIIC any T N2 M0
Stage IV any T any N M1

Clinical staging is based on the history and the physical examination, endoscopic findings, and biopsy results. Endoscopic tattooing, a process in which an agent is injected into the bowel wall submucosally at or near the site of the lesion, has been employed to facilitate intra operative identification of the tumor site. India ink is the agent most commonly used for this purpose and generally yields excellent results.

When a colon cancer is diagnosed by colonoscopy, synchronous cancers occur in 6% or fewer of patients. When present, it should raise the suspicion of possibly HNPCC which is associated with synchronous colon cancer.

If colonoscopy cannot be complete, an air-contrast barium enema study should be performed to evaluate the remainder color. A chest x-ray is routinely obtained to rule out metastases and prepare for operation. There is some debate regarding the utility of preoperative CT scans in the management of primary colon cancer. The rationale includes evaluation of potential metastatic disease and assessment of the local extent of disease.

In cases of rectal cancer, locoregional staging may significantly affect therapeutic decision making. Such staging includes determination of the depth of invasion of the rectal wall and the degree of egional node involvement. Modalities commonly used include CT, MRI and endoscopic ultrasonography (EUS). EUS has proved to be to most accurate technique for evaluating muscularis propria involvement and perirectal tissue invasion.

Definitive pathologic staging is carried out after surgical exploration and examination of the resected specimen.

Survival is correlated with the stage of the tumor. The AJCC staging system has subdivided stage II into stages IIA and IIB, and stage III into stages IIIA, IIIB and IIIC on the basis of both the extent of wall penetration and the number of nodes involved. The degree of lymphatic invasion and the extent of vascular invasion are important adjuncts to the TNM staging system. Certain histologic types, including signet-ring and mucinous carcinomas, are associated with poor outcomes. Carcinoembryonic antigen (CEA) increase correlates with either disease that has metastasized to the liver or with very large tumors. Patients with disease confined to the colonic mucosa or submucosa will have increased CEA in 30%–40% of cases. It is therefore not useful for screening but can be used to follow patients with colon cancer. In patients with increased CEA preoperatively and localized disease that is resectable, the CEA should decrease after surgery. If the CEA level does not decrease, then occult metastases may be present and may be an indication for adjuvant therapy.

Management of Colon Cancer

Surgical Therapy

Surgery remains the primary modality of treatment, and standard resection is the only therapy required for early-stage cancer.

The patient needs to be prepared for the procedure and the anesthetic so as to minimize perioperative and postoperative complications. Particular attention needs to be given to the patient's medical comorbidities. There have been metaanalyses that have concluded that mechanical bowel cleansing before colorectal surgery has no significant impact on perioperative infection rates. Despite these recent studies, we would still recommend that some type on colonic cleansing occur before surgery because it is easier to manipulate the bowel if it is not filled with stool.

The ideal extent of a bowel resection is defined by removing the blood supply and the lymphatics at the level of the origin of the primary feeding arterial vessel. Five centimeters of normal bowel on either side of the primary colon tumor is adequate to minimize anastomotic recurrences.

The standard extent of resection for various colon cancers has been defined. For tumors of the cecum and the ascending colon, a right hemicolectomy that includes the right branch of the middle colic artery at its origin should be performed. For tumors of the transverse colon, an extended right or left colectomy or a transverse colectomy may be performed. For tumors of the splenic flexure region, a left hemicolectomy is performed, and for sigmoid tumors, a sigmoid colectomy is performed.

The Clinical Outcomes of Surgical Therapy (COST) Study Group trial showed no difference between the laparoscopic and open approaches. In this multi-institutional study, the rates of recurrent cancer were similar after laparoscopically assisted colectomy and open colectomy, suggesting that the laparoscopic approach is an acceptable alternative to open surgery for colon cancer.

Obstructing and perforated cancers are associated with poor prognosis and with increased surgical morbidity. Patients with perforated colon cancer are managed with emergency laparotomy, washout, and resection of the primary lesion. A diverting stoma is usually indicated, with either a Hartmann pouch or a mucous fistula constructed distally. Select patients may be managed of primary anastomosis, with or without diverting stoma.

Sentinel Node Assessment

Saha described the application of sentinel node identification for colorectal cancer patients with proposed benefits of a high rate of node identification and pathologic upstaging. Subsequent evaluation of the technique, including some modifications, has demonstrated false-negative rates approaching 60%, and limitations in rectal cancers. Finally, there is insufficient evidence that the technique is sufficiently accurate to alter the extent if surgical resection. Therefore, at the present time, routine lymph node mapping cannot be recommended.

Adjuvant Therapy

The stage of disease at presentation remains the most important prognostic factor for colon cancer patients.

Stage I disease carries an excellent prognosis of more than 95% 5 year survival rate, and surgical treatment alone is considered sufficient, adjuvant therapy is not indicated.

The role of adjuvant chemotherapy for Stage II node-negative disease is still controversial. At this time, the use of adjuvant chemotherapy for Stage II node-negative disease remains an unanswered question, mainly because the prognosis for Stage II node-negative disease is good overall (5 year survival of 80%), and many patients would face unnecessary treatment. For the time being, patients with Stage II colon cancer at high risk for tumor recurrence might be considered for adjuvant treatment on an individual basis, or might be entered in a clinical trial.

Overall 5 year survival from curative surgery for Stage III colon cancer is 30%-60%. Recurrences are often systemic, hence the need for systemic adjuvant treatment in these high risk patients. Adjuvant chemotherapy improves survival by approximately 10%-15%. 5-Fluorouracil (5-FU)/leucovorin (LV)-based adjuvant chemotherapy for Stage III disease is the standard of care.

The newer chemotherapeutic agents currently under study or in use for treatment of metastatic disease (e.g., irinotecan, capecitabine, oxaliplatin) are undergoing evaluation for their usefulness in the adjuvant treatment of patients with Stage II and Stage III disease.

At this time, the precise role of adjuvant radiotherapy in the treatment of colon cancer remains undefined. There are no data to support a systemic recommendation for therapy or a well-recognized adjuvant regimen. The potential risks of adjuvant radiotherapy for colon cancer, particularly radiation damage to surrounding organs (e.g., small bowel) are significant. Treatment for individuals deemed at high risk for local recurrence after curative surgery for colon cancer should be individualized.

Management of Rectal Cancer

Surgical Therapy

The surgical approach is dependent on the location of the tumor, its depth of invasion, and whether, in the preoperative evaluation, metastases have been discovered. Presently, a surgeon has three major curative options: local excision, sphincter-saving abdominal surgery, and APR.

Surgical Principles

Total Mesorectal Excision

The mesorectum is defined as the lymphovascular, fatty and neural tissue that is circumferentially adherent to the rectum, starting at the level of the sacral promontory, where the superior hemorrhoidal vessel divides into right and left branches. The mesorectum tapers and then diminishes just below Waldeyer's fascia (the investing fascia of the levators) around the elevator ani muscles at the level of the distal third of the rectum.

Total mesorectal excision involves precise sharp dissection and removal of the entire rectal mesentery, including that distal to the tumor, as an intact unit, emphasizing autonomic nerve preservation, complete hemostasis, and avoidance of violation of the mesorectal envelope. The field of rectal cancer spread is limited to this envelope and its total removal encompasses virtually every tumor satellite. The reduction of positive radial margins can be reduced in cases resected by TME.

Distal and Radial Margins

Data from randomized prospective trial conducted by the National Surgical Adjuvant Breast and Bowel Project demonstrated no significant differences in survival or local recurrence when comparing distal rectal margins of < 2 cm, 2- 2.9 cm and > 3 cm. As a result, a 2 cm distal margin has become acceptable for resection of rectal carcinoma although a 5 cm proximal margin is still recommended. Even smaller distal margins may be acceptable in certain patients from whom there is no other option for sphincter preservation.

The discussion concerning the distal margin should not be confused with issues regarding a TME and the radial margin. It is now clear that the status of the radial margin is perhaps the most critical determining prognosis.

Each patient with rectal cancer should be viewed individually and a technical plan for their resection customized to their stage, gender, age and body habitus. In all of the technical choices for a radical resection, a TME should be performed.

The morbidity associated with radical resection can be substantial. Anastomotic leakage rates vary widely, ranging from less than 10% to more than 30%. Postoperative urinary and sexual dysfunction resulting from inadvertent damage to the pelvic hypogastric and splanchnic nerves are recognized complications of rectal resection. Even with incorporation of autonomic nerve-preserving techniques in TME, urinary and sexual dysfunction remains recognized complications in 0-12 and 10-35 per cent of patients respectively.

Surgical Options

Abdominoperineal Resection (APR)

Principles of APR include: removal of the whole pelvic mesocolon, removal of the zone of upward spread in the rectal mesentery, wide perineal dissection, an abdominal anus (colostomy) and removal of the lymph nodes along iliacs. Candidates for an APR are patients whose tumors are either into the anal sphincter or are so close to the anal sphincter that a safe distal margin cannot be obtained.

Low Anterior Resection (LAR) with Sphincter Preservation

An LAR involves dissection and anastomosis below the peritoneal reflection with ligation of the superior and middle hemorrhoidal arteries.

Local Excision

There are three approaches to local excision of rectal cancer: transanal, transcoccygeal and transsphincteric. Recently, a newer technique, transanal endosocpic microsurgery (TEM) has provided a minimally invasive option for local excision which also allows the surgeon to reach lesions that are located more proximally and would have required a transcoccygeal or transsphincteric approach in the past.

Tumors amenable to local excision should be < 4 cm in diameter and occupy < 40% of the bowel circumference. The distance of the tumor from the dentate line is important, because it will dictate which approach should be taken. Tumors < 5 cm from dentate line are amenable to resection via a transanal procedure, whereas tumors in the middle third of the rectum may require a transcoccygeal approach or transanal endoscopic microsurgery (TEM). The best candidates have either a T1N0 or a T2N0 lesion. For T2 lesions, local excision alone is not sufficient as therapy alone, and either preoperative or postoperative adjuvant therapy should be added.

Retrospective reviews report a local recurrence rate of 5%-33% and survival rates of 57%-100%. Superficial tumors and negative margins at the time of resection have low recurrence rates and a very good prognosis.

The addition of adjuvant or neodjuvant radiation has been shown to decrease these local recurrence rates, and there is increasing evidence that chemoradiation may have a beneficial effect on survival.

Laparoscopic Total Mesorectal Excision (LTME)

The application of laparoscopy for the treatment of intraabdominal malignancies including proctectomy for rectal cancer is now being performed. The main questions about laparoscopically total mesorectal excision (LTME) are whether it provides the same TME specimen as traditional open techniques, and whether there is any other unique biologic alteration in the laparoscopic procedure that leads to a change in survival or in recurrence patterns.

With respect to objective outcomes, LTME is associated with improved short-term results compared with open total mesorectal excision with respect to morbidity, recovery period, and postoperative pain. Long-term outcome data of LTME are not available yet; however, we know that the long-term survival of laparoscopic colectomy for colonic cancer is at least equal to open surgery.

Adjuvant Therapy

Many prospective trials have demonstrated the beneficial effect of preoperative and postoperative radiation therapy in patients with rectal cancer who had surgery with curative intent. Benefits of radiotherapy in the treatment of rectal cancer can be divided under four categories: first, radiotherapy lowers local failure and improves survival; second, radiotherapy allows surgery in nonresectable rectal cancer; third, it facilitates sphincter-preserving procedures and finally, it may offer a totally curative approach without major surgery. It can be used alone or in combination with chemotherapy.

The German CAO/ ARO/ AIO trial randomized patients with T3-4, N0, or any T, N1 rectal cancer to neoadjuvant chemoradiation followed by surgery and additional postoperative chemotherapy or postoperative chemoradiation. The results suggest that preoperative chemoradiation is the preferred adjuvant treatment in patients with locally advanced rectal cancer.

Postoperative adjuvant radiation therapy alone decreases local recurrence, although not to the same extent as neoadjuvant treatment, and does not improve survival.

A non-resectable rectal cancer is defined as a tumor that cannot be resected without a very high risk of local recurrence. Approximately, 10-15% of all patients with rectal cancer fall into this category; half of those patients have no metastases, indicating that there is potential for a curative procedure. Based on tumor characteristics, surgery alone is unlikely to be curative and it is indicated to offer radiotherapy.

Survival after Rectal Cancer Excision

Survival rates for colorectal cancer have shown improvement over recent decades with the combination of better surgery and adjuvant therapy. Overall 5-year survival rates after major surgery for rectal cancer are as follows: Stage I, 85%-100%; Stage II, 60%-80%; and Stage III, 30%-50%.

Follow Up

Recommendations on the use of surveillance colonoscopy after resection of colorectal cancer were produced jointly by the US Multi-Society Task Force on Colorectal Cancer and the American Cancer Society (ACS).

Patients undergoing curative resection for colon or rectal cancer should undergo a colonoscopy 1 year after the resection (or 1 year following the performance of the colonoscopy that was performed to clear the colon of synchronous disease). If the examination performed at 1 year is normal, the interval before the next subsequent examination should be 3 years. If that colonoscopy is normal, the the interval before the next subsequent examination should be 5 years. Following the examination at 1 year, the intervals before subsequent examinations may be shortened if there is evidence of hereditary nonpolyposis colorectal cancer or if adenoma findings warrant earlier colonoscopy.

Periodic examination of the rectum (proctoscopy and selective endorectal ultrasound) for the purpose of identifying local recurrence usually performed at 3 to 6 month intervals for the first 2 or 3 years, may be considered after low anterior resection of rectal cancer.

Serial CEA testing every 3 months for the first postoperative year or two and every 6–12 months thereafter, serial chest x-ray every 6–12 months is recommended. Based on the available evidence, there is no role for the routine use of liver function tests, hemoglobin, CT scanning, MRI, or PET scanning in asymptomatic patients

References

[1] J. Jesus Villaobos Perez, Marco A. Olivera Martinez, Aurora Loaeza del Castillo, ma. Luisa Villalobos, Gonzalo Torres Villalobos. Estudio de 25 años de cancer del aparato digestivo en cuatro instituciones de la Ciudad de Mexico. *Rev. Gastroenterol Mex.* 2006; 71(4):460-472

[2] Mario Grassini, Carlo Verna, Paolo Niola, Monica Navino, Edda Battaglia, Gabrio Bassotti Appropriateness of colonoscopy: Diagnostic yield and safety in guidelines *World J. Gastroenterol.* 2007 March 28; 13(12): 1816-1819

[3] Ramona M McLoughlin, Colm A O'Morain Colorectal cancer screening *World J. Gastroenterol.* 2006 November 14; 12(42): 6747-6750

[4] Peter Boyle, J S Langman ABC of colorectal cancer: *Epidemiology BMJ* 2000; 321; 805-808

[5] Heidi Nelson, Nicholas Petrelli, Arthur Carlin, Jean Couture, James Fleshman, Jose Guillem, Brent Miedema, David Ota, Daniel Sargent Guidelines 2000 for Colon and Rectal Cancer Surgery *J. Natl. Cancer Inst.* 2001;93:583–96

[6] T. M. Young-Fadok, R. D. Fanelli, R. R. Price, D. B. Earle. Laparoscopic resection of curable colon and rectal cancer: an evidence-based review *Surg. Endosc.* (2007) 21: 1063–1068

[7] K. A. Forde. Colonoscopic screening for colon cancer. *Surg. Endosc.* (2006) 20: S471–S474

[8] Kenneth E. Hung, MD, PHD and Daniel C. Chung, MD. Colorectal Cancer Screening: *Today and Tomorrow Southern Medical Journal* 2006;99(3): 240-246

[9] Victor Tovar-Guzman, M.Sc., Mario Flores-Aldana, M.Sc., Jorge Salmeron-Castro, Ph.D.,Eduardo Cesar Lazcano-Ponce, Ph.D. Epidemiologic Panorama of Colorectal Cancer in Mexico, 1980-1993 *Dis. Colon Rectum.* 1998;41: 225-231.

[10] Joel S. Levine, M.D., and Dennis J. Ahnen, M.D. Adenomatous Polyps of the Colon. *N. Engl. J. Med.* 2006;355:2551-7.

[11] Arch-Ferrer J, Barreto-Andrade JC, Takahashi T, García-Osogobio S, León-Rodríguez E. Tratamiento quirúrgico del cáncer colorrectal. Experiencia de 10 años en el *INCMNSZ Rev. Gastroenterol. Mex.* 2001; 66(4): 187-192

[12] Mitchell I. Chorost, Rajiv Datta, Rosemary C. Santiago, Byrne Lee, Jyoti Bollman, Michael Leitman, Bimal C. Ghosh. Colon Cancer Screening: Where Have We Come From and Where Do We Go? *Journal of Surgical Oncology* 2004;85:7–13

[13] Chung DC, Rustgi AK: The hereditary nonpolyposis colorectal cancer syndrome: genetics and clinical implications. *Ann. Intern. Med.* 2003;138:560

[14] Slattery Ml, Levin TR, Ma K, et al. Family history and colorectal cancer: predictors of risk. *Cancer Causes Control* 2003;14:879

[15] Johns LE, Houlston RS. A systematic review and meta-analysis of familial colorectal cancer risk. *Am. J. Gastroenterol.* 2001;96:2992

[16] Baron JA, Beach M, Mandel JS, et al Calcium supplements for the prevention of colorectal adenomas. Calcium Polyp Prevention Study Group. *N Engl. J. Med,* 1999; 340: 101

[17] Durán O, González Ojeda A, Cisneros FJ, Hermosillo JM. Experiencia en el manejo del cáncer colorrectal en el Centro Médico Nacional de Occidente. *Cirujano General* 2000; 22: 153-158

[18] Weeks JC, Nelson H, Gelber S, et al. Short-term qualityof- life outcomes following laparoscopic-assisted colectomy vs. open colectomy for colon cancer: a randomized trial. *JAMA* 2002;287:321–8.

[19] Breukink SO, Pierie JP, Grond AJ, et al. Laparoscopic versus open total mesorectal excision: a case-control study. *Int. J. Colorectal. Dis.* 2005;20:428–33.

[20] Lacy AM, Garcia-Valdecasas JC, Delgado S, et al. Laparoscopy-assisted colectomy versus open colectomy for treatment of non-metastatic colon cancer: a randomized trial. *Lancet* 2002; 359:2224–9.

[21] S. O. Breukink, H. J. van der Zaag-Loonen,E. M. C. Bouma, J. P. E. N. Pierie, C. Hoff, T. Wiggers, W. J. H. J. Meijerink Prospective Evaluation of Quality of Life and Sexual

Functioning After Laparoscopic *Total Mesorectal Excision Dis. Colon Rectum* 2006; 50: 147–155

[22] Quah HM, Jayne DG, Eu KW, Seow-Choen F. Bladder and sexual dysfunction following laparoscopically assisted and conventional open mesorectal resection for cancer. *Br. J. Surg.* 2002; 89: 1551–1556.

[23] Jayne DG, Brown JM, Thorpe H, Walker J, Quirke P, Guillou PJ. Bladder and sexual function following resection for rectalcancer in a randomized clinical trial of laparoscopic versus open technique. *Br. J. Surg.* 2005;92:1124-1132

[24] Clinical Outcomes of Surgical Therapy Study Group. A comparision of laparoscopically assisted and open colectomy for colon cancer. *N Engl. J. Med.* 2004; 350 (20):2050-2059

[25] Tellez-Avila FI, Garcia-Osogobio SM.The carcinoembryonic antigen: apropos of an old friend. *Rev. Invest Clin.* 2005 Nov-Dec;57(6):814-9.

[26] Saha S, Wiese D, et al. Technical details of sentinel lymph node mapping in colorectal cancer and its impact on staging. *Ann. Surg. Oncol.* 2000;7:120–124.

[27] Nicholls RJ, York-Mason A, Morson BC, et al. The clinical staging of rectal cancer. *Br. J. Surg.* 1982; 69:404–409.

[28] Colon and rectum. In: American Joint Committee on Cancer.: AJCC Cancer Staging Manual. 6th ed. New York, NY: Springer, 2002, pp 113-124.

[29] Compton CC, Greene FL: The staging of colorectal cancer: 2004 and beyond. CA *Cancer J. Clin* 2004; 54 (6): 295-308.

In: Topics in Prevalent Diseases
Editors: N. C. Chavez-Tapia and M. Uribe
ISBN 978-1-60456-959-9

Chapter 4

Acquired Immune Deficiency Syndrome in Minorities

Karina F. Zihlmann and Jorge Casseb

Trends in HIV/AIDS and the Role of Minority Populations

The first cases of acquired immunodeficiency syndrome (AIDS) were reported in the United States in June 1981, and the number of cases and deaths among persons with AIDS increased rapidly during the 1980s (Janssen et al., 2003). During 1981–2001, an estimated 1.3–1.4 million persons in the United States were infected with human immunodeficiency virus (HIV) (Fleming et al. 2002), and 816,149 cases of AIDS and 467,910 deaths were reported to CDC (CDC, 2001). During the late 1990s, after the introduction of combination antiretroviral therapy, the numbers of new AIDS cases and deaths among adults and adolescents declined substantially. From 1995 to 1998, the annual number of incident AIDS cases declined 38% from 69,242 to 42,832, and deaths from AIDS declined 63% from 51,670 to 18,823. The annual numbers of incident AIDS cases and deaths have remained stable since 1998, at approximately 40,000 and 16,000, respectively (CDC 2001).

Since the early 1990s, an estimated 40,000 new HIV infections have occurred annually in the United States. During 1999–2001, in the 25 states that had HIV reporting since 1994, the number of persons who had HIV infection newly diagnosed increased 14% among MSM and 10% among heterosexuals. The number of persons in the United States living with HIV continues to increase, and of an estimated 850,000–950,000 persons living with HIV, an estimated 180,000–280,000 (25%) persons are unaware of their serostatus (MacKellar et al. 2002). In 2003, an estimated 1 million persons in the United States were living with HIV infection (Glynn et al. 2005). Approximately 25% were unaware of their infection (Glynn et al., 2005); however, that percentage might have been greater among persons at high risk for HIV infection, including racial/ethnic minority populations (MacKellar et al. 2005; CDC, 2002).

The AIDS epidemic is occurring among black and Hispanic populations disproportionately to their percentage of the U.S. population and effective HIV prevention programs should be racially, ethnically, and culturally relevant and sensitive (Holman et al. 1991).

HIV infection among racial and ethnic minorities is an ongoing health crisis. The disproportionate impact of HIV infection on racial and ethnic minorities has affected communities already struggling with many social and economic challenges, such as poverty, substance abuse, homelessness, and unequal access to health care and unequal treatment once in the health care system (Cargill et al. 2005).

Participation of racial and ethnic minorities in HIV clinical trials, as in other disease states, has been very poor. Racial and ethnic minorities have been chronically underrepresented in HIV clinical trials, despite their overrepresentation in the HIV epidemiology. This underrepresentation seems to be the result of a combination of factors including (a) provider bias in referring to clinical trials, (b) mistrust of clinical research, (c) past poor experience with the health care system, and (d) the conspiracy theories of HIV disease. The paucity of minority health care professionals and minority investigators in HIV research further affects minority participation in clinical research (Cargill et al. 2005).

The care and management of racial and ethnic minorities who have HIV infection has been complicated by the unequal access to health care and the unequal treatment once enrolled in health care. Health insurance status, lack of concordance between the race of the patient and the provider, and satisfaction with the quality of their care all impact on treatment outcomes in this population (Cargill et al. 2005). Inclusion of women and racial/ethnic minorities is a requirement for federally supported clinical research, but data on clinical research participation from women and racial/ethnic minorities with HIV are few. HIV-infected women were more likely than HIV-infected men with comparable modes of HIV acquisition to have participated in a study. Self-reported participation in clinical research studies was higher among women than men, but racial/ethnic minority men were less likely to report study participation (Sullivan et al. 2007).

In addition, the provider must be aware of the many comorbid conditions that may affect the delivery of care to minority patients living with HIV infection: depression, substance and alcohol abuse, and posttraumatic stress disorders. The impact of these comorbid conditions on the therapeutic relationship, including treatment and adherence, warrants screening for these disorders and treating them when identified. Because the patient provider relationship has been repeatedly identified as a predictor of higher adherence, developing and maintaining a strong therapeutic alliance is critical (Cargill et al. 2005).

Although there are many barriers to discussing HIV risk behaviors and prevention strategies in an office visit, including time constraints and potential provider discomfort in discussing these matters, clinical visits represent an important opportunity to reinforce HIV prevention and possibly decrease further HIV transmission. Multidisciplinary HIV care teams and research staff with training in cultural competency and cultural sensitivity may also be helpful (Cargill et al. 2005).

Racial and Ethnic Minorities

The strong linkages established early on of HIV/AIDS with gay men and other so called "risk groups", seem to have blinded social researchers and others to the factors of racial, class and gender relations that frame AIDS as a social and not a bio-medical problem alone. It is an increasingly acknowledged reality today that through out the world those most deeply affected by the HIV epidemic are also the most severely disadvantaged. As in the case of most other stigmatized health conditions, fundamental structural inequalities, social prejudices and social exclusion explain why women, children, sexual minorities and people of colour are disproportionately impacted by AIDS and the accompanying stigma and discrimination (Shalini et al. 2002). Although, some amount of empirical evidence now exists on linking poverty and gender to HIV/AIDS, there are not enough data on the relationship between HIV/AIDS, ethnicity and race (UNAIDS/WHO, 2001).

AIDS related stigma and discrimination are complex social processes. They usually build upon and reinforce pre-existing fears, prejudices and social inequalities pertaining to poverty, gender, race, sex and sexuality, and so on (Shalini et al, 2002). In this sense, racist attitudes and racial discrimination linked to HIV/AIDS status are only playing into, and reinforcing, already existing racial stereotypes and inequalities concerning people of colour in general. Just like other forms of stigma, AIDS related stigma also results in social exclusion, scapegoating, violence, blaming, labeling and denial of resources and services meant for the consumption of all (Shalini et al. 2002).

Since it is primarily the disliked sectors of society – gay and bisexual men, injecting drug users, and sex workers – who have been most closely associated with the epidemic since its early onset, the former derives from fear of AIDS as a communicable and lethal illness while the latter refers to the use of AIDS as a vehicle for expressing hostility toward groups that are already stigmatized in society. Racism and racial discrimination linked to HIV status may be categorized as "Symbolic" stigma as the already stigmatized and marginalized racial groups are stigmatized further on account of their association with HIV (Shalini et al. 2002).

The linkage between race and HIV/AIDS cannot be seen in isolation from the dimensions of gender, class, and sexual orientation. Concerning gender differences in patterns of HIV infection vary widely around the world. In regions where the HIV transmission is mainly heterosexual, more young women are infected than men. In most of Africa infection rates among young women are at least twice that among young men (UNAIDS, 2000). In some parts of Kenya and Zambia, teenage girls have rates of 25% compared with 4% among teenage boys (UNAIDS and WHO, 1999). The gendered dimension of the HIV epidemic is closely related to patriarchal values and norms and to the fact that women bear the major consequences of the epidemic on account of loss of livelihood, economic pressures, care of sick family members and stigma of AIDS (UNAIDS, 2000). Women and young girls thus lack the necessary information resources and the power to make choices such as, in matters of contraceptive use, by which they may reduce their risk of infection. Lack of adequate education and training for earning livelihood further marginalize women, particularly those from disadvantaged racial and ethnic backgrounds. In situations of armed conflict, migration and crisis displacement, once again it is the women who bear the consequences of sexual assault and rape.

Poverty is yet another dimension that combines with race and gender to multiply HIV related risk several times over. Worldwide the AIDS epidemic is most severe in the poorest countries and among people of colour (UNAIDS/ WHO, 1999). The reason is that conditions of poverty, hunger, powerlessness, and ignorance provide fertile ground for the spread of HIV and most Black people and other ethnic minorities live in these very conditions. Poverty increases chances of taking personal risks. While poverty enhances the risk of HIV, HIV also accentuates poverty.

Geographical Dimensions of the Problem

HIV/AIDS epidemiological data is generally reported by countries and by risk groups and not by ethnicity/race due to the political sensitivity (PAHO/WHO and UNAIDS, 2001). It is also argued that race/ethnicity based data may further serve to perpetuate stigma linked to those groups and that in part the problem may also be a "definitional" one with respect to racial categories (UNAIDS and WHO, 2001). However, only a few countries provide specific data about racial/ethnic dimensions of the problem. These figures may not present the true racial profiling of HIV prevalence but they are suggestive of levels of social inequalities related to race, gender and class.

Although Afro-Americans make up for only 13% of the US population, they accounted for an estimated 54% of all new infections in 2000. Reports also suggest that AIDS has become the leading cause of death among African-Americans aged 25 to 44 in the US (CDC, 2000). In 2003, an estimated 1.2 million persons in the United States were living with human immunodeficiency virus (HIV) infection 47% of whom were non-Hispanic blacks (Glynn, 2005). During 2001--2004, in nearly every demographic and transmission category, Blacks had the highest average rates for all transmission categories. The number of cases and diagnosis rates among blacks were higher than those for all other racial/ethnic populations combined. Among males, blacks had the largest or second-largest percentage of cases in every transmission category; among females, blacks had the largest percentage of cases in all transmission categories. Moreover, among both males and females, blacks represented the largest percentage of HIV/AIDS diagnoses in every age group. (Prejean et al, 2006)

In Canada, the proportion of reported AIDS cases has steadily increased among ethnic groups. Between 1991 and 1999, for example, the proportion of White AIDS cases declined from 88.6% to 66.1%, while a corresponding rise was registered among various ethnic groups. According to one report, of the cumulative AIDS diagnoses reported to December 1998, 78.6% were reported by ethnicity. This trend was found to be particularly significant after 1994 among the Aboriginal persons and among Black people. Statistics reported for Canada for the year 2000 further reveals that whereas the Aboriginals and Blacks comprise 2.8% and 2.0% of Canada's population respectively, they accounted for nearly 9.2% and 8.3% of all reported cases of AIDS in that year (Canada Bureau of HIV/AIDS, STD and TB, 2001). In the Honduras, HIV infection among the Black Caribbean minority known as "Garifunas" is six times that of Honduran national average, at 8.2% in men and 8.5% in women. Among men and women in their 20s, HIV infection was reported to be a high of 16% (PAHO/WHO and UNAIDS, 2001, p.36). In Australia, significantly higher proportion of

HIV infection is reported among indigenous women (26%) than among the non-indigenous women (8%) (Commonwealth of Australia, 1997). Within Europe, HIV infection rates among African people in France especially among women, are reported to be increasing (Bungener, Marchand-Gonod, and Jouvent, 2000).

Recent statistics also reveal a narrowing gender gap in HIV infection rates. Globally women accounted for 40% of all new infections in 2001 and of the total AIDS deaths in 2001, 37% occurred among women (UNAIDS, 2002). Within minority racial and ethnic groups too, women are found to be increasingly at greater risk of infection and targets of greater levels of stigma and discrimination. The UNAIDS report for 2002 notes that "... young, disadvantaged women (especially African-American and Hispanic) are increasingly vulnerable to infection" (UNAIDS, 2002 p.40). In most parts of Africa, HIV prevalence among women is climbing faster than among men. In Botswana, for example, median HIV prevalence among pregnant women increased from 38.5% in 1997 to 44.9% in 2001 while in Zimbabwe the prevalence rate rose from 29% in 1997 to 35% in 2000 (UNAIDS, 2002 p.23).

Racial Discrimination Related to HIV/AIDS Status

Throughout the world HIV/AIDS related stigma is known to have triggered a range of negative and unsupportive reactions. Various contexts - family, community, work place, health care setting – have been identified where stigma and discrimination is known to occur (UNAIDS, 2002).

In the beginning of the epidemic, travel restrictions were placed on "foreigners" most of whom belonged to racial/ethnic, minorities and the HIV infected foreigners continue to be denied permission to enter the US. African-Americans, in general, have reported greater levels of stigma and discrimination in the health care sector due to their HIV status compared to Whites. In an evaluation of TASO (The AIDS Support Organizations) in Uganda, 58% of the clients reported fear of stigma as the main reason for non-disclosure of their serostatus to others (Kaleeba et al. 1997).

Although direct evidence of racial discrimination due to HIV/AIDS is not so readily available, there are findings among racial minorities that are inextricably related to racism and other forms of discrimination in society (WHO, 2001). Similar sharp disparities are reported in Brazil where infant mortality among Afro-Americans is 62/1000 compared to among Whites, which is 37/1000 (FOASE, 2000 apud Shalini, 2002). Access to health insurance too is generally poorer for racial groups.

More specifically in relation to HIV/AIDS, there is some evidence to show why racial minorities may be particularly vulnerable to HIV/STIs risk. In most countries men and women from indigenous groups and racial minorities generally have fewer opportunities for schooling and employment than the majority population. Consequently there is greater gravitation towards drug abuse and paid sex work. In the US city of Baltimore, for instance, over one half of drug injectors never graduated from secondary school and 97% of these were African-Americans (PAHO/WHO and UNAIDS, 2001).

Despite insufficient direct evidence linking racial discrimination to HIV/AIDS, given wide health disparities between White majority population and the people of colour, it is not too difficult to appreciate how racism, class and gender intensify these already existing inequalities in the context of HIV/AIDS (Shalini, 2002).

International Response

As early as 1983, 12 countries had adopted legal instruments on AIDS. By 1995 this number had increased to 120 (Paget, 1998). The legislatures largely reflect the conflict between protection of public health and protection of individual health. But even where supportive legislation exists, fear of social exclusion and blame, and prevents positive people from accessing legal action.

Today HIV/AIDS is largely recognized as a human rights issue (UNAIDS, 2002). At the international level the strategy has been to integrate principles of non-discrimination, confidentiality, participation, equality and beneficence into existing international human rights instruments, national legislatures, NGO work and AIDS related research and intervention initiatives (UNAIDS, 2002).

The London Declaration on AIDS Prevention in 1988 was the first international statement to call for destigmatizing HIV/AIDS. Subsequently Resolution WHA 41.24 of the 41st World Health Assembly of 1988, made recommendations to Member States to protect human rights of affected individuals. In 1989 the UN Center for Human Rights organized the first international consultation on HIV/AIDS and Human Rights. This was followed by a second consultation in 1996 in which a set of twelve International Guidelines on HIV/AIDS and Human Rights were drafted. Significantly many HR Instruments have now included "HIV/AIDS status" under the more general phrase "Health status". For example a General Comment adopted by the committee to monitor the International Covenant on Economic, Social and Cultural Rights, enumerates the grounds for non-discrimination in health by proscribing "any discrimination in access to health care and the underlying determinants of health as well as to means and entitlements for their procurement on the grounds of race, colour, sex, language, …birth, …health status (including HIV/AIDS) …or other status, which has the intention or effect of nullifying or impairing the equal enjoyment or exercise of the right to health". Further, Resolution 49/1999 of the UN commission on HR reaffirms that "…the term 'or other status' in non-discrimination provisions in international human rights texts should be interpreted to cover health status including HIV/AIDS". The UN commission on HR Resolution 2001/33 on 'Access to medication in the context of pandemics such as, HIV/AIDS' recognizes people's right to highest standards of health care.

The UN General Assembly special session on HIV/AIDS, June 2001, endorsed the establishment of a Global AIDS Fund to strengthen AIDS work in developing countries and with disadvantaged populations. The UNGASS also called upon States to enact, strengthen and enforce legislation to eliminate all forms of AIDS related discrimination and confront stigma, silence and denial by 2003. The need is to recognize and make explicit the inclusion of race –based discrimination a ground for legal action

In the specific context of the racial dimensions of HIV/AIDS the World Conference against Racism, Racial Discrimination, Xenophobia and Related Forms of Intolerance, held at Durban in September 2001, marks the strong resolve of the international community to challenge the racial linkages of the AIDS epidemic. At the regional level, the South African Development Community's Code on HIV/AIDS and Employment seeks to protect rights of HIV positive workers (UNAIDS, 2000).

Gender-specific Aspects of HIV/AIDS: Human Rights Dimensions, Women's Rights, Sexual and Reproductive Rights, Children and Vulnerable Groups in the Context of Prevention, Care and Access to Treatment

Although the epidemic is disproportionately affecting all racial and ethnic minorities, within these minority populations women are particularly affected. Despite several published recommendations for the inclusion of HIV prevention in the clinical care setting, studies have documented how few providers actually achieve this goal, especially those who care for disadvantaged patients (Cargill et al. 2005).

The HIV epidemic represents one of today's most profound challenges in improving global health. Women represent a growing proportion among people living with HIV and AIDS, and the ratio of infected men to women is particularly skewed among young people. At the end of 2006, in sub-Saharan Africa, for every HIV infected young man (15-24 years old) there were nearly three infected young women. Halting further expansion of the HIV pandemic within the next decade is a top priority of governments and civil society the world over, and one of eight Millennium Development Goals set by the United Nations. Reaching this goal will hinge upon the success of prevention efforts in reducing women's risk of HIV and other sexually transmitted infections (STIs).

Despite billions of dollars spent on programs designed to modify risky behavior, the annual number of incident HIV infections and other STIs has not declined (HRW, 2006, Kaiser Family Foundation, 2005). Over 80% of HIV infections occur through sexual contact with an infected partner (Gopalan, 2006); infections that could have been prevented through the adoption of safer sexual practices such as delayed sexual debut, abstaining from unprotected sex, and/or avoiding multiple and concurrent partnerships. Efforts to apply this knowledge to the development of interventions that lead to population-level reductions in HIV transmission have, however, had limited success.

Since HIV has a high potential for heterosexual transmission by vaginal intercourse, HIV has affected women. For example, in Brazil, half of the new cases are reported among women (Ministry of Health – Brazil, 2007). In one study done in USA, where 611 participants were interviewed from eight Infectious Diseases clinics in five southeastern states in 2001 to 2002. Sixty four percent of participants were African-American, 31% were female, and 43% acquired HIV through heterosexual sex; 25% had private health insurance. Eighty-one percent were on antiretroviral therapy, and 46% had HIV RNA viral loads (VL) <400. Women and racial/ethnic minorities were less likely to be on antiretrovirals and to have VL <400. Probable psychiatric disorders (54%) and history of childhood sexual (30%) and physical abuse (21%) were common (Pence et al. 2007).

The HIV epidemic represents one of today's most profound challenges in improving global health. Women represent a growing proportion among people living with HIV and AIDS, and the ratio of infected men to women is particularly skewed among young people.

At the end of 2006, in sub-Saharan Africa, for every HIV infected young man (15-24 years old) there were nearly three infected young women. Halting further expansion of the HIV pandemic within the next decade is a top priority of governments and civil society the world over, and one of eight Millennium Development Goals set by the United Nations. Reaching this goal will hinge upon the success of prevention efforts in reducing women's risk of HIV and other sexually transmitted infections (STIs) (Krishnan, S, 2007).

HIV/AIDS and Gender-based Violence: A Problem to Be Faced

The gender-based violence is rooted in gender inequality, and has a lethal dynamic by itself and in combination with HIV/AIDS (The Center for Women's Global Leadership- US, 2005). Around the world, women are facing a catastrophic assault on their bodies, rights and health as well as the high prevalence of HIV. Increasingly, women are dealing with the way violence puts them at greater risk of contracting HIV while women who are HIV+ are more likely to be targets of violence because of additional layers of discrimination and stigma.

Elements of the AIDS testing and treatment machinery may bring danger of violence connected to disclosure of HIV+ serostatus or coercive testing in the guise of VCT (voluntary counseling and testing), or the insidious treatment of women as vectors of disease, as in the case of PMTCT (prevention of mother-to-child transmission) programs that fail to treat pregnant HIV+ women as patients or clients with rights, or only as, and nothing more than, child-bearers.

A Zambian nongovernmental organization (NGO) revealed that it records eight cases of rape of young girls every week at its centre in the capital, Lusaka. The statistics were released by the Young Women's Christian Association (YWCA) and Katembu Kaumba, YWCA's executive director, referred the organization's shelter in Lusaka also recorded 10 cases of rape of adult women every week. Government actors are generally unwilling to address abuses committed by soldiers, police and other agents of the state, as well as the sexual violence that takes place within the family, community and other traditionally "private spheres" (Rothschild et al. 2006).

Social Factors and Risks to Women

Race, ethnicity, language, sexuality, age, and many other social factors have a significant and differential impact on the effect of both gender-based violence and HIV/AIDS on the lives of women and girls in various communities.

The resolution *2005/84* notes that "an estimated 95 per cent of all people infected with HIV live in the developing world, mostly in conditions of poverty, underdevelopment, conflict and inadequate measures for the prevention, care and treatment of HIV infection, and that marginalized groups in these societies are even more vulnerable to HIV infection and the impact of AIDS" (The Center for Women's Global Leadership- US, 2005).

Gender inequality and violence against women often inhibits women's and girls' ability to take full advantage of crucial services. Age is a key factor in determining risk and vulnerability to both gender-based violence and to HIV/AIDS: a recent study by the WHO found that as many as 30% of women in some locations reported that their first sexual experience was coerced or forced (WHO, 2006). The younger the women were at the time of sexual initiation, the higher the chance that it was violent. Moreover, HIV/AIDS is fast becoming *a girls' epidemic*: The WHO notes that young people (aged 15-24) account for half of all new HIV infections, and of infected youths, two-thirds are female. In parts of sub-Saharan Africa, teen girls are six times more likely to be infected than male peers. The burden of care also falls on girls who may leave school to care for sick relatives (WHO, 2006).

Furthermore, age-related risks do not only correspond to youth. Patterns of wife-inheritance in some communities have been noted to fuel the spread of HIV (HRW, 2006). In some communities, older women, in particular, may be targeted for rape in connection to HIV/AIDS. For instance, during a recent trip, UN special envoy on HIV/AIDS in Africa, Stephen Lewis, reported "a significant number of women aged 65 to 80 were also raped. The men who did it were confident they could have unprotected sex with them without getting AIDS" (HRW, 2006).

In the United States, the Kaiser Family Foundation reports that "racial and ethnic minorities have been disproportionately affected by HIV/AIDS since the beginning of the epidemic, and minority Americans now represent the majority of new AIDS cases (71%) and of those estimated to be living with AIDS (64%) in 2003" with African-Americans and Latinos accounting for a disproportionate share of new AIDS diagnoses (Kaiser Family Foundation, 2005). Moreover, women of color are particularly hard hit with African American women accounting for 67% of estimated new AIDS diagnoses among women in 2003, while Latinas account for 16% (Kaiser Family Foundation, 2005).

Discrimination and a hostile legal and political environment seriously circumscribe efforts to address the health and rights of marginalized communities. Cases such as HIV outreach workers being arrested on sodomy charges, or as sex workers (using evidence of carrying condoms as an indication of prostitution) are simply the tip of the iceberg (Gopalan, 2006). In a recent article in Medical News Today, Anjali Gopalan of the Naz Foundation India Trust, an organization working on HIV care and prevention with diverse communities commented "The police harass health outreach workers working on HIV prevention among the gay community".

Various forms of "minority" status also indicate risk. The estimated HIV prevalence rate among self identified gay men in South Africa may be as high as 30%, while the rates for transgender individuals may be even higher. Amongst sex workers, available data from 2000 shows that slightly over 50% of sex workers were HIV-positive (UNAIDS, 2006). In Nepal, an HIV prevalence rate among men who have sex with men of 3.9 %, exists alongside a long-term and consistent pattern of serious violence and abuse of transgender persons (ILGA, 2004). Moreover, while women who have sex with women are generally considered to be a "low risk" group, the calculation changes when lesbians are targeted for violence. For example, due to the high incidence of rape, HIV/AIDS rates among black South African lesbians are reportedly as high as in the general population (Samelius and Wagberg, 2005).

Other institutional issues, such as profiling of particular groups (including in but not limited to situations related to the war on terrorism), historic and persistent discriminatory practices against racial and ethnic minorities by the police and other state actors, among other circumstances, can lead to perpetrators of violence against women in racially diverse communities acting with virtual impunity. Agents of the state often are protected against appropriate investigation and punishment (The Center for Women's Global Leadership- US, 2005).

Obstacles and Strategies: Gender-sensitive and Human Rights-based Responses

One of the key obstacles and challenges to comprehensively addressing the intersection of gender-based violence and HIV/AIDS is the lack of adequate human and financial resources. However, while more funding is crucial, it will only mitigate, but not arrest, either HIV/AIDS or violence against women, nor will it achieve gender equality, without a clear understanding and analysis of the impact of policy, programming and services (The Center for Women's Global Leadership- US, 2005).

The current framework for HIV/AIDS funding (inclusive of the acronyms of VCT [voluntary counseling and testing], ABC [abstain, be faithful, use condoms], PMTCT [prevention of mother-to-child transmission] among others) fails to interrogate its gender bias, and therefore, often fails to reduce HIV infections among women, or mitigate its more general impact on women and girls. This includes, for example, PMTCT programs that treat women only in the context of childbearing, VCT programs that fail to understand that "voluntary" can become coercion in a context of gender inequality and a pervasive threat of violence, or that ABC initiatives generally ignore the fact that many women and girls are not in a position to negotiate the conditions of a sexual encounter. The current axiom of universal access to prevention, treatment, support and care will not reach its goals nor halt the feminization of the pandemic without a gender-sensitive realignment fully anchored in human rights norms and standards. Nor will a "results-based" focus that emphasizes quantity over quality necessarily protect the rights of women (The Center for Women's Global Leadership- US, 2005).

Governments have begun establishing programs to facilitate access on prevention of mother-to-child transmission (PMTCT). While the benefits of PMTCT programs are immense—for individual women, their children, and societies alike—it is crucial that governments implement these programs with respect for their human rights. PMTCT programs are primarily conceived as prevention programs for infants and in many contexts, the women are forgotten after they deliver healthy infants. These encompass their right to privacy and to physical integrity, including their right not to be tested without their informed choice or consent or to have their HIV status disclosed without their permission.

The use of media has, in several cases, provided promising results. Cultural stereotypes involving sex workers and other sexually active women, and myths involving condom use and the virtues of machismo, are systematically undermined—and reframed. Special attention is given to the experiences of HIV+ women when designing responses and services.

Governments, multilateral institutions and donors must engage in a dialogue with civil society in order to draw important lessons that will allow for governments and donors to provide the resources for scaling up effective gender and human rights based strategies, and to support the social movements within which these new, innovative and/or effective strategies are grown (The Center for Women's Global Leadership- US, 2005).

Actions and Strategies toward Minorities

As the HIV/AIDS epidemic neared the end of its first decade in the late 1980s, the US Centers for Disease Control and Prevention (CDC) recognized the disparate impact on racial and ethnic minority communities. In response, a program was initiated to build capacity to prevent the further spread of HIV and other STDs in these communities (Taveras et al. 2007).

During 1984, CDC assessed the educational activities to AIDS of community-based organizations and public health agencies in some cities in the United States and they noted that the challenge of the epidemic lay in finding effective strategies for disseminating relevant information needed to be appropriate to the lifestyle, language, and environment of a particular risk group (Bailey ,1991).

The CDC created the Minority AIDS Initiative (MAI) in 1998 to address the disproportionate rates of HIV/AIDS among racial and ethnic minorities in the United States. At CDC, steps are currently underway to develop a comprehensive strategy to prevent and reduce the burden of HIV/AIDS among racial and ethnic minorities (Eshel et al. 2008).

Since that time, the program has expanded in scope, intensity of efforts, and funding. Today, the CDC's Capacity Building Assistance (CBA) Initiative serves communities across the nation by building community, organizational, and HIV prevention program/intervention capacity designed to reduce the number of new HIV infections among at-risk populations (Taveras et al. 2007).

Stable HIV-associated morbidity and mortality, concerns about possible increases in HIV incidence, and the recent availability of a simple, rapid HIV test combined with strong prevention collaborations among communities heavily affected by HIV. An emphasis on greater access to testing and on providing prevention and care services for persons infected with HIV can reduce new infections and lead to reductions in HIV-associated morbidity and mortality (Janssen et al. 2001). In addition, simplifying prenatal and other testing procedures can lead to more effective prevention to perinatal and other HIV transmission.

Conclusion

Prevention and care systems need to address the HIV epidemic's shift into poor, minority, and female populations. High levels of trauma and probable psychiatric disorders indicate a need to assess for and address these conditions in HIV clinical care. There are several promising strategies that may improve health care quality for racial/ethnic minorities, but a lack of studies specifically targeting disease areas and processes of care for which disparities have been previously documented.

References

Aissata, De Diop (2001). Panel discussion at the CSW 45th session, 6-16, March 2001, Geneva.

Anjali Gopalan of the Naz Foundation India Trust, "Gay Rights Groups in India Protest Arrest of MSM, HIV/AIDS Advocates Say Antiquated Laws Hinder Prevention," Medical News Today, 13 January 2006, at http://www.medicalnewstoday.com/medicalnews.php?newsid=36093

Bailey ME. Community-based organizations and CDC as partners in HIV education and prevention. *Public Health Rep.* 1991 Nov-Dec;106(6):702-8

Bungener, C., Marchand-Gonod, N., and Jouvent, R. (2000). African and European HIV-positive women: Psychological and psychosocial differences. *AIDS Care,12*(5), 541-548.

Cargill VA, Stone VE. HIV/AIDS: a minority health issue. *Med Clin North Am.* 2005 Jul;89 (4):895-912.

Canada Bureau of HIV/AIDS, STD and TB (2001). AIDS/HIV ethnicity in Canada (HIV Epi Update May 2001).

CDC. Advancing HIV prevention: new strategies for a changing epidemic---United States, 2003. *MMWR* 2003;52:329—32. Page converted: 4/17/2003

CDC. HIV/AIDS Surveillance report, 2001;13(2).

CDC. Unrecognized HIV infection, risk behaviors, and perceptions of risk among young black men who have sex with men---six U.S. cities, 1994--1998. *MMWR* 2002;51:733--6.

Centers for Disease Control and Prevention – CDC (2000). Young people at risk: HIV/AIDS among America's youth. Atlanta, Georgia.

Common Wealth of Australia (1997). The national indigenous Australian's Health Strategy 1996/7 – 1998/9

Cynthia Rothschild, Mary Anne Reilly and Sara A. Nordstrom, Strengthening Resistance: Confronting Violence Against Women and HIV/AIDS. New Jersey, USA: Center for Women's Global Leadership, 2006, p. 7. Hereafter referred to as "Strengthening Resistance."

D Aguirre, Bienestar Human Svcs; A Mares-DelGrasso, C Emerson, J Tsang, J Pincus, K Jafa-Bhushan, K Bowles, H Clark, MPH, B Song, PS Sullivan, JD Heffelfinger, J Cleveland, E Tai, Rapid HIV Testing in Outreach and Other Community Settings --- United States, 2004--2006

Date last reviewed: 11/28/2007. *MMWR-Weekly*.November 30, 2007 / 56(47);1233-1237

Eshel A, Moore A, Mishra M, Wooster J, Toledo C, Uhl G, Agüero LW. Community stakeholders' perspectives on the impact of the minority AIDS initiative in strengthening HIV prevention capacity in four communities. *Ethn. Health.* 2008 Jan;13(1):39-54.

Farmer, P. and Kim, J.Y. (1991). Anthropology, accountability and the prevention of AIDS. *Journal of Sex Research, 28,*203-221.

Fleming P, Byers RH, Sweeney PA, Daniels D, Karon JM, Janssen RS. HIV prevalence in the United States, 2000. [Abstract]. In: Program and abstracts of the 9th Conference on Retroviruses and Opportunistic Infections, Seattle, Washington, February 24--28, 2002. Alexandria, Virginia: Foundation for Retrovirology and Human Health

Glynn M, Rhodes P. Estimated HIV prevalence in the United States at the end of 2003 [Abstract T1-B1101]. Programs and abstracts of the 2005 National HIV Prevention Conference; June 12--15, 2005; Atlanta, GA. Available at http://www.aegis. com/ conferences/nhivpc/2005/t1-b1101.html.

Glynn MK, Rhodes P. Estimated HIV prevalence in the United States at the end of 2003 [Abstract T1-B1101]. Presented at the 2005 National HIV Prevention Conference, Atlanta, GA; June 14, 2005.

Goffman, E. (1963). Stigma: Notes on the Management of a Spoiled Identity. New York: Simon and Schuster. Health Canada (1999). HIV and AIDS in Canada. Surveillance report to December 31, 1998. Ottawa.

Gopalan, A. Gay Rights Groups in India Protest Arrest of MSM, HIV/AIDS Advocates Say Antiquated Laws Hinder Prevention. *Medical News Today.* 2006. Jan. Naz Foundation India Trust. Available in http://www.medicalnewstoday.com/medicalnews.php?newsid =36093

Holman, PB, Jenkins, WC, Gayle, JA, Duncan, C, Lindsey, BK. Increasing the involvement of national and regional racial and ethnic minority organizations in HIV information and education. *Public Health Rep.* 1991 Nov–Dec; 106(6): 687–694.

Holman, PB, Jenkins, WC, Gayle, JA, Duncan, C, Lindsey, BK. HIV/AIDS: a minority health issue. *Med. Clin. North Am.* 2005 Jul;89(4):895-912.

HRW. Double Standards: Women's Property Rights Violations in Kenya (New York, 2003); International Center for Research on Women, "Reducing Women's and Girls' Vulnerability to HIV/AIDS by Strengthening their Property and Inheritance Rights." *Information Bulletin*., May 2006 (ICRW: Washington, DC, 2006).

Hutchinson AB, Farnham PG, Dean HD, Ekwueme DU, del Rio C, Kamimoto L, Kellerman SE. The economic burden of HIV in the United States in the era of highly active antiretroviral therapy: evidence of continuing racial and ethnic differences. *J. Acquir. Immune Defic. Syndr.* 2006 Dec 1;43(4):451-7.

ILGA. International Lesbian and Gay Association. CALL FOR ACTION 39 members of Blue Diamond Society arrested. Nepal, Ago, 2004. Disponível no endereço: http: //www.ilga.org/news_results.asp?LanguageID=1andFileCategory=52andZoneID=3andFileID=287

Janssen RS, Holtgrave DR, Valdiserri RO, Shepherd M, Gayle HD, DeCock KM. The serostatus approach to fighting the HIV epidemic: prevention strategies for infected individuals. *Am. J. Pub. Health* 2001;91:1019--24.

Janssen, MD, IM Onorato, MD, Div of HIV/AIDS Prevention--Surveillance and Epidemiology; RO Valdiserri, MD, TM Durham, MS, WP Nichols, MPA, EM Seiler, MPA, HW Jaffe, MD, National Center for HIV, STD, and TB Prevention, CDC. Weekly - April 18, 2003 / 52(15);329-332 . Advancing HIV Prevention: New Strategies for a Changing Epidemic - United States, 2003

Kaiser Family Foundation, "The HIV/AIDS Epidemic in the United States." HIV/AIDS Policy Fact Sheet, 2005, p. 2

Kaleeba, N., Kalibala, S., Kaseje, M., Ssebbanja, P., Anderson, S., van Praag, E., Tembo, G. and Katabira, E. (1997). Participatory evaluation of counseling medical and social services of The AIDS Support Organisation (TASO) in Uganda, *AIDS Care, 9,* 13-26.

Krishnan, S. Religion and Ethics newsweekly: An online companion to the weekly television news program. January, 05, 2007. Episode n. 1019. Avaiable in http://www.pbs.org/wnet/religionandethics/week1019/profile.html

MacKellar DA, Valleroy LA, Secura GM, Behel SK. Unrecognized HIV infection, risk behaviors, and mis-perceptions of risk among young men who have sex with men---6 United States cities, 1994--2000. [Abstract]. In: Final program and abstracts of the XIV International AIDS Conference, Barcelona, Spain, July 5--12, 2002.

MacKellar DA, Valleroy LA, Secura GM; Young Men's Survey Study Group, et al. Unrecognized HIV infection, risk behaviors, and perceptions of risk among young men who have sex with men: opportunities for advancing HIV prevention in the third decade of HIV/AIDS. *J. Acquir. Immune Defic. Syndr.* 2005;38:603--14.

Ministry of Health - Brazil. *Boletim Epidemiológico Aids e DST.* Ano IV - nº 1 - 27ª - 52ª - semanas epidemiológicas - julho a dezembro de 2006. Ano IV - nº 1 - 01ª - 26ª - semanas epidemiológicas - janeiro a junho de 2007. Brasilia, 2007.

Paget, D.Z. (1998). HIV/AIDS and the legislature: An international comparison. *AIDS Care, 10*, 565-573.

PAHO.,WHO/UNAIDS (2001). HIV and AIDS in the Americas: An epidemic with many faces. Geneva.

Pence, BW, Barroso, J, Leserman,J, Harmon,J, Salahuddin, N. Measuring fatigue in people living with HIV/AIDS: psychometric characteristics of the HIV-related fatigue scale. *AIDS care.* 2008. Aug, 20 (7), p 829-37.

Prejean, PhD, AJ Satcher, MPH, T Durant, PhD, X Hu, MS, LM Lee, PhD, Div of HIV/AIDS Prevention, National Center for HIV, STD, and TB Prevention, CDC. Weekly . February 10, 2006 / 55(05);121-125. Racial/Ethnic Disparities in Diagnoses of HIV/AIDS --- 33 States, 2001—2004.

Randall, V.R. (2001). Race Relations – Result – 2001. The University of Dayton. http://academic.udayton.edu/race/surveys/relations01.htm.

Rothschild, C, Reilly, MA and Nordstrom, SA. Strengthening Resistance: Confronting Violence Against Women and HIV/AIDS. New Jersey, USA: Center for Women's Global Leadership, 2006, p. 7.

Shalini Bharat. Tata Institute of Social Sciences, Mumbai, India. Racism, Racial Discrimination and HIV/AIDS. "UNESCO/OHCHR Workshop To Develop Educational Material to Foster Tolerance and to Eliminate Prejudice" at Paris, France, February 19-20, 2002.

Sullivan PS, McNaghten AD, Begley E, Hutchinson A, Cargill VA.Enrollment of racial/ethnic minorities and women with HIV in clinical research studies of HIV medicines. *J. Natl. Med. Assoc.* 2007 Mar;99(3):242-50.

Samelius, L and Wagber, E. Sexual Orientation and gender identity issues in development. A Study of Swedish policy and administration of Lesbian, Gay, Bisexual and Transgender issues in international development cooperation Swedish International Development Agency (SIDA). Sida Health Division, november, 2005. Avaiable in http://www.ilga-europe.org/europe/guide/country_by_country/sweden/sexual_orientation_and_gender_identity_issues_in_development

Taveras S, Duncan T, Gentry D, Gilliam A, Kimbrough I, Minaya J. The evolution of the CDC HIV prevention capacity-building assistance initiative. *J. Public Health Manag. Pract.* 2007 Jan;Suppl:S8-15.

The Center for Women's Global Leadership (US), in collaboration with Action Aid International (South Africa), Action Canada for Population and Development/ACPD (Canada), Center for Health and Gender Equity/CHANGE (US), Center for Reproductive Rights (US), Fundación para Estudio e Investigación de la Mujer /FEIM (Argentina), Gestos- Soropositividade, Comunicação e Gênero (Brazil), International AIDS Women's Caucus, International Women's Health Coalition/IWHC (US), Latin American and Caribbean Women´s Health Network/LACWHN. This paper is a reference to *Resolution 2005/84* (adopted by consensus on 21 April 2005) for the *Commission on Human Rights* to gender-specific aspects of HIV/AIDS in its human rights dimensions such as women's rights, sexual and reproductive rights and health, HIV positive women's and development organizations, children and vulnerable groups in the context of prevention, care and access to treatment as described in the Guidelines on HIV/AIDS and Human Rights for the Human Rights Council. http://www2.ohchr.org/english/issues/hiv/docs/cwgl.doc

UNAIDS (2002). Report on the global HIV/AIDS epidemic. July Geneva: UNAIDS.

UNAIDS, 2006. Report on the global AIDS epidemic, p. 516. Geneva.

UNAIDS/WHO (1999). AIDS epidemic update. Geneva.

UNAIDS/WHO (2001). Fighting HIV related intolerance: Exposing the links between racism, stigma and discrimination.

UNAIDS/WHO (2001). Fighting HIV related intolerance: Exposing the links between racism, stigma and discrimination.

UNAIDS/WHO. Epidemiological Fact Sheet South Africa

WHO (2001). Health and freedom from discrimination. Geneva: WHO.

Williams, D. (1997). Race, socio-economic status, and health: The added effects of racism and discrimination. *Annals of the NY Academy of Sciences, 986*, 173-188.

World Health Organization (WHO) 2006, Multi-country study on women's health and domestic violence against women, p. 51. Accessed at http://www.who.int/gender/violence/who_multicountry_study/en/

In: Topics in Prevalent Diseases
Editors: N. C. Chavez-Tapia and M. Uribe
ISBN 978-1-60456-959-9

Chapter 5

Ischemic Heart Disease in Minorities

Fernando Lanas and Pamela Serón
Facultad de Medicina, Universidad de La Frontera, Temuco, Chile

Background

Cardiovascular Diseases

Cardiovascular diseases (CVDs) are caused by disorders of the heart or blood vessels; they include ischemic heart disease (IHD), stroke, peripheral artery disease, hypertensive heart disease and congenital malformations, among others. CVDs are the main cause of death in the world and they will be the leading cause of death for a long time. In year 2005, 17.5 million people died due to CVDs in the world, representing a 30 % of the total mortality. Of those, 7.6 millions were due to acute myocardial infarction (AMI) and 5.7 millions to stroke. Most of these deaths, 80%, occurred in developing countries. Twenty millions are expected to die for CVDs in year 2015, mainly for AMI and stroke [1;2].

The most important cardiac disease for its frequency and mortality is IHD. The main abnormality in IHD is the inability of coronary arteries to deliver enough blood flow and oxygen to a certain part of the cardiac muscle, determining an abnormal function of the heart. Atherosclerosis, with a deposit of lipidic substances in the coronary arterial wall, with atheroma plaques reducing the blood flow is the main cause of IHD. The clinical manifestations of IHD are acute coronary syndromes (AMI with or without ST segment elevation and unstable angina), chronic stable angina and cardiac sudden death. Sudden death is a consequence of a cardiac event in 60 to 70 % of the cases and IHD is the most frequent cause of these cardiac events.

Ischemic Heart Disease Epidemiology

At the beginning of the 20th century a major change in the mortality pattern in developed countries was observed, chronic disease became predominant as cause of death. Developing countries have followed the same tendency during the second half of the century. Infant mortality and infectious diseases have declined, allowing more individuals to reach middle or advance age where chronic diseases, including IHD, are predominant. In developed countries cardiovascular death rate has decreased due to better control of risk factors at individual and community level, for example, USA adjusted mortality rate due to chronic diseases has been decreasing steadily since 1950, the risks of sudden cardiac death and no sudden coronary heart disease mortality have decreased by 49% to 64% over the past 50 years [3]. However, this decline has not been homogeneous, with less improvement in ethnic minorities group. In developing countries, cardiovascular mortality has increased so the greater burden of CVDs is observed in people of those countries[4].

Risk Factors for Ischemic Heart Disease

CVD risk factors were developed from de pioneer epidemiologic study of Framingham [5]. The Framingham cohort started in 1948 providing evidence that CVDs are related with cholesterol serum levels, smoking and elevated blood pressure in a consistent, progressive, strong and independent relationship. Subsequent observations from Framingham and other epidemiological studies have identified other risk factors (table 1). New risk factors, known as emerging risk factors, have been added to the traditional ones, they include psychosocial risk factors like stress and depression, blood levels of homocistein, fibrinogen, protein C and others.

Table 1. Risk factors for ischemic heart disease

Non modifiable risk factors -Age -Gender -Family history of coronary artery disease
Modifiable risk factors Dyslipidemia Hypertension Smoking Diabetes mellitus Lack of physical exercise Overweight/ Obesity Diet

The effect of these risk factors in IHD in different populations and ethnic groups has been a topic of debate. The INTERHEART study assessed the effects of traditional and emerging risk factors in AMI in different populations of the world. It included nearly 15 thousand cases of first AMI and 15 thousand controls in 52 patients in all continents. Their main conclusions were that the strength of risk factors was similar in all regions and mayor ethnic groups and that known risk factors explain 90% of the risk of AMI. Those risk factors were: abnormal blood lipids (measured as a ratio of apolipoprotein B/A1), smoking, hypertension, abdominal obesity, psychosocial factors like stress and depression, diabetes mellitus and the absence of protective factors like exercise, daily consumption of fruits and vegetables and alcohol [6].

Ischemic Heart Disease in Minorities

Several definitions exist for ethnic minorities, although there is no consensus on appropriate terms for the scientific study of health by ethnicity, the one used in this chapter is that an ethnic minority group is a population of not European origin, and not white, living in a developed country [7]. These groups may present marked differences with the natural population of the country regarding prevalence, morbidity and mortality for IHD. Important differences in mortality due to CVD and IHD between the European origin population and the ethnic minorities exist in North America and Europe.

CVD remains by far the leading cause of death in the United States [8]. The difference between African American and non Hispanic Whites is the one more studied in USA. African Americans have the highest overall IHD mortality rate and the highest out-of-hospital coronary death rate of any ethnic group in the United States, particularly at younger ages [9]. The cardiovascular mortality, adjusted for age, is 40% higher in the African American population compared with Whites. These results are confirmed with several publications, among them the data from the Multiple Risk Factor Intervention Trial (MRFIT) [10], where the age-adjusted Black-to-White CVD hazard ratio over 25 years was 1.35. In 2001, life expectancy at birth was 5.5 years higher in Whites compared with African Americans. [11]. Levine [12] using historical information from the National Center for Health Statistics and the Census Bureau found that there has not been reduction in death inequalities adjusted for age, or life expectancy, between African American and Whites since 1945. The age-adjusted all-cause mortality for African Americans in 1998 was similar to the Whites in 1969 (a 29-year lag). The relationship in mortality between African American and Whites increased form 1979 to 1998 from 1.13 to 1.43 in men and from 1.45 to 1.66 in women.

"Hispanic paradox" has been called the observation that Hispanics have lower all-cause and cardiovascular mortality rates despite increased rates of diabetes and obesity and lower socioeconomic status. In a study done in New Mexico about mortality for IHD between 1958 and 1982 it was found that rates for Hispanics in New Mexico were lower than for non-Hispanic Whites and rates for American Indians were the lowest among the three groups. These data support previous observations that Hispanics and American Indians in the Southwest are at decreased risk for mortality from IHD in comparison with U.S. Whites [13]. Latin populations have been reported to have a lower than expected prevalence of CVD when compared to Caucasian populations despite a lower socioeconomic status and education [14]. However, some studies contradict these observations: death rates from IHD in USA in 2001 in Asian or Pacific Islander was 103 for 100.000 inhabitants, in American Indian or Alaska Native 114, in Hispanic 149.9, in Whites 176.5 and in African Americans 211,6[15]. Also in the San Antonio Heart Study the age- and gender-adjusted hazard ratios for coronary heart disease mortality comparing Mexican Americans with non-Hispanic Whites was 1.60, after adjusting for possible confounders, among diabetic individuals not using insulin, the authors found excess risk of all-cause, cardiovascular and coronary heart disease mortality associated with being Mexican American; however, in no diabetic individuals and insulin-using diabetic individuals, Mexican Americans and non-Hispanic Whites appeared to be at similar risk of mortality [16]. Furthermore, other studies suggest that the Hispanic paradox derives from inconsistencies in counts of Hispanic-origin deaths and populations [17]

Native population in Hawaii has higher cardiovascular mortality than other ethnic groups living in Hawaii. The adjusted mortality rates due to heart disease are 66% greater in Native Hawaiians than Caucasians in the state. However, Hispanics and Japanese descendents have a lower cardiovascular mortality than non Hispanic Whites. In the Multiethnic Cohort, a large population-based study of adult men and women living in Hawaii and California, compared to White males, age-adjusted death rates for AMI were highest in Native Hawaiians (RR = 1.62) and in African Americans (RR = 1.54). In contrast, rates for Latino men were similar to those of Whites (RR=0.94) while mortality rates of Japanese-American men were significantly lower than the rates for Whites (RR = 0.63). The results were similar in women. However, between the Asian groups there are differences in mortality, with higher percentage in Asian Indians and Hawaiians and lower in Vietnamese and Korean minorities [18].

Similar disparities in mortality for IHD have been reported in immigrants in England and Wales [19;20]. A study compared adult mortality between 1970-72 and 1989-92 using census data. IHD was the leading cause of death for all population groups with the exception of women immigrants from West Africa, who were relatively young. Standardized mortality ratios for IHD were highest than the national average for South Asian men and women and east African men and lowest for Caribbean and west African immigrants, differences between men by country of birth were even greater for the youngest age group. Also death rates for IHD are lower in Chinese minorities living in England and Wales (table 2) [21]. In the UK, mortality from IHD in both South Asian men and women is 1.5 times that of the general population, and South Asians have not benefited to the same extent from the general decline in deaths caused by IHD over the last few decades. In striking contrast, African Caribbean's in the UK have a significantly lower risk of heart disease compared to the majority population. This is particularly true in men, where both, morbidity and mortality from heart disease, is about half that of the general population. The reduction observed in women is of the order of 20–30% [19].

The effect of residence duration between different ethnic groups in mortality has been studies by Harding in England in populations from the Indian subcontinent and Afro Caribbean's [22]. A cohort of South Asian migrants between 25 and 54 years was followed since 1971 to 2000. All cause mortality increased with the increase of the residence duration in 1.07 hazard ratio for year in the youngest (25-34 years) and 1.02 in those between 45-54 years. CVD and IHD were the fundamental cause of this increased risk, with increments of cardiovascular mortality in the youngest group of 1.09 and 1.02 in the oldest. Similar results were observed in a cohort of migrants Caribbean's followed from 1971 to 2000: Circulatory disease mortality in Caribbean migrants increased with increasing duration of residence and age at migration in the oldest age cohort [23].

Table 2. Standardized mortality rates (95% confidence intervals) for ischemic heart disease (ICD-9 410-414) by country of birth 1989-92, England and Wales (from Gill et al. 2005) (21)

	India	Pakistan	Bangladesh	China*	Caribean	Africa**
Men	142 (137, 147)	148 (138, 158)	151 (136, 167)	44 (36, 54)	62 (58, 67)	58 (47, 70)
Women	158 (148, 168)	111 (93, 130)	91 (60, 133)	43 (30, 60)	86 (77, 96)	61 (37. 94)

* including Hong Kong and Taiwan ** West and South

The biological, social and environmental determinants of IHD have important differences between these ethnic groups and these health disparities have a mayor role in health outcomes. Health disparities refers to differences of health indicators (like incidence, prevalence, mortality, burden of disease) in different population groups, defined by race, ethnicity, gender, level of education, socioeconomic status and geographic location of residence. The different health status of minorities can be partially explained by: 1.-differences in prevalence of risk factors, 2.-economical and social factors, 3.-factors related with health care or 4.-biological differences between ethnic groups.

1. Prevalence of Risk Factors

Risk factors are characteristics of individuals associated with the presence or prognosis of a condition. They are related with life style, social or environmental conditions or genetics. The results of INTERHEART study demonstrated that cardiovascular risk factors have the same association strength between the mayor ethnic groups in the world. However, given the different prevalence in risk factors among different populations, the population attributable risk varies [6]. In a similar way we can expect that differences in mortality between the population of a country and groups of immigrants of another ethnicity can be explained by differences in prevalence of risk factors.

Traditional risk factors predict IHD in African Americans as well as in Whites in USA, but the prevalence and influence of these risk factors differs by ethnicity. Indeed, increased cardiovascular risk among the Atherosclerosis Risk in Communities Study showed that clustering of risk factors (obesity, hypertension, diabetes, smoking and hypercholesterolemia), was markedly greater in African American men and women, with any risk factor being markedly more common among White subjects [18;24]. The Dallas Heart Study showed that risk factors, such as cigarette smoking, hypertension, and diabetes mellitus, were significantly more common among African Americans than among Whites [25]. African

American males in USA have more smoking than Whites and African American women have more obesity than Whites. The relationship between total cholesterol and IHD risk is similar in African Americans and Whites, as demonstrated by the MRFIT study. Dyslipidemia is as common among African Americans as it is among White individuals, although the pattern tends to be somewhat different in these ethnicities. Mean levels of low density lipoprotein cholesterol (LDL-C) tend to be lower in African Americans, although LDL-C levels are more frequently elevated in that population group (due to a cluster of patients with high LDL-C). Mean levels of high-density lipoprotein cholesterol (HDL-C) are higher among African American men than among White men, whereas mean HDL-C levels are similar between African American and White women. Triglyceride levels are lower in both African American men and women compared with their White counterparts (10). In the Genoa study, prevalence of dyslipidemia was significantly greater among Whites than African Americans (women, 64.7% vs. 49.5%; and men, 78.4% vs. 56.7%; $P<0.001$ for both) [26].

In USA a comparison of median values of waist perimeter and cholesterol was made between Whites, African Americans and Mexican-Americans, using data from NHANES III, conducted between 1988 and 1994. In men the waist perimeter was higher in Whites (96.6 cm), than in Mexican Americans (93.8 cm) and African Americans (92.3 cm). Interestingly in women it was observed the opposite situation: lowest perimeters were observed in White women (87.9) cm and the higher in African American women (92.9), having the Mexican Americans an intermediate value (90.6 cm). LDL cholesterol values were lower in Mexican American men than in African American, and Whites, with a similar tendency in women. However, HDL cholesterol was more elevated in African American, and White women and lower in Mexican American men and White men [27].

The prevalence of risk factors and cardiovascular events were assesses in the Multiethnic Cohort Study in 139,406 individuals with different ethnic background: African-American, Native Hawaiian, Japanese-American, Latino and White men and women initially free from CVD followed prospectively between 1993–1996 and 2003 was studied (Table 3).

Table 3. Age standardized distribution of risk factors prevalence in the Multiethnic Cohort Study

	White		Afro-American		Native Hawaiian		Japanese American		Latino	
	men	women	men	women	men	women	men	women	men	women
Obesity	15.5	17.0	21.4	35.3	31.8	30.3	7.8	6.3	19.5	26.7
Hypertension	31.0	34.6	51.9	59.4	48.9	50.0	42.1	37.9	33.2	39.1
Diabetes	5.4	4.9	13.3	13.1	15.7	13.6	10.4	8.5	14.2	13.7
Smoking past	50.4	38.5	45.4	33.5	47.1	32.3	53.6	22.4	47.3	22.9
Smoking current	15.9	16.6	27.8	20.6	20.6	19.7	15.9	9.2	18.4	10.3

Adapted from Henderson 2007 [28].

Obesity, defined by BMI≥30.0 was least common in Japanese Americans men and women but was more common in African Americans and Native Hawaiians. Hypertension was reported between a third and slightly more than a half of men in the different ethnic groups from the lowest proportion in Whites to the highest proportion in African Americans (51.9%). In women, Japanese, Americans and Latinas reported the lowest proportions of hypertension, with very high rates in Native Hawaiians (50.0%) and African Americans. (59.4%) Similar large differences were seen for diabetes in men and women: the disease was most frequently reported by African Americans, Native Hawaiian and Latinos, at more than 2.5 times the frequency in Whites. Current smoking was more frequent in the African Americans but the Native Hawaiians had more current smokers with a greater than 20 pack-years history. The pattern of smoking by ethnic group in women was vastly different from that in men. Approximately two-thirds of Japanese-American and Latino women had never smoked compared to 45% of the other ethnic groups. Native Hawaiians have increased rates of obesity, a higher prevalence of diabetes, higher serum cholesterol and the highest cardiovascular mortality rate of any group in Hawaii [28]. In the Multiethnic Cohort Study during this period compared with Whites the relative risk of dying for AMI was markedly increased in African Americans and Native Hawaiians and lower in Japanese Americans. Latinos has a risk similar to Whites (Table 4). After adjustment for risk factor prevalence African Americans men excess relative risks of mortality changes to 6% deficit and in Native Hawaiians it was reduced from 62% to 17%. However, the lowest risk observed in Latinos was increased from -6 to -26% and in Japanese Americans from -37% to -51%. In women, in comparison with Whites, there was an excess of mortality of 147% in African Americans. After adjustment for risk factors prevalence it was reduced to an excess of 48%. Similarly, the excess risk in Hawaiian women was reduced from 82% to 24% Rates for Japanese Americans and Latinos were similar and approximately 35% lower than in Whites.

Table 4. Prevalence of risk factors and cardiovascular events in different ethnic groups

	Whites	African Americans	Native Hawaiians	Japanese Americans	Latin Americans
Men AMI RR	1.00	1.54 (1.22–1.96) P=0.001	1.62 (1.17–2.25) P = 0.004	0.63 (0.49–0.80) P=0.001	0.94 (0.74–1.20) P = 0.614
RR adjusted for risk factors	1.00	0.98 (0.76–1.26) P = 0.884	1.08 (0.77–1.52) P = 0.651	0.45 (0.35–0.58) P=0.001	0.74 (0.57–0.96) P = 0.022
Women AMI RR	1.00	2.47 (1.87–3.25) P=0.001	1.82 (1.17–2.82) P = 0.008	0.65 (0.47–0.90) P = 0.009	1.06 (0.75–1.49) P = 0.752
RR adjusted for risk factors	1.00	1.45 (1.07–1.95) P = 0.015	1.13 (0.72–1.77) P = 0.600	0.57 (0.40–0.81) P = 0.002	0.72 (0.50–1.04) P = 0.081

Adapted from Henderson 2007 [28]. RR= relative risk

This analysis demonstrated that differences in prevalence of risk factors accounts for a large proportion of the differences in mortality between ethnic minorities. However, the fact that differences persist after adjustment suggest the presence of unmeasured determinants for cardiovascular mortality that are distributed unequally across these populations. [29]. This is confirmed by the observations of Agyemang that after controlling for the established risk factors of blood pressure, serum cholesterol, cigarette smoking, and diabetes, African Americans continued to exhibit higher mortality rates from cardiovascular causes when compared to their Caucasian counterparts [30].

Ethnic minorities also differ from European descendents in the time trend in risk factors prevalence. Smoking has decreased less in Black Americans compared with Whites, and overweight and obesity has increased in the former group. Compared to non-Hispanic Whites, all minorities except Alaskan natives have a 2- to 6-fold increased risk of acquiring diabetes mellitus and the prevalence is rising in some groups, including African Americans, Hispanic Americans, and American Indians [31].

In Canada, South Asians, compared with Chinese and Europeans, had an increased prevalence of glucose intolerance, higher total and LDL cholesterol, higher triglycerides, and lower HDL cholesterol, and much greater abnormalities in novel risk factors including higher concentrations of fibrinogen, homocysteine, lipoprotein (a), and plasminogen activator inhibitor-1 [32]. Anand studied the prevalence of risk factors, atherosclerosis, and CVD in population-based study among people of Aboriginal and European ancestry in Canada. Conventional and new CVD risk factors were measured, atherosclerosis was measured by B-mode carotid ultrasonography and clinical CVD was defined by history or electrocardiography findings. Aboriginal people had higher rates of smoking, obesity, abdominal obesity, glucose intolerance, and substantially higher concentrations of fibrinogen, and plasminogen activator inhibitor-1. Aboriginal people also had significantly more carotid atherosclerosis and had a higher frequency of CVD (18.5% *vs.* 7.6%) compared with Europeans.

Differences in prevalence of risk factors in minorities have been studied in Europe also. There are wide variations by country of birth and ethnic group in the prevalence of IHD risk factors in England. These ethnic differences have been extensively studied in South Asian migrants. Classical risk factors, such as smoking, blood pressure, obesity, and cholesterol vary substantially between subgroups of South Asians—such that in some cases, levels are equivalent or lower than, a comparable European population. For example, while smoking is less common compared to the general population among Indian, Pakistani and Bangladeshi women, the proportion of Bangladeshi men who smoke (44%) is the highest of any ethnic group [33]. However, levels of insulin, glucose intolerance, abdominal obesity and fasting triglyceride are uniformly elevated in South Asian compared to Europeans. These factors are key features of the metabolic syndrome, a group of disturbances including hyperinsulinaemia, hyperglycemia, and associated frank diabetes, and dyslipidaemia, characterized by elevated triglyceride and a reduction in high density lipoprotein (HDL) cholesterol concentrations. As the elevated risk of IHD is shared by all South Asian subgroups, a possible explanation is that factors related with metabolic syndrome account for the susceptibility of South Asians to IHD.

In England and Wales, in Caribbean migrants, IHD incidence is lower and stroke incidence higher than the national average. A study using the Health Survey for England 1999 compared risk factors between migrant Caribbean and Irish origin people, who has higher incidence of IHD and stroke. Caribbean men were more likely to smoke but had higher mean HDL-cholesterol than men in the general population. Caribbean women had greater body mass indices and lower mean triglyceride levels. These findings were independent of differences in socio-economic position. Previously, Caribbean-born migrants to Britain had generally favorable lipid profiles in line with lower IHD rates, despite obesity and diabetes. This study suggest that UK-born Caribbean appear to be losing this more favorable lipid pattern [34].

A comparison of CVD risk factors in the UK between Europeans, African Caribbean and South Asians shows that African Caribbean men are less centrally obese than their European counterpart. Both minorities have an increased risk of glucose intolerance and diabetes, and raised fasting and post-load insulin, indicating a greater degree of insulin resistance. However, very low density lipoprotein, small dense LDL, and triglyceride concentrations are substantially lower in African Caribbean than in Europeans, and triglycerides does not increase to the same extent in the presence of glucose intolerance [34]. High standardized mortality ratios for IHD and cerebrovascular disease in South Asian men and women are consistent with the high rates of IHD in this group worldwide and are associated with increased prevalence of central obesity and insulin resistance. It is not clear why Afro-Caribbean people, in whom prevalence of diabetes and hypertension are high, have relatively low rates of IHD [20].

2. Economical and Social Factors

Ethnic minorities usually differ from the white population in several conditions that can be related with the risk of CVDs as income, education and environment.

Income: In the MRFIT cohort the age-adjusted Black-to-White CVD hazard ratio was 1.35 (10). However, after adjusting for the risk and income of the groups the hazard ratio was 1.05. CVD mortality rates were dramatically lower in cases of favorable risk profiles. The authors conclude that differences in risk can be explained by social and economic factors and differences in prevalence of risk factors. However, other studies suggest that differences in mortality ratios for migrants compared with the general population are not simply due to socioeconomic inequalities. The low mortality from all causes for Caribbean immigrants to England could largely be attributed to low mortality from IHD, which is unexplained for differences in family income or socioeconomic level. The low mortality from all causes that was observed in Caribbean immigrants cannot be explained by a favorable social class distribution because a higher proportion of people of Afro-Caribbean ethnic origin are manual workers (70%) compared with the whole population (52%).

Education: Income is closely related with education, which is related with the prevalence of risk factors and life stile. Cause-specific risks of death were estimated in USA from the National Health Interview Survey data and from linked vital statistics. Using these risk estimates, potential years of life lost and potential gains in life expectancy related to specific causes were calculated. Persons without a high-school education lost 12.8 potential life-years per person in the population, as compared with 3.6 for persons who graduated from high school. IHD contributed most to the difference according to education in potential life-years lost, with all CVDs accounting for 35.3 %. The pattern of disparities according to level of income was similar to that according to level of education. African Americans lost more potential life-years per person than Whites, 7.0 and 5.2 respectively, as a result of deaths from any cause (ratio, 1.35). CVDs accounted for one third of this disparity, in large part due to differences in prevalence of hypertension. Although many conditions contribute to racial disparities in potential life-years lost, a few conditions account for most of these disparities: hypertension, HIV, diabetes mellitus and trauma. When adjusted for age, sex, and race, the number of potential life-years lost from all causes of death was 3.5 times as great for persons with less education than for persons with more education. Persons with less education and those with more education lost 12.8 and 3.6 potential life-years before 75 years of age per person, respectively, a difference of 9.2 years. Less-educated persons lost more potential life-years than more educated persons for every specific cause examined. IHD contributed most to the educational disparity in life-years lost, 11.7 % of the total difference in life-years lost. When adjusted for age, sex, and level of education, the number of potential life-years lost from all causes of death was 35 percent greater for African Americans than for Whites [35].

Risk factors distribution changes between ethnic minorities educational level. Among men who had not completed a high school education, White men have a high prevalence of obesity and abdominal obesity, whereas among men who had completed a high school education, this prevalence is high among Whites and Mexican Americans. In contrast, African American women have a high prevalence of obesity and abdominal obesity regardless of educational status. Generally, the prevalence of hypertension was high among African Americans regardless of sex or educational status. The prevalence of hypercholesterolemia was generally high among White and Mexican American men and White women in both education groups. The prevalence of low concentrations of HDL cholesterol and hypertriglyceridemia was most favorable among African American participants, although among the most educated women, Whites and African Americans had a similar prevalence of low concentration of HDL cholesterol. The prevalence of measured levels of glycosylated hemoglobin > 7% was highest in African American men, except among the most educated. Among men who had not completed a high school education, the prevalence of elevated concentrations of C-reactive protein was high among White men. Among men who had completed high school, the prevalence of elevated concentrations of C-reactive protein was highest among African American men. Among women who had not completed high school, the prevalence was variable among the 3 racial or ethnic groups, whereas among women who had completed high school, African American and Mexican American women tended to have a high prevalence of elevated concentrations of C-reactive protein [36].

Neighborhood: The risk factor levels found in some ethnic minority groups might be partly due to their greater susceptibility to the adverse neighborhood environment in which many ethnic minority people live. A study to investigate associations between neighborhood-level environmental stressors, including crime, housing density, nuisance from alcohol and drug misuse, quality of green space and social participation, and blood pressure and hypertension among different ethnic groups was done in Amsterdam, the Netherlands. Dutch, Turkish and Moroccans living in 15 neighborhoods in Amsterdam were studied. Amongst Moroccans, high density housing and nuisance from drug misuse were associated with a higher systolic BP, while high quality of green space and social participation were associated with a lower systolic BP and lower rate of hypertension. Among Turkish, high level of crime and nuisance from motor traffic were associated with a higher diastolic BP. Similar associations were observed among the Dutch group, but none of the differences were statistically significant. Another study conducted in USA also showed a stronger neighborhood deprivation effect on cardiovascular risk factors in African Americans than in White Americans [37]. These results are indications that the impact of the neighborhood environment on ill health is greater in ethnic minority population groups than in natural populations.

3. Factors Related with Health Care

Possible additional explanations for risk factor differences involve differences in health-related behaviors. For example, socioeconomic deprivation in early life, like fetal growth restriction, poor nutrition in childhood, or infections acquired in childhood, are more likely experienced by ethnic minorities and it has been shown to have a strong association with risk factors prevalence and the risk of stroke. Among men at low risk factor levels, the influence of early life deprivation may be particularly important. Also adverse environmental conditions (deprivation, poor working conditions, lack of social support, unhealthy lifestyle, etc) in the country of origin may have long term effects on immigrants and may persist or develop in the host country [20].

There is growing international concern that the ethnic origin of a patient may unfairly affect access to medical care such that equal treatment is not provided for equal need. In recent years, it has become clear that the healthcare system in the United States does not provide the same quality of care for minority populations that it does for the majority White population. The Institute of Medicine report "Unequal Treatment" confirmed that racial and ethnic disparities in healthcare are not entirely explained by differences in access, clinical appropriateness, or patient preferences. Additionally, there is increasing evidence that provider behaviors and practice patterns contribute to disparities in care and that healthcare organizational processes also compromise quality.

Access to health care: There is evidence that for both, acute and chronic disease, South Asian people in UK are less likely to receive appropriate and timely care. In both instances, South Asians have to wait significantly longer before being brought to the attention of a specialist, and are less likely to receive diagnostic and intervention services, despite being more likely to have disease. Language was considered an important barrier for access to health care in a study about the knowledge and attitudes of South Asians about risk factor of coronary artery disease [38]. Chest pain may be experienced, understood, interpreted and described differently in different cultures. That the history given by South Asians on admission to hospital with an AMI is more likely to be classified as non-typical, compared to Europeans, supports this hypothesis. In the USA African Americans also request health care latter and receive a less intense treatment due to barriers to access health care. For example, African American men may receive less health care at early stages of disease development, possibly owing to employment, insurance, or other circumstances that effectively limit their access. There is evidence that African American and White men are highly segregated within the US health care system, with African American men more likely to visit doctors who are not board certified and less likely to have access to high quality specialists, high-quality diagnostic imaging, and other important ancillary resources.

Death due to "symptoms, signs, and ill-defined conditions" included in the Manual of the International Classification of Diseases, Injuries, and Causes of Death is an indicator of access and use of health services. The frequency of this categorization of cause of death was studied in New Mexico's minority populations, using state vital records data for 1958-1982. Death rates attributed to symptoms, signs, and ill-defined conditions in all three major ethnic groups in New Mexico exceeded the national rate for Whites. Males American Indians had the highest rates (115.6 per 100,000), followed by Hispanics (58.3 per 100,000), and non-Hispanic Whites (49.2 per 100,000); the national rates were 41.3 and 13.1 per 100,000 males for African Americans and Whites, respectively. Comparable differences were observed among females [39].

Differences in treatment intensity of cardiovascular risk factors can explain part of the different risk in ethnic minorities. Goff assess the implementation of the Third Report of the Adult Treatment Panel of the National Cholesterol Education Program in the Multi-Ethnic Study of Atherosclerosis [40]. He determined the prevalence, treatment, and control of dyslipidemia, including ethnic and gender differences. Participants were evaluated for CVD risk and self-reported use of lipid-lowering therapy. Control to ATP III goal was observed in 75.2% of participants with treated dyslipidemia and 40.6% of participants with dyslipidemia. African American and Hispanic Americans had prevalence of dyslipidemia that was comparable to that of non-Hispanic Whites but were less likely to be treated and controlled. Relative to non-Hispanic Whites, Chinese Americans were less likely to qualify for drug treatment, but no differences in treatment and control rates were observed. Ethnic disparities were attenuated substantially by adjustment for healthcare access variables. These results are supported by the GENOA study: treatment with lipid regulating drugs was significantly more common among Whites than African Americans (women, 25.4% vs. 16.4%; men, 32.6% vs. 12.8%) [26].

Lower control of diabetes in minorities in USA has been demonstrated in a comparison of risk factors control in a cohort of veterans with diabetes mellitus. African Americans and Hispanics had poorer glycemic control and received less intensive insulin treatment, particularly African-Americans with A1c $\geq$ 8.0% who received over 25 units of insulin less per day than non-Hispanic Whites. However, no difference for control of other CVD risk factors was found [41]. In the Third National Health and Nutrition Examination Survey, Non-Hispanic black women and Mexican-American men were disproportionately represented among those in poor glycemic control [42]. There are evidence that control of hypertension is lower in African Americans compared with non-Hispanic Whites, Chinese and Hispanics [43].

Delay in consultation after the beginning of symptoms in acute coronary syndrome (ACS) is associated with poor outcome because the benefice of some interventions is greater when is delivered early in the onset of the disease, i.e., thrombolysis or angioplasty. African Americans patients in USA can have a delay in consult 3 times greater than Whites in the presence of an acute coronary syndrome [44-46]. Similar observations in Canada have reported that South Asians have a longer time between symptoms and consultation in AMI than Canadians of European origin [47]. However, when given an identical chest pain scenario, South Asians in UK are equally likely to indicate that the pain is related to the heart, and 2–3 times more likely to state that they would seek immediate medical assistance compared to Europeans. Several causes can explain the delay in consultation: lower access to health care, knowledge and beliefs in relation with coronary heart disease, symptoms perception, etc. Lower socio economic level influence access to health care, because patient with worse health insurance coverage delay consultation due to involved costs. Even when minority patients arrive on time to the emergency unit they may have a delay in diagnosis due to differences in clinical characteristics of the ACS. Atypical symptoms in ACS has been reported as more frequent in African American compared with White individuals, leading to lower diagnosis of ACS in African Americans in emergency units [48-50]. Electrocardiography abnormalities that are more frequent in African Americans can contribute to this underdiagnosis of ACS. Non diagnostic abnormalities of ST segment, T wave changes and early repolarization are described more often in African Americans, African American patients have more AMI without ST elevation and unstable angina than Whites [51], conditions where the diagnosis is less evident than in AMI with ST elevation [44;52].

Optimal management: During the last years important advances in ACS treatment has reduced mortality significantly. African American patients with ACS have a high risk; however, they receive less treatments and reperfusion therapies, like thrombolysis and angioplasty, than Whites. The reasons for this undertreatment include more comorbidity that precludes the use of therapy, like severe hypertension or renal failure, the process of health care (type of hospital, physicians and patient preferences) and possible physician bias. Management of non-ST-segment elevation acute coronary syndromes in Hispanic patients was assessed using data from the CRUSADE Quality Improvement Initiative (53). Clinical characteristics, process of care, and outcomes of Hispanics presenting with ACS at US hospitals was described. Hispanics were more likely to be uninsured (12.5% vs. 5.1%). During hospitalization, Hispanics were more often managed conservatively, undergoing stress tests more frequently (13.0% vs. 10.1%), with less use of cardiac catheterization within 48 hours (48.7% vs. 55.5%) or percutaneous coronary intervention (39.6% vs. 46.4%) at any time.

Hispanics received similar discharge treatments but were less frequently referred for cardiac rehabilitation (38.5% vs. 49.2%, $P < .0001$). Adjusted in hospital mortality was similar in both groups [53]. Individuals from ethnic minorities are under represented in rehabilitation programs, as well as women and elderly people, although they benefit similarly to other patients. Reported causes for non-participation include lack of physician referral, lack of affordability of service, problems with insurance coverage, lack of support from a spouse or other care, gender-specific attitudes, individual factors, such as anxiety or poor motivation, and logistical and financial limitations; cardiac complications occurred more frequently in the ethnic minority subgroup compared with other patients and were more often a reason for discontinuation of the rehabilitation program [51;54].

Patients who are considered appropriate for revascularization but who do not receive it are less likely to survive and more likely to have angina than those who are revascularized. In the US, African Americans patients has less possibilities of having coronary angiography and revascularization procedures performed, they also were significantly less likely than Whites to undergo primary angioplasty for AMI [55]. This can be attributed to differences in severity of the disease or patient preferences. However, in the Coronary Artery Surgery Study, surgery was recommended to 47% of the African American patients and to 59% of the Whites, having similar coronary lesions. In addition, in UK a study of angiography showed that while revascularization was the intended management for equivalent proportions of South Asians and Europeans, fewer South Asians actually received the intervention. This effect was particularly striking in older people, women and those of lower socioeconomic status, suggesting that difficulties in understanding and navigating the health care system may be responsible for lower uptake rates [56-58]. In a tertiary cardiac centre in London, rates of revascularization in South Asian and White patients undergoing coronary angiography were compared in relation to the appropriateness of revascularization and clinical outcome. Appropriateness of revascularization was rated by nine experts with no knowledge of ethnicity of patient [59] There was no difference between South Asian and White patients in the proportions deemed appropriate for revascularization (72% *vs.* 68%) or in the proportions for whom the physician's intended management was revascularization (39% *vs.* 41%). Among patients appropriate for revascularization, age adjusted rates of coronary angioplasty and coronary artery bypass grafting were lower in South Asian than in White patients. These differences were smaller but still present after adjustment for socioeconomic status and after restriction of analysis to those patients for whom the intended management was revascularization [60]. Existing data suggest that although physicians think that their decision of not provide advanced care (angioplasty or CABG) to minority patients is based in disease severity and prognosis, they unconsciously project negative racial stereotypes in minority patients, and those stereotypes determined his treatment recommendations.

Differences in outcome of treatments can influence differences in mortality for IHD between minorities and predominant population. The importance of differences in clinical characteristics between ethnic groups on operative mortality of coronary artery bypass grafting was studied using data from the California CABG outcomes reporting program. Based on a multivariate model, the predicted operative mortality for Hispanics (3.2%), Asians (3.3%), and African-Americans (3.6%) was higher than that of Caucasians (2.8%). However, observed operative mortality was similar across ethnic groups, although there was a trend toward higher mortality in Asians compared with Caucasians (3.5% vs. 2.8%) [61].

4. Biologic Differences

The human population is not homogeneous in terms of disease susceptibility; the basis for ethnic differences in CVD susceptibility is not fully understood but it is likely that environmental factors interact with genetic factors to contribute to CVDs, either by determining presence or severity of risk factors, as well as the susceptibility to environmental or lifestyle risk factors [62]. Differences in cardiovascular 'intermediate' phenotypes occur among populations; for example, plasma lipid levels differ significantly between African-Americans and non-Hispanic Whites, African Americans hypertensive have lower renin values, increased plasmatic volume and increased salt sensitivity when compared with Whites. Also plasma levels of C-reactive protein vary substantially between people of different ethnic origins [32].

The South Asian disadvantage in terms of IHD does not simply involve risk factor status. Coronary vessels are generally smaller than in Europeans, and although appropriate for the smaller body frame, increase the technical difficulty of invasive techniques. The type of coronary atherosclerosis may also differ by ethnicity. A reappraisal of angiography studies indicates that, compared to Europeans, South Asians in the UK are more likely to have triple vessel disease, several lesions on angiography and non-discrete lesions [63]. Differences in the prevalence and severity of coronary artery calcification, using electron-beam tomography, as a measure of atherosclerosis, have been reported, in different ethnic groups: Caucasians, African-American, Hispanics, and Asians. African-American men were least likely to have any coronary calcium while African-American women had significantly higher OR of any calcification. Asian men and women had significantly lower OR of any calcification. There was no significant difference in prevalence or severity of atherosclerosis between Hispanics and Caucasians, in men or women [64]. Although there are differences in conventional and novel risk factors between ethnic groups, this variation and the degree of atherosclerosis only partly explains the higher rates of CVD among ethnic minorities. The increased risk of cardiovascular events could be due to factors affecting plaque rupture, the interaction between prothrombotic factors and atherosclerosis, or as yet undiscovered risk factors. [32].

Several studies have demonstrated that the genotype frequencies of single nucleotide polymorphisms (SNPs) in candidate genes for CVDs differ among populations. A few studies will be summarized as examples. Lanfear [65] found higher frequencies of disease-associated genotypes in African-Americans, than in European-Americans, for polymorphisms in *GJA4*, *SERPINE1* (*PAI-1*) and *MMP3*. Two nonsense mutations in *PCSK9* that lead to lower plasma levels of low-density lipoprotein cholesterol are relatively common in African-Americans (2%) but rare in European-Americans (<0.1%). Significant differences in allele frequencies were noted in the polymorphisms of *IL2*, *IL6*, and *IL10* among Blacks, Whites, and Asians. In a meta-analysis, Ioannidis assessed 43 validated gene-disease associations across 697 study populations of various ethnicities and found that frequencies of polymorphisms in seven CVD genes – *APOE*, *ACE*, *ITGB3*, *MTHFR*, *F2*, *PON1*, and *PON2* – varied significantly between ethnicities [66].

Apolipoprotein E (apoE) plays a key role in the metabolism of cholesterol and triglycerides: apoE mediates the catabolism of remnants of chylomicrons and VLDL via a "remnant" receptor and also the binding of chylomicron remnants, VLDL, and intermediate density lipoproteins to the LDL receptor. It has been estimated that apoE polymorphism may account for 2–16% of the variability of LDL cholesterol levels, a contribution incomparable with any other gene in the general population. Compared with e3 homozygotes, carriers of the e2 allele have lower circulating cholesterol and higher triglyceride levels, whereas the e4 allele is associated with higher levels of total and LDL cholesterol [67]. Several studies have demonstrated that apoE allele frequency varies across ethnic groups; the e4 allele frequency varies among Europeans, with a high frequency among Northern Europeans [68], whereas certain Asian [69] and American Indian [70] groups appear to have reduced frequencies of the e2 and e4 alleles. The relationship of apoE isoforms and coronary artery disease was studies in 224 African Americans and 326 Caucasians undergoing coronary angiography. Among African Americans, CAD was present in 9 of 34 e2 carriers (26%), significantly smaller in proportion compared with 39 of 82 e3 carriers and 43 of 92 e4 carriers (48% and

47%, respectively), suggesting a protective effect of the e2 allele. No such difference was seen in Caucasians. In African Americans, LDL cholesterol was lower in e2 carriers than in e3 and e4 carriers (106 vs. 127 and 134mg/dl, respectively). After adjusting for lipid levels, the association between apoE2 and IHD was no longer significant. Thus, the protective effect of apoE2 seen in African Americans could be explained by a favorable lipid profile in e2 carriers, whereas in Caucasians, the absence of such a protective effect could be attributable to the lack of effect of apoE2 on the lipid profile [71].

Conclusion

Although, further research is needed to understand the causes and to evaluate strategies designed to reduce disparities in risk factors prevalence and health care quality, there is clear evidence that minorities ethnic groups living in developed countries have an excess risk for developing IHD, they receive less effective treatment and have a worst prognosis [72]. In order to reduce, and in the future, eliminate disparities in cardiovascular care and outcomes the following elements of a comprehensive programs of education and advocacy has been recommended [51]:

1. increasing provider and public awareness of the disparities in treatment;
2. decreasing patient delays in seeking medical care for AMI and other cardiac disorders;
3. more timely and appropriate therapy for ACSs;
4. improved access to preventive, diagnostic, and interventional cardiovascular therapies;
5. more effective implementation of evidence-based treatment guidelines; and
6. improved physician-patient communications

To reach these goals requires a systems change, that includes a change in the quality of health care delivered to minorities that considers patient preferences, healthcare utilization, adherence, culture, lifestyles, and personal behaviors, eliminating prejudice, discrimination, and bias in all major public and private health settings [36]. There are several promising strategies that may improve health care quality for racial/ethnic minorities, Some quality improvement strategies have already demonstrated favorable results: bypassing the physician to offer preventive services directly to patients, provider education, use of a structured questionnaire to assess health behaviors, remote simultaneous translation [72]. The high prevalence of modifiable risk factors in ethnic minorities provides great opportunities for the prevention of IHD. Patients at high risk should be targeted for intensive risk reduction measures, early recognition/diagnosis of ischemic syndromes, and appropriate referral for coronary interventions and cardiac surgical procedures. Use of evidence-based therapies for management of patients who have ACSs and better understanding of various available treatment strategies are of utmost importance.

References

[1] Murray CJL, Lopez AD. The Global Burden of Disease: A Comprehensive Assessment of Mortality and Disability From Diseases, Injuries, and Risk Factors in 1990 and Projected to 2020. 2006.

[2] Murray CJ, Lopez AD. Alternative projections of mortality and disability by cause 1990-2020: Global Burden of Disease Study. *Lancet* 1997 May 24;349(9064):1498-504.

[3] Fox CS, Evans JC, Larson MG, Kannel WB, Levy D. Temporal trends in coronary heart disease mortality and sudden cardiac death from 1950 to 1999: the Framingham Heart Study. *Circulation* 2004 Aug 3;110(5):522-7.

[4] Yusuf S, Reddy S, Ounpuu S, Anand S. Global burden of cardiovascular diseases: Part II: variations in cardiovascular disease by specific ethnic groups and geographic regions and prevention strategies. *Circulation* 2001 Dec 4;104(23):2855-64.

[5] Dawber TR, Kannel WB, Revotskie N, Kagan A. The epidemiology of coronary heart disease--the Framingham enquiry. *Proc. R Soc. Med.* 1962 Apr;55:265-71.

[6] Yusuf S, Hawken S, Ounpuu S, Dans T, Avezum A, Lanas F, et al. Effect of potentially modifiable risk factors associated with myocardial infarction in 52 countries (the INTERHEART study): case-control study. *Lancet* 2004 Sep 11;364(9438):937-52.

[7] Bhopal R. Glossary of terms relating to ethnicity and race: for reflection and debate. *J. Epidemiol. Community Health* 2004 Jun;58(6):441-5.

[8] National Vital Statistics Reports. National Vital Stadistic Report 2003 December 30 [cited 2005 Mar 1];52(2003):1-45. Available from: URL: http://www.cdc.gov/nchs/data/products/ pubs/pubd/nvsr/52/52-23.htm

[9] Clark LT. Issues in minority health: atherosclerosis and coronary heart disease in African Americans. *Med. Clin. North Am.* 2005 Sep;89(5):977-1001, 994.

[10] Thomas AJ, Eberly LE, Davey SG, Neaton JD, Stamler J. Race/ethnicity, income, major risk factors, and cardiovascular disease mortality. *Am. J. Public Health* 2005 Aug;95(8):1417-23.

[11] Anderson RN, Smith BL. Deaths: leading causes for 2001. *Natl. Vital. Stat. Rep.* 2003 Nov 7;52(9):1-85.

[12] Levine RS, Foster JE, Fullilove RE, Fullilove MT, Briggs NC, Hull PC, et al. Black-white inequalities in mortality and life expectancy, 1933-1999: implications for healthy people 2010. *Public Health Rep.* 2001 Sep;116(5):474-83.

[13] Becker TM, Wiggins C, Key CR, Samet JM. Ischemic heart disease mortality in Hispanics, American Indians, and non-Hispanic whites in New Mexico, 1958-1982. *Circulation* 1988 Aug;78(2):302-9.

[14] Sorlie PD, Backlund E, Johnson NJ, Rogot E. Mortality by Hispanic status in the United States. *JAMA* 1993 Nov 24;270(20):2464-8.

[15] Health, United States, 2003. National Center for Health Statistics (NCHS), Centers for Disease Control and Prevention (CDC), editors. 2003.

[16] Hunt KJ, Resendez RG, Williams K, Haffner SM, Stern MP, Hazuda HP. All-cause and cardiovascular mortality among Mexican-American and non-Hispanic White older

participants in the San Antonio Heart Study- evidence against the "Hispanic paradox". *Am. J. Epidemiol.* 2003 Dec 1;158(11):1048-57.

[17] Smith DP, Bradshaw BS. Rethinking the Hispanic paradox: death rates and life expectancy for US non-Hispanic White and Hispanic populations. *Am. J. Public Health* 2006 Sep;96(9):1686-92.

[18] Ferdinand KC. Coronary artery disease in minority racial and ethnic groups in the United States. *Am. J. Cardiol.* 2006 Jan 16;97(2A):12A-9A.

[19] Chaturvedi N. Ethnic differences in cardiovascular disease. *Heart* 2003 Jun;89(6):681-6.

[20] Wild S, McKeigue P. Cross sectional analysis of mortality by country of birth in England and Wales, 1970-92. *BMJ* 1997 Mar 8;314(7082):705-10.

[21] Gill PS, Kai J, Bhopal RS, Wild S. Health care needs assessment: black and minority ethnic groups. In: Raftery J, Stevens A, Mant J, editors. *Health care needs assessment. The epidemiologically based needs assessment reviews.*Abingdon: Radcliffe Medical Press; 2005.

[22] Harding S. Mortality of migrants from the Indian subcontinent to England and Wales: effect of duration of residence. *Epidemiology* 2003 May;14(3):287-92.

[23] Harding S. Mortality of migrants from the Caribbean to England and Wales: effect of duration of residence. *Int. J. Epidemiol.* 2004 Apr;33(2):382-6.

[24] Hutchinson RG, Watson RL, Davis CE, Barnes R, Brown S, Romm F, et al. Racial differences in risk factors for atherosclerosis. The ARIC Study. Atherosclerosis Risk in Communities. *Angiology* 1997 Apr;48(4):279-90.

[25] Jain T, Peshock R, McGuire DK, Willett D, Yu Z, Vega GL, et al. African Americans and Caucasians have a similar prevalence of coronary calcium in the Dallas Heart Study. *J. Am. Coll Cardiol.* 2004 Sep 1;44(5):1011-7.

[26] O'Meara JG, Kardia SL, Armon JJ, Brown CA, Boerwinkle E, Turner ST. Ethnic and sex differences in the prevalence, treatment, and control of dyslipidemia among hypertensive adults in the GENOA study. *Arch Intern. Med.* 2004 Jun 28;164 (12): 1313-8.

[27] Zhu S, Heymsfield SB, Toyoshima H, Wang Z, Pietrobelli A, Heshka S. Race-ethnicity-specific waist circumference cutoffs for identifying cardiovascular disease risk factors. *Am. J. Clin. Nutr.* 2005 Feb;81(2):409-15.

[28] Henderson SO, Haiman CA, Wilkens LR, Kolonel LN, Wan P, Pike MC. Established risk factors account for most of the racial differences in cardiovascular disease mortality. *PLoS ONE* 2007;2(4):e377.

[29] Ferdinand KC. Ethnic, gender, and age-related differences in the treatment of dyslipidemia. *Am. J. Manag Care* 2006 Nov;12(15 Suppl):S400-S404.

[30] Agyemang C, Bhopal RS. Is the blood pressure of South Asian adults in the UK higher or lower than that in European white adults? A review of cross-sectional data. *J. Hum. Hypertens* 2002 Nov;16(11):739-51.

[31] Burke JP, Williams K, Gaskill SP, Hazuda HP, Haffner SM, Stern MP. Rapid rise in the incidence of type 2 diabetes from 1987 to 1996: results from the San Antonio Heart Study. *Arch Intern. Med.* 1999 Jul 12;159(13):1450-6.

[32] Anand SS, Yusuf S, Vuksan V, Devanesen S, Teo KK, Montague PA, et al. Differences in risk factors, atherosclerosis, and cardiovascular disease between ethnic groups in Canada: the Study of Health Assessment and Risk in Ethnic groups (SHARE). *Lancet* 2000 Jul 22;356(9226):279-84.

[33] Erens B, Primatesta P, Prior G (eds). Health Survey for England: The Health of Minority Ethnic Groups '99 Vols. 1 & 2, ix-633. The Stationery Office. London, 2001.

[34] Abbotts J, Harding S, Cruickshank K. Cardiovascular risk profiles in UK-born Caribbeans and Irish living in England and Wales. *Atherosclerosis* 2004 Aug; 175 (2): 295-303.

[35] Wong MD, Shapiro MF, Boscardin WJ, Ettner SL. Contribution of major diseases to disparities in mortality. *N Engl. J. Med.* 2002 Nov 14;347(20):1585-92.

[36] Mensah GA, Mokdad AH, Ford ES, Greenlund KJ, Croft JB. State of disparities in cardiovascular health in the United States. *Circulation* 2005 Mar 15;111(10):1233-41.

[37] Cubbin C, Hadden WC, Winkleby MA. Neighborhood context and cardiovascular disease risk factors: the contribution of material deprivation. *Ethn. Dis.* 2001; 11 (4): 687-700.

[38] Farooqi A, Nagra D, Edgar T, Khunti K. Attitudes to lifestyle risk factors for coronary heart disease amongst South Asians in Leicester: a focus group study. *Fam. Pract.* 2000 Aug; 17 (4):293-7.

[39] Becker TM, Wiggins CL, Key CR, Samet JM. Symptoms, signs, and ill-defined conditions: a leading cause of death among minorities. *Am. J. Epidemiol.* 1990 Apr;131(4):664-8.

[40] Goff DC, Jr., Bertoni AG, Kramer H, Bonds D, Blumenthal RS, Tsai MY, et al. Dyslipidemia prevalence, treatment, and control in the Multi-Ethnic Study of Atherosclerosis (MESA): gender, ethnicity, and coronary artery calcium. *Circulation* 2006 Feb 7;113(5):647-56.

[41] Wendel CS, Shah JH, Duckworth WC, Hoffman RM, Mohler MJ, Murata GH. Racial and ethnic disparities in the control of cardiovascular disease risk factors in Southwest American veterans with type 2 diabetes: the Diabetes Outcomes in Veterans Study. *BMC Health Serv. Res.* 2006;6:58.

[42] Harris MI, Eastman RC, Cowie CC, Flegal KM, Eberhardt MS. Racial and ethnic differences in glycemic control of adults with type 2 diabetes. Diabetes Care 1999 Mar;22(3):403-8.

[43] Kramer H, Han C, Post W, Goff D, ez-Roux A, Cooper R, et al. Racial/ethnic differences in hypertension and hypertension treatment and control in the multi-ethnic study of atherosclerosis (MESA). *Am. J. Hypertens* 2004 Oct;17(10):963-70.

[44] Asher CR, Topol EJ, Moliterno DJ. Insights into the pathophysiology of atherosclerosis and prognosis of black Americans with acute coronary syndromes. *Am. Heart J.* 1999 Dec;138(6 Pt 1):1073-81.

[45] Cooper RS, Simmons B, Castaner A, Prasad R, Franklin C, Ferlinz J. Survival rates and prehospital delay during myocardial infarction among black persons. *Am. J. Cardiol.* 1986 Feb 1;57(4):208-11.

[46] Crawford SL, McGraw SA, Smith KW, McKinlay JB, Pierson JE. Do blacks and whites differ in their use of health care for symptoms of coronary heart disease? *Am. J. Public Health* 1994 Jun;84(6):957-64.

[47] Gupta M, Doobay AV, Singh N, Anand SS, Raja F, Mawji F, et al. Risk factors, hospital management and outcomes after acute myocardial infarction in South Asian Canadians and matched control subjects. *CMAJ* 2002 Mar 19;166(6):717-22.

[48] Johnson PA, Lee TH, Cook EF, Rouan GW, Goldman L. Effect of race on the presentation and management of patients with acute chest pain. *Ann. Intern. Med.* 1993 Apr 15;118(8):593-601.

[49] Taylor HA, Jr., Canto JG, Sanderson B, Rogers WJ, Hilbe J. Management and outcomes for black patients with acute myocardial infarction in the reperfusion era. National Registry of Myocardial Infarction 2 Investigators. *Am. J. Cardiol.* 1998 Nov 1; 82(9):1019-23.

[50] Venkat A, Hoekstra J, Lindsell C, Prall D, Hollander JE, Pollack CV, Jr., et al. The impact of race on the acute management of chest pain. *Acad. Emerg. Med.* 2003 Nov;10(11):1199-208.

[51] Clark AM, Hartling L, Vandermeer B, McAlister FA. Meta-analysis: secondary prevention programs for patients with coronary artery disease. *Ann. Intern. Med.* 2005 Nov 1;143(9):659-72.

[52] Nakamura Y, Moss AJ, Brown MW, Kinoshita M, Kawai C. Ethnicity and long-term outcome after an acute coronary event. Multicenter Myocardial Ischemia Research Group. *Am. Heart J.* 1999 Sep;138(3 Pt 1):500-6.

[53] Cohen MG, Roe MT, Mulgund J, Peterson ED, Sonel AF, Menon V, et al. Clinical characteristics, process of care, and outcomes of Hispanic patients presenting with non-ST-segment elevation acute coronary syndromes: results from Can Rapid risk stratification of Unstable angina patients Suppress ADverse outcomes with Early implementation of the ACC/AHA Guidelines (CRUSADE). *Am. Heart J.* 2006 Jul; 152 (1): 110-7.

[54] Jeger RV, Jorg L, Rickenbacher P, Pfisterer ME, Hoffmann A. Benefit of outpatient cardiac rehabilitation in under-represented patient subgroups. *J. Rehabil. Med.* 2007 Apr; 39 (3):246-51.

[55] Casale SN, Auster CJ, Wolf F, Pei Y, Devereux RB. Ethnicity and socioeconomic status influence use of primary angioplasty in patients presenting with acute myocardial infarction. *Am. Heart J.* 2007 Nov;154(5):989-93.

[56] Ferguson JA, Tierney WM, Westmoreland GR, Mamlin LA, Segar DS, Eckert GJ, et al. Examination of racial differences in management of cardiovascular disease. *J. Am. Coll Cardiol.* 1997 Dec;30(7):1707-13.

[57] Sonel AF, Good CB, Mulgund J, Roe MT, Gibler WB, Smith SC, Jr., et al. Racial variations in treatment and outcomes of black and white patients with high-risk non-ST-elevation acute coronary syndromes: insights from CRUSADE (Can Rapid Risk Stratification of Unstable Angina Patients Suppress Adverse Outcomes With Early Implementation of the ACC/AHA Guidelines?). *Circulation* 2005 Mar 15; 111 (10): 1225-32.

[58] Wu AH, Parsons L, Every NR, Bates ER. Hospital outcomes in patients presenting with congestive heart failure complicating acute myocardial infarction: a report from the Second National Registry of Myocardial Infarction (NRMI-2). *J. Am. Coll Cardiol.* 2002 Oct 16;40(8):1389-94.

[59] Hemingway H, Crook AM, Dawson JR, Edelman J, Edmondson S, Feder G, et al. Rating the appropriateness of coronary angiography, coronary angioplasty and coronary artery bypass grafting: the ACRE study. Appropriateness of Coronary Revascularisation study. *J. Public Health Med.* 1999 Dec;21(4):421-9.

[60] Feder G, Crook AM, Magee P, Banerjee S, Timmis AD, Hemingway H. Ethnic differences in invasive management of coronary disease: prospective cohort study of patients undergoing angiography. *BMJ* 2002 Mar 2;324(7336):511-6.

[61] Yeo KK, Li Z, Amsterdam E. Clinical characteristics and 30-day mortality among Caucasians, Hispanics, Asians, And African-Americans in the 2003 California coronary artery bypass graft surgery outcomes reporting program. *Am. J. Cardiol.* 2007 Jul 1; 100 (1): 59-63.

[62] Kullo IJ, Ding K. Patterns of population differentiation of candidate genes for cardiovascular disease. *BMC Genet.* 2007;8:48.

[63] Chambers JC, Eda S, Bassett P, Karim Y, Thompson SG, Gallimore JR, et al. C-reactive protein, insulin resistance, central obesity, and coronary heart disease risk in Indian Asians from the United Kingdom compared with European whites. *Circulation* 2001 Jul 10;104(2):145-50.

[64] Budoff MJ, Nasir K, Mao S, Tseng PH, Chau A, Liu ST, et al. Ethnic differences of the presence and severity of coronary atherosclerosis. *Atherosclerosis* 2006 Aug; 187 (2): 343-50.

[65] Lanfear DE, Marsh S, Cresci S, Shannon WD, Spertus JA, McLeod HL. Genotypes associated with myocardial infarction risk are more common in African Americans than in European Americans. *J. Am. Coll Cardiol.* 2004 Jul 7;44(1):165-7.

[66] Ioannidis JP, Ntzani EE, Trikalinos TA. 'Racial' differences in genetic effects for complex diseases. *Nat. Genet.* 2004 Dec;36(12):1312-8.

[67] Dallongeville J, Lussier-Cacan S, Davignon J. Modulation of plasma triglyceride levels by apoE phenotype: a meta-analysis. *J. Lipid Res.* 1992 Apr;33(4):447-54.

[68] Gerdes LU, Klausen IC, Sihm I, Faergeman O. Apolipoprotein E polymorphism in a Danish population compared to findings in 45 other study populations around the world. *Genet Epidemiol.* 1992;9(3):155-67.

[69] Asakawa J, Takahashi N, Rosenblum BB, Neel JV. Two-dimensional gel studies of genetic variation in the plasma proteins of Amerindians and Japanese. *Hum. Genet.* 1985; 70 (3):222-30.

[70] Kataoka S, Robbins DC, Cowan LD, Go O, Yeh JL, Devereux RB, et al. Apolipoprotein E polymorphism in American Indians and its relation to plasma lipoproteins and diabetes. The Strong Heart Study. *Arterioscler. Thromb Vasc. Biol.* 1996 Aug; 16(8):918-25.

[71] Anuurad E, Rubin J, Lu G, Pearson TA, Holleran S, Ramakrishnan R, et al. Protective effect of apolipoprotein E2 on coronary artery disease in African Americans is mediated through lipoprotein cholesterol. *J. Lipid Res.* 2006 Nov;47(11):2475-81.

[72] Beach MC, Gary TL, Price EG, Robinson K, Gozu A, Palacio A, et al. Improving health care quality for racial/ethnic minorities: a systematic review of the best evidence regarding provider and organization interventions. *BMC Public Health* 2006;6:104.

In: Topics in Prevalent Diseases
Editors: N. C. Chavez-Tapia and M. Uribe
ISBN 978-1-60456-959-9

Chapter 6

Stroke in Minorities

Fahmi Yousef Khan
Department of Medicine, Hamad Medical Corporation, Doha, Qatar

Introduction

There are definitive and persistent patterns of inequality in stroke incidence and prevalence, stroke risk factors and subtypes, stroke severity, and mortality. Few studies in multiethnic societies, have attempted to explore race/ethnic-based differences in the incidence, risk factors, subtypes, utilization of procedures, or services and outcome of stroke. The evidence that the incidence of stroke in Black communities is worse than in non-Black communities comes mainly from the United States (US) and suggests that minority groups have higher rates or more severe strokes; later on many studies had been conducted to address risk factor profiles in Black and white groups. Noteworthy, epidemiological studies for ethnic issues of stroke have been performed predominantly in the US and United Kingdom (UK) to understand risk factor associations with stroke subtypes for different ethnic groups, which is required to improve primary and secondary preventive strategies as well as stroke management guidelines. Different national clinical guidelines for stroke were established in many countries to provide a framework for optimum standardized care for all patients after stroke. However, these guidelines do not take into account the variability of risk factors, both physiological and behavioral, for people from different ethnic backgrounds and how they might have an impact on the care of such people after stroke. This chapter is designed to provide information about stroke in minorities (race/ethnic-based) in a standardized format that contributes to a better understanding of this conflicting issue.

Incidence of Stroke in Minorities

There are differences in cerebrovascular disease incidence between ethnic and racial groups. In US, race/ethnicity-specific stroke incidence rates for Blacks and Hispanics have rarely been reported because of under-representation of these minority groups in past studies. [1] The increased incidence and prevalence of stroke among Blacks and Hispanics as compared with Whites had been reported in earlier studies [2-5] as well as in more recent studies. [1,6,7] The incidence of stroke in the Blacks and Hispanics is found to be approximately twice compared with Whites;[1,7] furthermore, Mexican Americans (MAs), the largest and fastest growing subgroup of Hispanic Americans, have been shown to have an increased risk for ischemic stroke compared with non-Hispanic Whites (NHWs), especially at younger ages. [8,9] In UK, ethnic based incidence of stroke in residents aged less than 75 years was identified by a community stroke register in south London in 1989-90. [10] Afterward, the south London stroke register (SLSR) was established to investigate ethnic differences in the natural history of stroke. [11] The incidence of stroke among Blacks and South Asians (especially male Bangladeshis) is found to be higher than in Whites. [10-13] Interestingly, the incidence of stroke in Black Caribbeans in South London is higher than Black population of Barbados (a Caribbean island). The risk in Barbados approaches that in the white population in South London and strokes occur at an older age. [14] Moreover, stroke incidence among the Black population of Barbados is lower than among African-origin populations in the US and UK [15]. In Martinique (French West Indies), the incidence of first-ever stroke in very old Black Caribbean patients seems similar to that in white patients. [16] In Canada, South Asian Canadians had the highest rates of cardiovascular disease, Canadians of European origin had intermediate rates, and Chinese Canadians had the lowest rates. [17,18] Although many studies have documented that immigrants from South Asia living in Western countries have a higher burden of cardiovascular disease than other ethnicities, less attention has been paid to the enormous burden of cardiovascular disease in the Indian subcontinent itself.

In New Zealand (NZ), the incidence of ischemic stroke and ICH is higher for NZ/non-white (Maori/Pacific and Asian/other people), compared with NZ/Europeans. [19,20]

On the other hand, studies from Gulf area showed high frequencies of stroke among Arab subgroup of patients compared with the South Asians. [21]

The ethnic differences in the incidence of stroke may in part be attributed to different risk factor profiles among the ethnic groups. Table 1 presents summary of ethnic disparity in stroke incidence among different ethnic groups.

Table 1. Summary of ethnic disparity in stroke incidence

• In the US and UK, the incidence of stroke in the Black population is approximately twice as high compared with the local white populations.
• Mexican Americans have been shown to have an increased risk for ischemic stroke compared with non-Hispanic Whites, especially at younger ages.
• South Asians have high incidence of stroke compared with white population in UK and Canada.
• The incidence of ischemic stroke and ICH is higher for NZ/non-white (Maori/Pacific and Asian/other people), compared with NZ/Europeans

Risk Factors Variations

Data on risk factor profiles for stroke in minorities are sparse; some studies showed predominance of certain risk factors in certain ethnic groups. In US, the link between ethnicity and risk factors had been discussed early by some authors. [3,6,22] However, recent studies have found more consistent data about the relative proportions of ischemic risk factors among races. Hypertension, diabetes mellitus, hypercholesterolemia, heavy alcohol use, and current smoking are significantly more prevalent in Hispanics and Blacks than in Whites; whereas atrial fibrillation is significantly more prevalent among Whites than Blacks and Hispanics. [2,7] furthermore, MAs are more likely to have diabetes and less likely to have atrial fibrillation when compared with NHWs. [9] In UK, hypertension and diabetes are significantly more prevalent in Blacks than in Whites whereas atrial fibrillation, alcohol excess and current smoking are significantly more prevalent among Whites than Blacks. [23] Compared to other ethnic groups, British South Asian patients have more hyperlipidaemia, [24] moreover, a recent study has shown high level of lipoprotein (a) [Lp (a)] with high apolipoprotein (Apo) B to AI ratio among south Asians living in Britain. [25] In Canada, South Asians have an increased prevalence of glucose intolerance, higher total and low-density lipoprotein cholesterol, higher triglycerides and lower high-density lipoprotein cholesterol, compared with other ethnicities. South Asians have also greater abnormalities in prothrombotic markers such as raised fibrinogen, PAI-1, lipoprotein (a), and homocysteine concentrations than other groups. [17]

Table 2. Summary of risk factors among different ethnic groups

• Hispanics and American Blacks have higher frequencies of hypertension, diabetes mellitus, hypercholesterolemia, heavy alcohol use, and current smoking than Whites.
• Atrial fibrillation is more prevalent among Whites than Blacks and Hispanics.
• MAs are more likely to have diabetes and less likely to have atrial fibrillation when compared with NHWs.
• Hypertension and diabetes are significantly more prevalent in Blacks than in Whites whereas atrial fibrillation, alcohol excess and current smoking are significantly more prevalent among Whites than Blacks.
• South Asians have an increased prevalence of hyperlipedemia compared with white population in UK and Canada.
• Obesity and diabetes are significantly higher in NZ/non-white than in NZ/European, but smoking is higher in NZ/European than NZ/non-white.
• Obesity and diabetes are significantly more prevalent in Arabs than in south Asians living in Qatar, furthermore, carotid artery stenotic lesions and ventricular wall motion abnormalities are observed with a higher frequency in the Arab subgroup of patients compared with the South Asians.

In NZ, obesity and diabetes are significantly higher in NZ/non-white than in NZ/European, but smoking is higher in NZ/European than NZ/non-white. [19,20] In Gulf area, significant differences between the Arab and South Asian subgroup of patients are observed with respect to number of risk factors and occurrence of obesity and diabetes. Obesity and diabetes are significantly more prevalent in Arabs than in south Asians; [21] moreover, carotid artery stenotic lesions, ventricular wall motion abnormalities and stroke recurrence are observed with a higher frequency in the Arab subgroup of patients compared with the South Asians.

As observed, there is a similarity in the physiological cerebrovascular risk factors (hypertension and diabetes) between the UK and US Black populations supporting the theory of genetic disposition, on the other hand un-correspondence in the behavioral risk factors (smoking and alcohol intake) between these two groups suggests that the acculturation process also plays a significant role in determining the incidence of stroke in a given Black population; moreover, increased risk of stroke for minor ethnicities in different countries support the view that within populations of similar genetic stock living in different settings, disease risk varies, and this variation is likely to be driven by environmental factors. Table 2 presents summary of risk factors of stroke among different ethnic groups.

Stroke Subtypes Differences

The proportionate distribution of ischemic stroke subtypes was different in some race-ethnic group. An understanding of risk factor associations with stroke subtypes for different ethnic groups is required to improve primary and secondary preventive strategies. In US, Whites had a significantly greater proportion of cardioembolic stroke than Hispanics and Blacks, although the absolute incidence rate of cardioembolic stroke was lowest in Whites. Hispanics and Blacks had a significantly greater proportion of intracranial atherosclerotic stroke than Whites. The proportions of lacunar, extracranial atherosclerotic and cryptogenic stroke were not significantly different among the 3 race-ethnic groups. [2,7] Greater proportion of cardioembolic stroke among Whites compared with Hispanics and Blacks is due to higher rates of atrial fibrillation among this group, whereas greater proportion of intracranial atherosclerotic stroke among Hispanics and Blacks can be explained partially by high rates of hypertension, diabetes, hypercholesterolemia, heavy alcohol use, and current smoking in this group. In UK, many studies have described stroke subtypes in different ethnic groups; the results of these studies have often been contradictory. Hajat, *et al.* [23] have found no difference in clinical subtypes between Black and White populations, while the SLSR shows an increased risk in the Black population across all Oxfordshire Community Stroke Project (OCSP) subtypes except POCI and unclassified groups. [11] Although the reasons for the increased risk in UK Black population are unclear, demographic factors such as socioeconomic status do seem to play a significant independent part. In NZ, compared with NZ/Europeans, Maori/Pacific people are at greater risk of embolic stroke, Asian/other people are at greater risk of lacunar stroke, and both groups are at greater risk of ischaemic stroke due to other determined and undetermined causes (TOAST criteria). [19] In Canada, despite high LDL cholesterol among south Asians, Europeans had more atherosclerosis than South Asians. [17]

Utilization of Procedures, or Services

Stroke is an equal-opportunity disease and therefore deserves equal access to definitive diagnostic studies. There are contradictory evidences for ethnic and racial disparities in acute and postacute stroke care in western countries. Inequality in quality health care for minorities has been addressed in several recent articles. In US, disparities in health care for minorities reached national attention with the studies of Schulman and associates in examining the practice patterns of physicians in both minorities and women in cardiovascular evaluations. [26] Johnston and coworkers have presented evidence of the disparate use of rtPA in Blacks. [27] Oddone and colleagues have presented racial variations in the rates of carotid angiography and endarterectomy in patients with stroke and transient ischemic attack. [28] Kennedy BS et al have found lower rates of initial carotid endarterectomy (CEA) use but higher rates of in-hospital death and stroke in NonWhites than Whites. [29] On the other hand, Goldstein et al [30] investigated race/ethnic-based differences in utilization of stroke-related procedures or services among patients admitted to Veterans Administration (VA) hospitals with acute ischemic stroke. Aside from cerebral angiography and ECG, they found no race/ethnic-based disparities in the utilization of a variety of stroke-related procedures and services. Why ECG and angiography were obtained more frequently in nonWhites is uncertain.

In UK, Socioeconomic health inequalities have been studied for a long time but the publication of the Black Report in the UK provoked the attention of policy makers for the existence of important health inequalities and resulted in an increased awareness of these issues in health care in general. [31] Hsu, et al. [32] has examined trends involving stroke management in groups from the Indian subcontinent. Their important finding was that South Asian stroke patients were not admitted acutely to hospital compared with their white counterparts. Moreover, Bourke, et al. [33] have found variations in the management of acute stroke because of ethnicity; measurement of total cholesterol concentrations was much more likely to be performed in white Europeans compared with Bangladeshis. White Europeans were more likely to be given warfarin and lipid lowering drug compared with Bangladeshis. Prescribing more warfarin for White Europeans may be explained by the greater incidence of atrial fibrillation in that group, but prescribing more lipid lowering drugs for them is uncertain. In NZ, the proportions of investigations which were done for ischemic stroke patients did not differ significantly between the ethnic groups. [19]

Evidence for health disparities in stroke care across settings, regions, and the continuum of care varies considerably. Overall there are variations in the management of acute stroke because of ethnicity and these variations could have substantial consequences on secondary rates of cerebrovascular and cardiovascular disease. Whether the reasons for this disparity are attributable to inequity or iniquity of care need to be further investigated perhaps along with the development of ethnicity specific protocols. [33]

Case Fatality Rate

Although stroke is the third leading cause of death in developed countries, few studies have addressed racial/ethnic differences in stroke mortality. [34,35] In US, as reported previously[36], all racial/ethnic minority populations aged 35–64 years experienced higher mortality rates for stroke than did the White population. Recent figures on the age-standardized rates of ischemic stroke death for Blacks have been reported as 30% higher than those for Whites. The mortality rates with ICH for Blacks and Asian/Pacific Islanders are higher than those of Whites, whereas the rates from subarachnoid hemorrhage are higher for all ethnic minorities. [37] Risks of death among US Hispanics for ischemic stroke have been considerably lower than those in non-Hispanic Whites, slightly lower in cases of ICH, but slightly higher for subarachnoid hemorrhage. [38] In UK, Studies on case fatality rates in different ethnic populations have had conflicting results; Balarajan, *et al.* had found highest stroke mortality rates among Black Caribbean people compared with other ethnic groups, [12,39] whereas no significant differences have been found in case fatality rates between ethnic groups according to Stewart, et al. [40]

Data on case fatality rates in other countries either is sparse or conflicting. However, the degrees to which there are ethnic disparities in overall patient outcomes are questions demanding further consideration.

In general, differences in mortality rates for stroke between minority populations and Whites may reflect socioeconomic status, and variations in risk factors such as obesity, uncontrolled high blood pressure, diabetes, and cigarette smoking. Other factors that influence death rates include the lack of access to medical care, which may include lack of health insurance, differential access to or acceptance of invasive procedures, transportation difficulties, and lack of knowledge about early warning signs of stroke.

Summary

Evidence for ethnic disparities in stroke incidence, risk factors, subtypes and mortality has continued to mount in recent years. Race-ethnic differences in ischemic stroke subtype distribution and incidence are thought to be due to variations in risk factor burden and possibly in genetic susceptibility. Risk factors differences between white and other ethnic groups should be taken into consideration when measures for primary and secondary prevention of stroke are devised. Data on ethnic disparities in utilization of procedures and/or services as well as case fatality rates have been conflicting. Overall, the management of stroke and its risk factors in many racial/ethnic minority populations remains lamentable. Case fatality rates due to stroke, among American Blacks are higher than other ethnic groups. It was suggested that part of the reported excess stroke mortality among Blacks in the United States may be a reflection of racial/ethnic differences in stroke incidence.

Accordingly, more targeted research on race/ethnic disparities in the incidence, risk factors, subtypes, utilization of procedures and/or services and outcome of stroke in multiethnic societies must be conducted to identify specific differences between and within subpopulations related to lower socioeconomic or educational levels or to adverse environmental factors.

References

[1] Sacco RL, Boden-Albala B, Gan R, Chen X, Kargman DE, Shea S, Paik MC, Hauser WA. Stroke Incidence among White, Black, and Hispanic Residents of an Urban Community. *Am. J. Epidemiol.* 1998;147:259-68.

[2] Haerer AF, Anderson DW, Schoenberg BS. Survey of major neurologic disorders in a biracial United States population: The Copiah County Study. *South Med. J.* 1987; 80: 339-43.

[3] Gross CR, Kase CS, Mohr JP, et al. Stroke in south Alabama: incidence and diagnostic features—a population based study. *Stroke* 1984;15:249-55.

[4] Heyman A, Karp HR, Heyden S, et al. Cerebrovascular disease in the bi-racial population of Evans County, Georgia. *Stroke* 1971;2:509-18

[5] Alter M, Sobel E, McCoy RL, et al. Stroke in the Lehigh Valley: incidence based on a community-wide hospital register. *Neuroepidemiology* 1985;4:1-15

[6] Kittner SJ, McCarter RJ, Sherwin RW, et al. Black-white differences in stroke risk among young adults. *Stroke* 1993; 24(suppl 1):I13—15

[7] White H, Boden-Albala B, Wang C, Elkind MS, Rundek T, Wright CB, Sacco RL. Ischemic Stroke Subtype Incidence Among Whites, Blacks, and Hispanics-The Northern Manhattan Study. *Circulation.* 2005;111:1327-1331

[8] Lisabeth LD, Risser Jan MH, Devin L. Brown DL, et al. Stroke Burden in Mexican Americans: The Impact of Mortality Following Stroke. Ann Epidemiol 2006;16:33–40.

[9] Lisabeth LD, Smith MA, Brown DL, et al. Ethnic Differences in Stroke Recurrence. *Ann. Neurol.* 2006; 60:469–475

[10] Wolfe C, Taub N,Woodrow J, Richardson E,Warburton F, Burney P. Does the incidence, severity, or case fatality of stroke vary in southern England? *J. Epidemiol. Community Health* 1993;47:139-43.

[11] Wolfe CD, Rudd AG, Howard R, et al. Incidence and case fatality rates of stroke subtypes in a multiethnic population: the South London Stroke Register. *J. Neurol. Neurosurg. Psychiatry* 2002; 72: 211–16.

[12] Balarajan R. Ethnicity and variations in the nation's health. *Health Trends* 1995; 27: 114–19.

[13] Razzaq AA, Khan BA, Baig SM. Ischemic stroke in young adults of South Asia. *J. Pak. Med. Assoc.* 2002;52:417–22.

[14] Wolfe CD, Corbin DO, Smeeton NC, et al. Estimation of the Risk of Stroke in Black Populations in Barbados and South London. *Stroke*. 2006;37:1986-1990

[15] Corbin DO, Poddar V, Hennis A, Gaskin A, Rambarat C, Wilks R, Wolfe CD, Fraser HS. Incidence and Case Fatality Rates of First-Ever Stroke in a Black Caribbean Population-The Barbados Register of Strokes. *Stroke*. 2004; 35:1254-1258

[16] Olindo S, Cabre P, Deschamps R, et al. Acute Stroke in the Very Elderly Epidemiological Features, Stroke Subtypes, Management, and Outcome in Martinique, French West Indies. *Stroke*. 2003;34:1593-1597

[17] Anand SS, Yusuf S, Vuksan V, Devanesen S, Teo KK, Montague PA, *et al.* Differences in risk factors, atherosclerosis, and cardiovascular disease between ethnic groups in Canada: the Study of Health Assessment and Risk in Ethnic groups (SHARE). *Lancet* 2000; *356* : 279-84.

[18] Sheth T, Nair C, Nargundkar M, Anand S, Yusuf S. Cardiovascular and cancer mortality among Canadians of European, South Asian, and Chinese origin from 1979 to 1993: an analysis of 1.2 million deaths. *Can. Med. Assoc. J.* 1999; 161: 132–38.

[19] Feigin V, Carter K, Hackett M, Barber PA, McNaughton H, Dyall L, Chen MH, Anderson C;Auckland Regional Community Stroke Study Group. Ethnic disparities in incidence of stroke subtypes: Auckland Regional Community Stroke Study, 2002-2003. *Lancet Neurol.* 2006;5:130-9

[20] Bonita R, Broad JB, Beaglehole R. Ethnic differences in stroke incidence and case fatality in Auckland, New Zealand. *Stroke.* 1997;28:758–761.

[21] Deleu D, Hamad AA, Kamran S, El Siddig A, Al Hail H, Hamdy SM. Ethnic variations in risk factor profile, pattern and recurrence of non-cardioembolic ischemic stroke. *Arch Med. Res*. 2006 ;37:655-62

[22] Kittner SJ, White LR, Losonczy KG, et al. Black-white differences in stroke incidence in a national sample: the contribution of hypertension and diabetes mellitus. *JAMA* 1990; 264:1267-70.

[23] Hajat C, Dundas R, Stewart JA, Lawrence E, Rudd AG, Howard R, Wolfe CD. Cerebrovascular Risk Factors and Stroke Subtypes:Differences Between Ethnic Groups. *Stroke* 2001;32;37-42

[24] Gunarathne A, Patel JV, Potluri R, Gill PS, Hughes EA, Lip GY. Secular trends in the cardiovascular risk profile and mortality of stroke admissions in an inner city, multiethnic population in the United Kingdom (1997-2005). *J. Hum. Hypertens*. 2007 Aug 2; [Epub ahead of print]

[25] Sharobeem KM, Patel JV, Ritch AE, Lip GY, Gill PS, Hughes EA. Elevated lipoprotein (a) and apolipoprotein B to AI ratio in South Asian patients with ischaemic stroke. *Int. J. Clin. Pract.* 2007 Nov;61(11):1824-8

[26] Schulman KA, Berlin JA, Harless W, Kerner JF, Sistrunk S, Gersh BJ, Dubé R, Taleghani CK, Burke JE, Williams S, et al. The effect of race and sex on physicians' recommendations for cardiac catheterization. *N Engl. J. Med.* 1999;340:618–626. Correction, 1999;340:14.

[27] Johnston SC, Fung LH, Gillum LA, Smith WS, Brass LM, Lichtman JH, Brown AN. Utilization of intravenous tissue-type plasminogen activator for ischemic stroke at academic medical centers: the influence of ethnicity. *Stroke*.

[28] Oddone EZ, Horner RD, Monger ME, Matchar DB. Racial variations in the rates of carotid angiography and endarterectomy in patients with stroke and transient ischemic attack. *Arch Intern. Med*. 1993;153: 2781–2782.

[29] Kennedy BS, Fortmann SP, Stafford RS. Elective and isolated carotid endarterectomy: health disparities in utilization and outcomes, but not readmission. *J. Natl. Med. Assoc.* 2007; 99:480-8
[30] Goldstein LB, Matchar DB, Hoff-Lindquist J, Samsa GP, Horner RD. Veterans Administration Acute Stroke (VASt) Study: lack of race/ethnic-based differences in utilization of stroke-related procedures or services. *Stroke*. 2003;34:999-1004.
[31] Putman K, De Wit L, Schoonacker M, et al. Effect of socioeconomic status on functional and motor recovery after stroke: a European multicentre study. *J. Neurol. Neurosurg. Psychiatry* 2007;78:593–599.
[32] Hsu RT, Ardron ME, Brooks W, et al. The 1996 Leicestershire community stroke and ethnicity study: differences and similarities between South Asian and white strokes. *Int. J. Epidemiol.* 1999;28:853–8
[33] Bourke J, Sylvester R, Sharma P. Ethnic variations in the management of patients with acute stroke. *Postgrad. Med. J.* 2006;82:13–15
[34] Howard G, Anderson R, Sorlie P, et al. Ethnic differences in stroke mortality between non-Hispanic Whites, HispanicWhites, and Blacks. The National Longitudinal Mortality Study. *Stroke* 1994;24:2120–5.
[35] Wein TH, Smith MA, Morgenstern LB. Race/ethnicity and location of stroke mortality: implications for population-based studies. *Stroke* 1999;30:1501–5.
[36] Age-specific excess deaths associated with stroke among racial/ethnic minority populations—United States, 1997. *MMWR Morb. Mortal Wkly Rep.* 2000;49:94–7.
[37] Ayala C, Greenlund KJ, Croft JB, Keenan NL, Donehoo RS, GilesWH, Kittner SJ, Marks JS. Racial/ethnic disparities in mortality by stroke subtype in the United States, 1995–1998. *Am. J. Epidemiol.*2001;154:1057–1063.
[38] Stansbury JP, Jia H, Williams LS, et al. Ethnic Disparities in Stroke Epidemiology, Acute Care, and Postacute Outcomes. *Stroke*. 2005;36:374-387
[39] Balarajan R. Ethnic differences in mortality from ischaemic heart disease and cerebrovascular disease in England and Wales. *BMJ* 1991;302:560-4.
[40] Stewart JA, Dundas R, Howard RS, et al. Ethnic differences in incidence of stroke: prospective study with stroke register. *BMJ* 1999;318:967–71.

In: Topics in Prevalent Diseases
Editors: N. C. Chavez-Tapia and M. Uribe
ISBN 978-1-60456-959-9

Chapter 7

Ethnicity and the Metabolic Syndrome

Roopa Mehta and Carlos A. Aguilar-Salinas
Departamento de Endocrinología y Metabolismo del Instituto Nacional de Ciencias Médicas y Nutrición Salvador Zubirán, Mexico City, Mexico

Abbreviations

IDF: The metabolic syndrome defined by the International Diabetes Federation criteria
ATP-III: The metabolic syndrome defined by the Adult Treatment Panel-III criteria
WHO: The metabolic syndrome defined by the World Health Organization Criteria

Introduction

The metabolic syndrome, a cluster of impaired glucose metabolism (insulin resistance), dyslipidemia, obesity and arterial hypertension is increasing in prevalence throughout the world. These metabolic risk factors are thought to share an underlying physiology. This hypothesis is supported by the observation that the individual components co- occur more often than would be expected by chance alone [1]. As yet the pathological basis of the metabolic syndrome remains controversial; insulin resistance and central obesity have been postulated to have etiological roles [2]. The importance of this condition rests in its association with cardiovascular disease (CVD) and type 2 diabetes mellitus (Figure 1). Individuals with the metabolic syndrome are twice as likely to develop cardiovascular disease and four times more likely to develop type 2 diabetes than subjects without it [1]. In addition, there appears to be a linear association between the number of metabolic syndrome criteria and the risk of CVD mortality [3] or type 2 diabetes. Hence the metabolic syndrome should be viewed as a concept which can be used to identify those persons at high metabolic risk [4].

The prevalence of the metabolic syndrome and the expression of the components of the syndrome vary greatly among ethnic groups. In addition, the metabolic syndrome is associated with varying disease risk according to ethnicity. The term ethnicity refers to groups of people sharing cultural factors including language, religion, diet and ancestry [5]. A person's race, on the other hand, is based on physical characteristics. Among ethnic groups, differences in the incidence and prevalence of disease states (e.g. diabetes mellitus, cardiovascular disease etc.) remain largely unexplained. A combination of genetic and environmental factors probably account for these discrepancies.

Despite the growing ethnic diversity in various countries, the majority of published literature regarding the metabolic syndrome focuses on the white population. Several organizations have proposed definitions of the metabolic syndrome to aid in diagnosis and CVD prevention. Since these have been derived using Caucasian data, it is becoming increasingly evident that they need to be modified for ethnicity; this will ensure a more realistic estimate of disease risk in other populations.

In this chapter we will discuss the relationship between ethnicity and the metabolic syndrome with particular emphasis on the Hispanic population. This is the fastest growing minority in the United States, accounting for at least 13.7% of the total population [6]. The term Hispanic refers to people born in a country that was "conquered" by Spaniards and for whom Spanish is the mother tongue [5]. This ethnic group has one of the highest rates of the metabolic syndrome and its associated complications. In order to adequately manage the metabolic syndrome in multi- ethnic populations, studies incorporating different ethnic groups will become increasingly important. In particular, they may give us insight into the disease mechanisms involved. Perhaps ethnicity per se should be considered a potential risk factor that modifies the expression of the disease and the risk of complications.

Diagnostic Criteria for the Metabolic Syndrome

There is no universally accepted definition of the metabolic syndrome. As shown in table 1, five groups have presented alternative proposals: the World Health Organization (WHO) (1998 and 1999), the European Group for the study of Insulin Resistance (EGIR) (1999), the National Cholesterol Education Program Adult treatment panel III (NCEP ATP III) (2001 and 2004), the American Association of Clinical Endocrinologists/ American College of Endocrinology (AACE/ACE) (2003) and the International Diabetes Federation (IDF) (2005) [7,8,9,10,11]. The majority of clinical studies have used either the WHO or NCEP-ATP III criteria. Newer investigation is utilizing the IDF or NCEP-ATP-III definitions due to their easy application. All three groups include type 2 diabetes among their diagnostic criteria. However, many believe that since diabetes is a consequence of the syndrome, it should not be used as a component [1].

The WHO definition considers insulin resistance an essential component of the metabolic syndrome. This definition appears to be most useful in the research setting: authors have pointed out the impracticality of evaluating insulin resistance (i.e with euglycemic clamp or using plasma insulin concentrations) in population studies. The use of overall obesity or waist-hip ratio has also been criticized because waist circumference is a more direct measure of abdominal obesity [12]. Furthermore, the inclusion of microalbuminuria is controversial; it is not routinely measured and many consider this a consequence of the metabolic syndrome [13].

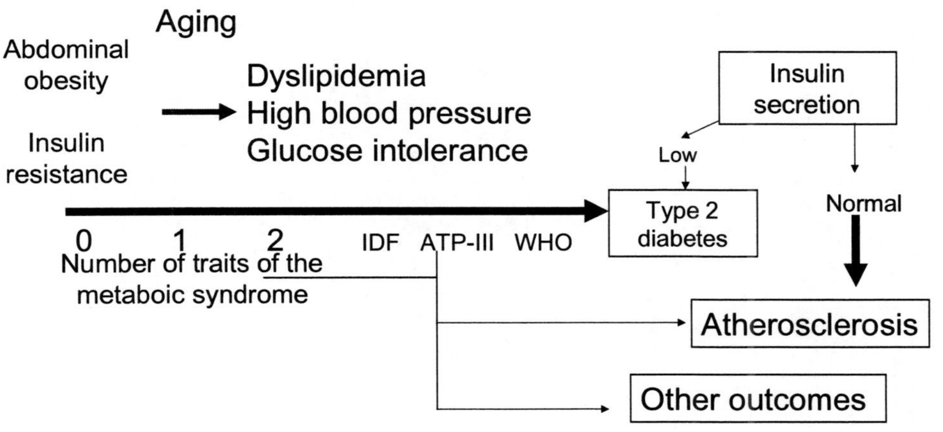

Figure 1. The metabolic syndrome: a precursor condition of type 2 diabetes and cardiovascular disease.

The EGIR has simplified the WHO definition: the most important change being the exclusion of diabetes as a component of the disease [13].

In 2001, the NCEP-ATP-III definition was proposed to allow the straightforward detection of the metabolic syndrome in the consulting room setting. It does not include a specific measure of insulin resistance and considers fasting plasma glucose an adequate measure of glycemic status. In addition, it gives all 5 diagnostic criteria equal weighting. This makes dyslipidemia a prominent feature of the syndrome (2 abnormal lipid criteria are included). This definition uses waist circumference as a measure of visceral obesity. However, the cut-off values were derived from data in Caucasians. This has been the most practical of the metabolic syndrome interpretations to date; the components being easy to measure in epidemiological studies. Recently, the American Heart Association/National Heart, Lung and Blood Institute modified this definition to include drug treatment of certain components (e.g. dyslipidemia) as equivalent to the diagnostic criteria [14].

The 2005 AACE/ACE proposal appears to be a more open definition. It includes numerous possible criteria, allowing greater physician discretion. This group, in accordance with the WHO, believes insulin resistance is the underlying cause of the metabolic syndrome. However, they do not include any surrogate marker for insulin resistance; nor is there any criterion for central obesity.

Finally, the IDF definition due to its recent introduction has not been as widely utilized as the previous definitions. It uses simple methods to assess criteria making it a practical tool for future studies. In contrast to the other definitions, this group gives central obesity, as measured by waist circumference, a prominent position [2]. Furthermore, it is the only definition to date which includes ethnicity specific waist circumference thresholds [13].

Although these definitions have many similarities, there are distinct differences (Table 1). Each group has put emphasis on a particular component of the metabolic syndrome depending on the prevailing etiological hypothesis at the time. Each definition identifies a different underlying abnormality. The WHO/ EGIR definitions diagnose a cohort with a greater degree of insulin resistance, whereas the NCEP ATP III / AHA/NHLB definitions put emphasis on abdominal obesity as the driving force of the disease [15, 16].

Table 1. Current definitions of the metabolic syndrome

	Blood pressure (mmHg)	Lipid factor	Hyperglycemia	Adiposity	Insulin resistance	Other	Main strength	Main weakness
World Health Organization*	> 140/90	TG≥150 or HDL-C < 35-40 mg/dl (one component)	Impaired glucose tolerance or type 2 diabetes	BMI >30 kg/m2 or waist/hip ratio > 0.85 (women)-0.9 (men)	Fasting insulin > 75th percentile, or HOMA-IR > 75th percentile, or M value < 25th percentile	Micro-Albumi nuria	The demonstration of insulin resistance	Lack of comparable insulin assays
National Cholesterol Education Program (3 positive components are required)	> 130/85 or drug therapy	TG≥150 mg/dl or drug treatment HDL-C< 40-50 mg/dl or drug treatment (2 components)	Fasting glycemia >110 and later >100 mg/dl or drug treatment	Waist circumference > 102 cm in men and > 88 cm in women	Not included	None	Easy access	Poor sensitivity for insulin resistance
European Group for the Study of Insulin Resistance**	> 140/90 or drug therapy	TG≥180 or HDL-C < 40 mg/dl or lipid lowering treatment (one component)	Fasting glycemia >110 mg/dl (non diabetics)	Waist circumference > 94 cm in men and > 80 cm in women	Fasting insulin > 75th percentile	None	The demonstration of insulin resistance, the exclusion of cases with type 2 diabetes	Lack of comparable insulin assays
American Assoc. Clinical Endocrinology (2 positive components are required)	> 130/85	TG≥150 mg/dl HDL-C< 40-50 mg/dl (2 components)	Fasting glycemia 110 –125 mg/dl or impaired glucose tolerance	Not included	Not included	None	Easy access, the exclusion of cases with type 2 diabetes	Poor sensitivity for insulin resistance
International Diabetes Federation***	> 130/85 or drug therapy	TG≥150 mg/dl or drug treatment HDL-C< 40-50 mg/dl or drug treatment (2 components)	Fasting glycemia >100mg/dl or previous diagnosis of type 2 diabetes	Central obesity as defined by waist circumference (ethnicity specific thresholds)	Not included	None	Easy access Ethnic specific thresholds	Poor sensitivity for insulin resistance. Thresholds selected based on cross-sectional data. Obesity obligatory component

*The presence of 2 or more components plus either type 2 diabetes,impaired glucose tolerance or insulin resistance is required.

** The presence of 2 or more components plus insulin resistance is required.

*** The presence of 2 or more components plus central obesity.

In addition, the arbitrarily derived criteria thresholds have also been changing as new research evidence has cropped up (e.g. arterial hypertension, fasting glucose etc.). Hence, the prevalence of the metabolic syndrome in a population can vary greatly depending on which definition is applied. This variability has meant that epidemiological studies are difficult to interpret and compare. The lack of agreement among definitions means that only about 30% of people are identified by most definitions [17].

The Impact of Ethnicity on Diagnostic Criteria

It is evident that certain ethnic groups are more susceptible to particular components of the metabolic syndrome [18]. This will result in over or underestimation of prevalence data according to definition applied. The impact of ethnicity is being taken more seriously as illustrated by the waist circumference adjustments proposed by the IDF. This is particularly relevant since waist circumference appears to be the most predictive parameter of the metabolic syndrome criteria. Increased waist circumference in the setting of normal body mass index (BMI) is found in various ethnic groups, notably Asians and Hispanics. In fact, compared to Caucasians, Asians and Hispanics have greater centripetal obesity and other metabolic abnormalities at any given BMI [19]. The NCEP-ATP-III definition would underestimate syndrome prevalence in these groups. It is worth mentioning that the WHO has recently revised its obesity guidelines for Asian populations; the recommended thresholds are waist circumference in men >90cm and in women >80cm [20]. A BMI threshold for overweight in Asians of >23kg/m^2 has also been endorsed but only for public health measures [21].

In certain populations these new waist circumference thresholds may still be inadequate. Recent data from the Mexican National Health and Nutrition Survey 2006 indicate that they may be too low for some age groups [22]. This is most striking in women over the age of 50 where a waist circumference >80cm identifies >90% of the population, lowering the specificity of this criterion significantly. A similar result is obtained using a waist circumference >90cm in men over the age of 50.

Hence, current anthropometric thresholds do no accurately reflect cardiovascular (CV) risk in certain ethnic groups; the same may be true for arterial hypertension, dyslipidemia and blood glucose levels [4]. Studies in the UK have shown high rates of arterial hypertension in the Afro-Caribean population but lower rates of CV mortality when compared with hypertensive South Asians or whites [23]. The discrepancy between hypertension and CV risk in this group suggests that arterial blood pressure cut off points may need to be altered or that a different weighting be given to arterial hypertension in this population. With regards to dyslipidemia, the African American population for example has a low prevalence of atherogenic dyslipidemia but the highest CV mortality of all ethnic groups in the US. In the Mexican population, >60% of adults fulfill the current ATP III HDL cholesterol criterion [22]. The CV and diabetic risk associated with blood glucose values also varies among populations. Tai *et al.* reported that South Asians are more insulin resistant for any given glucose level, indicating a greater diabetes risk affiliated with this criterion [24]. Additionally, the fasting plasma glucose parameter may not be an accurate measure of glucose metabolism. Dickinson et al. found that postprandial glucose response and not fasting plasma glucose varied among ethnic groups [25]. A glucose tolerance test is a better method for detecting abnormal glucose metabolism. The IDF consensus statement recently recommended this test in the presence of raised fasting plasma glucose [11].

Furthermore, since certain metabolic abnormalities tend to cluster in different ethnic groups, there may be combinations of syndrome criteria that are more appropriate for one population than another [4]. In Hispanics central obesity is often accompanied by abnormal glucose values; this combination may provide the greatest risk in this population. Perhaps more weight should be given to this combination of criteria in this group. Following on from this, changing metabolic syndrome definitions or diagnostic criteria alters prevalence rates in the same population. The most important question is whether these new prevalence rates really reflect the CV or diabetic risk of this group. Several groups have tested this hypothesis in Caucasians without any remarkable improvement in the identification of at-risk individuals. However, this remains to be explored in other ethnic groups.

In certain populations waist circumference does not contribute more to the identification of at risk persons. Therefore, some authors suggest it should be an optional component [16, 26]. In the Singapore Cardiovascular Cohort Study, subjects with the metabolic syndrome with or without central obesity had significant CV risk. This is reaffirmed in a recent population based survey in Korea where the IDF criteria failed to detect 44.9% of men and 16.6% of women identified as having the metabolic syndrome by the ATP III definition. This disparity is explained by the fact that this population has a high prevalence of metabolically abnormal non obese individuals [27]. These observations contrast with that found in Caucasians; in this group the lower waist circumference limits selected by the IDF identify a greater number of cases as abnormal compared to the ATP III criteria.

Finally, in addition to the effects of ethnicity, there are other concerns regarding the current metabolic syndrome proposals. The main misgivings are that continuous variables are assessed in a dichotomous fashion and that the definitions do not take into account that disease risk is a progressive function of abnormal metabolic parameters [28]. In order to overcome these problems, several authors (including us) have suggested describing the metabolic syndrome as a continuous variable and adapting it to the characteristics of the population being studied [29, 30]. Such a population based approach was recently applied to the results of the Mexico City study: this method had better prognostic power for incident diabetes than the NCEP ATP III definition (area under the ROC curve 0.746 vs. 0.697 respectively, $p<0.05$). It allows the detection of cases at the extremes of the range of diabetic risk and permits this risk to be estimated as a continuum.

In conclusion, it is evident that the present-day metabolic syndrome definitions are a work in progress. They must be adapted for differing populations. The majority of current data has been generated from cross-sectional studies and case- control studies. Longitudinal studies are needed to define appropriate ethnicity specific cut off points that will enable the accurate determination of CV or diabetic risk. Without doubt, the popular versions of the metabolic syndrome are useful tools to grossly identify individuals at risk of type 2 diabetes and/or cardiovascular mortality. They also provide the primary care physician with a workable framework which integrates the pathophysiology of the syndrome.

The Prevalence of the Metabolic Syndrome in Various Ethnic Groups

The prevalence of the metabolic syndrome is increasing worldwide but with significant ethnic and national differences. The best population data comes from the cross-sectional National Health and Nutrition Examination Surveys (NHANES) in the United States; NHANES III (1988-1994) and NHANES 1999-2002. In both surveys, the prevalence of the metabolic syndrome, estimated with the NCEP-ATP III definition, increases with age. Using NHANES III data, the rates were 6.7% in the 20-29 year group and 43.5% in the 60 to 69 year old group [31]. Significantly, the age-adjusted prevalence grows from 24.1% in NHANES III to 27% in NHANES 1999-2000 [3]. These figures were calculated using the original NCEP-ATP III criteria. When the revised definition is applied these figures increase to 28.0% and 31.9% respectively. In NHANES 1999-2002, the age-adjusted prevalence using the revised NCEP-ATP III definition and the IDF definition was 34.6% and 39.1% respectively [32]. The prevalence of the metabolic syndrome has increased the most in women aged 20-40 years. This contrasts with the reduction in prevalence, observed among older men (>age 60). The higher rates in women are probably due to the effect of pregnancies on body weight. In contrast, the lower prevalence in older males is related to survival bias. Thus, the metabolic syndrome definition helps us to detect adverse health changes in subsets of the population.

These population surveys clearly illustrate the growing epidemic of the metabolic syndrome. Between 1990 and 2000, the number of people affected in the United States is estimated to have increased from 50 million to 64 million using the revised NCEP ATP III criteria [33]. More worrying still is the increase in syndrome prevalence seen in children and adolescents; an increase from 4.2% (NHANES III) to 6.4% (NHANES 1999-2000) in adolescents [34,35]. In the United States, current estimates consider approximately 2 million adolescents affected by the metabolic syndrome [35].

The NHANES data has also been analyzed according to ethnicity: non-Hispanic whites (NHW), Mexican- Americans (MA) and African- Americans (AA). In NHANES III, Mexican- Americans had the highest prevalence rates of the metabolic syndrome (31.9%) [31]. The estimates in NHW and AA were 23.8% and 21.6% respectively. MA and AA women had higher rates than their male counterparts (26% and 57% higher respectively). In NHANES 1999-2002, there is a similar picture. Using the NCEP-ATP III criteria, the age adjusted prevalence in MA men and women is 40.3% and 44% respectively. The corresponding rates in NHW and AA men and women are 35.4% / 31.5% (NHW) and 24.5%/ 36.4% (AA) respectively.

These results can be explained by the significant ethnic differences in the components of the metabolic syndrome [36]. Mexican-Americans have the highest prevalence of low HDL, hypertriglyceridemia, obesity and fasting glucose/diabetes. African-Americans have a higher prevalence of arterial hypertension. They also have a high prevalence of obesity and diabetes but a less atherogenic lipid profile (higher HDL cholesterol). US whites on the other hand appear to be more predisposed to obesity and atherogenic dyslipidemia. When the IDF criteria are applied to the NHANES 1999-2002 data, not surprisingly prevalence rates increased further in all ethnic groups but particularly in MA. The prevalence rates in MA men superseded that of MA women on using the ethnicity specific thresholds: 50.6% *vs.*

46.2%. In NHW and AA the respective rates in men and women were 41.9%/ 34.4% (NHW) and 27.1%/ 38.8% (AA).

Ethnic differences in the prevalence of the metabolic syndrome have been confirmed by various authors. These rates range from 4% to 84% depending on the group being evaluated [37]. Two important studies in MA and AA show concordance with NHANES findings. The San Antonio Heart Study (SAHS) examined the prevalence of the metabolic syndrome as defined by the ATP III and WHO criteria in NHW and MA [15]. Using the former criteria the prevalence rates were 23% in NHW and 31 % in MA: the later criteria estimated rates of 21% and 30% respectively. The highest rates were identified in MA women. The ARIC study reported a 23% prevalence of the metabolic syndrome in AA using the original NCEP ATP III definition [38]. When the lower threshold for impaired fasting glucose is applied, the prevalence increases to 32%.

South Asians appear to be another group susceptible to the metabolic syndrome. This population has high rates of diabetes/insulin resistance, atherogenic dyslipidemia and central obesity. Deepa *et al.* estimated prevalence rates of 23.2% (WHO), 18.3% (NCEP ATP III) and 25.8% (IDF) in an urban South Indian population [39]. A UK population based study has also reported a high prevalence in South Asians (WHO, men 46%, women 31%; NCEP, men 29%, women 32%) [40].

Data from the 1998 Singapore National Health Survey found that the crude prevalence of the metabolic syndrome increased from 12.2% to 17.9% when using the ATP III criteria with a modified waist circumference threshold (>90cm in men , >80cm in women). The syndrome was more common in men than women (20.9% vs. 15.5%). It was also more common in South Asians (28.8%), than Malays (24.2%) or Chinese (14.8%) [41]. These results have been confirmed in a recent study in the same population; the prevalence of the metabolic syndrome was 17.7% by IDF criteria and 26.2% by AHA/NHLBI criteria. South Asians had higher rates than Chinese and Malays [26]. Yang *et al.* have estimated syndrome prevalence in China and reported rates of 16.5% using IDF criteria and 23.3% using NCEP ATP III criteria; with higher rates in women compared to men (23.3% vs. 10% IDF, 29.1% vs. 17.7% ATP III) [42]. This difference is accounted for by women having higher rates of central obesity and low HDL cholesterol, whereas men had significantly higher rates of arterial hypertension.

Finally, the Strong Heart Study (SHS) confirms the widespread prevalence of the metabolic syndrome in the Native American population. This study included three Native American populations; they found that the prevalence of the metabolic syndrome in men and women aged 45-49 years was 43.6% and 56.7% respectively. The overall prevalence of the metabolic syndrome in SHS participants aged 45-74 years was 55.2%. These figures are high if we consider that in men and women of all ages in NHANES III the rates were 20.0% and 23.1% respectively [43]. This population is renowned for high levels of central obesity, diabetes and low HDL cholesterol.

Cardiovascular Disease in the Hispanic Population

In this chapter, we have decided to focus on one particular ethnic group, the Hispanic people. This ethnic minority is growing rapidly in the United States; from 1990 to 2000 this population increased by 58%, more than 4 times the national average of 13% [44]. Interest in this group has been sparked by the high metabolic syndrome prevalence encountered in various reports. However it is important to remember that this is a heterogeneous population. The NHANES data and the majority of older studies include only MA; this is because this subgroup constitutes 66.9% of the United States Hispanic people. Findings in this subgroup are not applicable to all Hispanics. Furthermore, the results encountered in MA migrants differ from those reported in Mexican natives.

Mexico, similar to other countries in Latin America has undergone major alterations in the last decades. The economic growth and urbanization of the population has gone hand in hand with changes in health status. Whereas infectious diseases were once rife, now there appears to be an epidemic of chronic diseases, in particular cardiovascular disease and diabetes.

In the Global Burden of Disease Study, 31% of all deaths in 2000 in LA countries were attributed to CV disease. The WHO predicts that the CV mortality rate in Latin America will increase by >60% between 2000 and 2020; in the developed world this figure is estimated to be 5%. [45]. In the USA, CVD is the leading cause of death in Hispanic men and women (28% and 34% respectively) [46]. In Mexico, the CV mortality rate has risen significantly from 3.7% in the 1940s to 21% in the 1990s [47].

In the Mexican American population, there has been controversy regarding cardiovascular disease mortality data. This population is known to have high levels of obesity, triglycerides, diabetes, high blood pressure, lower socio-economic status and poorer access to health care. Despite this, several studies have reported lower cardiovascular and coronary heart disease mortality compared with non-Hispanic whites. [48,49] This so called "Hispanic Paradox" has been largely disproved and explained by discrepancies between studies including differing definitions of CVD, ethnic misclassification, inaccuracies in reported events and differences in the health status of the compared populations [50]. The Corpus Christi Heart Project reported a higher incidence of hospitalized myocardial infarction and greater case fatality after myocardial infarction in Hispanics [51]. The recent San Antonio Heart Study found that Mexican Americans were at greater risk of cardiovascular and coronary heart disease mortality than non-Hispanic whites. Hunt *et al.* compared US born MA, Mexico-born MA and NHW and reported a 50% higher risk of CVD and coronary hearth disease (CHD) mortality in diabetic US born MA. The Mexico-born MA had a similar risk to NHW [52]. Hispanics also have a significantly elevated cerebrovascular disease mortality rate than whites under the age of 60 years. In older age categories, they have significantly lower rates than whites. [46].

The Metabolic Syndrome in the Hispanic Population

The prevalence of the metabolic syndrome varies among Latin American populations. As mentioned earlier, most work has been carried out with people of Mexican ancestry (immigrants and nationals) and high prevalence rates have been recorded. NHANEs data and the San Antonio Heart Study clearly demonstrate this in Mexican Americans; using ATP III criteria, 31.9% and 31% respectively [15,31]. In Mexico, however, the National Survey of Chronic Diseases (1993) reported an age-adjusted prevalence of the NCEP-metabolic syndrome of 26.6% [53]. This figure falls between that reported in US Caucasians and Mexican Americans. The disease was more common in men than in women (age-adjusted prevalence 28.5 vs 25.2%, $p<0.05$). Furthermore, the age distribution of affected cases was shifted to younger age groups (20-29 years= 21.3%, 30-39 years=27.5%, 40-49years=24.6%, 50-59 years=17.7%, 60-69 years=8.7%, $p<0.001$). The WHO-metabolic syndrome criteria were also applied to this data. The age-adjusted prevalence of the metabolic syndrome was significantly lower (13.61%). The WHO criteria identified fewer cases than the ATP III criteria. The level of agreement between the diagnostic criteria was moderate (kappa=0.507). The same phenomenon has been reported in Mexican Americans (kappa=0.45), but is less common in other ethnic groups [15]. This lack of agreement was observed mainly in non diabetic subjects. The main reasons for this are: the requirement for insulin resistance in the WHO criteria and the higher lipid and blood pressure thresholds of this definition. In addition, the subjects diagnosed using the WHO recommendations had a worse metabolic profile compared those detected by the NCEP-III definition, indicating a higher risk for future complications.

Applying the results of the 1993 survey to the 2000 Mexican population census, close to 14 million Mexicans may be affected (ATP III definition). The recent Mexican National Health Survey (2000) has estimated a metabolic syndrome prevalence of 34% [54]. These are perturbing figures; no other chronic disorder (besides the individual components of the metabolic syndrome) affects a greater number of Mexican adults.

The major drawbacks of the surveys discussed above are their cross-sectional nature. To date, the Mexico City Study is the only population based study which provides us with longitudinal data [55]. Here, the age adjusted prevalence of the metabolic syndrome using the revised ATP III definition in men and women was 38.9%/ 65.4% in 1990-1992, 43.4%/ 65.7% in 1993-1995 and 39.9%/ 59.9% in 1997-1999 respectively. The authors reported that prevalence rates did not significantly change in men ($p=0.349$) but did decrease in women ($p<0.001$). Hence the prevalence of the metabolic syndrome did not increase as one would expect. These results are in marked contrast to the NHANES reports, where Ford et al. have described increased metabolic syndrome prevalence, particularly in MAs [32]. However, the interpretation of the data reported in the Mexico City study is controversial. Between 1990-1992 and 1997-1999, there was an increase in the prevalence of elevated waist circumference, fasting glucose and low HDL concentrations. This was counterbalanced by a decrease in prevalence of high blood pressure and hypertriglyceridemia explaining the discordant findings. Since arterial hypertension is an irreversible condition, it is unlikely that the lower number of "hypertensive" individuals was due to a lower prevalence rate. It is more probable that this result reflects better blood pressure control among affected cases.

Furthermore, it is clear that diabetic risk has increased in Mexico as a consequence of prevalent obesity and elevated glucose values.

Hence, the metabolic syndrome is common in the Mexican population. However, few studies have evaluated how this group compares with other Hispanic subgroups. Lorenzo *et al.* analyzed syndrome prevalence in population based studies from San Antonio (San Antonio Heart Study), Mexico City (Mexico City Study 1990-1992), Spain (Spanish Insulin Resistance Study) and Peru (Peruvian Insulin Resistance Study) [56]. The IDF criteria compared with ATP III criteria, calculated higher metabolic syndrome prevalence rates in all ethnic groups. The prevalence in men and women using ATP III criteria were: Lima 11.5%/25.6%, Mexico City 31.9%/56.3%, San Antonio MA 32.5%/36.1% and Spain 22.3%/30.7%. The corresponding results using IDF criteria were; Lima 26.0%/28.1%, Mexico City 54.4%/61%, San Antonio MA 46.3%/41% and Spain 27.7%/ 33.1%. As we can see the data confirm yet again the high prevalence in Mexican ethnic groups. Furthermore, each ethnic group had a characteristic risk profile: Mexico city residents had high triglyceride levels and low HDL and total cholesterol, Spanish subjects had high levels of arterial hypertension, fasting glucose, HDL cholesterol and total cholesterol, Peruvian subjects had low levels of arterial hypertension and total cholesterol but high HDL cholesterol levels, differences between the definitions were more significant in Mexican and Peruvian men because of the IDF ethnicity specific thresholds. The authors conclude that the IDF criteria are not suitable for the Mexico City subjects because 94.4% of the women had central obesity and 94.2% had low HDL cholesterol. Furthermore, the prevalence of the metabolic syndrome in native Mexicans is higher than would be expected for the level of central obesity alone. This is probably due to dietary factors; fat consumption is lower in Mexico City than in San Antonio but carbohydrate consumption is higher, resulting in a greater prevalence of hypertriglyceridemia and low HDL cholesterol.

Population studies in other Hispanic subgroups are scarce. A recent study in Venezuela reported a metabolic syndrome prevalence of 31.2%, with higher rates in men [57]. In this mixed race group, differences were only evident among men. Amerindians had the lowest prevalence (17%) followed by Blacks (27.2%), Whites (33.3%) and Mixed race men (37.4%). Low HDL cholesterol (65.3%), central obesity (42.9%) and arterial hypertension (38.1%) were the most frequent syndrome components. The authors concluded that the metabolic syndrome is highly prevalent in the Venezuelan population, the principal risk factor being dyslipidemia.

A study in Peruvian Andean Hispanics found a greater prevalence (as evaluated by the AHA/NHLBI definition) in women compared to men (23.2% vs, 14.3% respectively). This ethnic group is characterized by a high prevalence of dyslipidemia (low HDL cholesterol) and a relatively low prevalence of abnormal fasting glucose [58].

Factors Influencing the Epidemiology of the Metabolic Syndrome in Mexico

The high metabolic syndrome prevalence in Mexico is influenced by both genetic and environmental factors. Authors have speculated regarding the influence of genetic admixture to disease risk. The higher the contribution of Amerindian/or Black genes the higher the risk for type 2 diabetes mellitus. This is related to a survival/selection effect in which a population's predisposition to insulin resistance was protective in times of hardship. In our present day environment of abundance, this mechanism of safeguard has become detrimental to health [5]. Other authors propose that in addition to Native American admixture, the contribution of Spanish admixture may also be important [59].

Dickinson et al. suggest that certain populations may have a genetic predisposition to developing the metabolic syndrome. Lean young adults from 5 ethnic groups (European Caucasians, Chinese, South East Asians, South Asians and Arabic Caucasians) were fed white bread (75g of carbohydrate) and postprandial glucose levels and insulin sensitivity (using euglycemic clamp and HOMA) were measured [25]. Subjects were matched for age, BMI, waist circumference, birth weight, and current diet. South East Asians had the highest postprandial glucose values and were the most insulin resistant. In contrast the European and Arabic Caucasians were the most insulin sensitive with lower postprandial levels. This study clearly demonstrates that abnormal glucose metabolism is prevalent in certain ethnic groups from an early age and in the absence of obesity [60]. Although this study did not include Hispanics, it would be interesting to see if the same is true in this population.

Several candidate genes or genetic loci have been discovered which may increase risk of the metabolic syndrome. Chromosome 1q is thought to be linked to diabetes susceptibility: in fact linkage of the metabolic syndrome to 1q23-q31 has been reported in Hispanics, Amerindians, European-Caucasians and Chinese [61]. In addition, a Pro12Ala polymorphism of the PPAR gamma gene appears to affect glucose and lipid metabolism. It is speculated that this variant is associated with an increased risk for type 2 diabetes [62]. Finally, recent work has uncovered a possible role for the ATP-binding cassette transporter A1 (ABCA1) R230C variant in the metabolic syndrome [63]. Expression of this allele has been associated with early onset type 2 diabetes and low HDL cholesterol levels. Most significantly, it appears to be exclusive to the Amerindian and Amerindian-derived populations such as Mexican-Mestizos.

Attributing the high prevalence rates in Mexico to mainly genetic factors is tempting [60]. However, environmental factors are equally important in explaining the high obesity and dyslipidemia prevalence in this population. Weight at birth appears to be an important prognostic parameter. Low birth weight babies have a higher prevalence of abnormal glucose metabolism and non insulin dependent diabetes in adult life [64]. It is hypothesized that nutritional deprivation in utero induces changes in neuroendocrine function which ultimately contribute to insulin resistance and beta cell dysfunction. In Pima Indians, a U-shaped relationship between birth weight and diabetes is reported [65]. The low birth weight babies are more insulin resistant than those of normal weight; in high birth weight babies, the increased diabetic risk is due to gestational diabetes in the mother. Duration of breast-feeding during infancy is another important factor since this has been related to obesity in adulthood [66]. Gillman *et al.* demonstrated that those who received more breast milk than formula had lower levels of overweight during childhood and adolescence.

Mexican cultural beliefs must also be considered. Physical robustness is considered a sign of good health in this ethnic group. In addition, the traditional dietary habits are changing with the growing urbanization of the population. Food is being purchased more often from supermarkets than fresh-food markets. There is a higher consumption of refined carbohydrates (e.g. high-calorie soft drinks) and fat with an overall reduction in total carbohydrate intake [67]. Furthermore, physical inactivity is significant in this population. In the NHANES III survey 65% of MA men and 74% of MA women reported little or no physical exercise [5]. The Latin American INTERHEART Study reports a low proportion of physically active persons; only 22% of the control group underwent regular exercise [68]. The ENSANUT survey confirms these findings, only 35.2% of adolescents perform sufficient exercise and more than 50% spend >12 hours a week watching television [22].

In Mexico, several anti-poverty programs provide food and conditional economic aid to millions of homes (ENSANUT 2006) [22]. This strategy has proven to be successful to reverse undernourishment. However, these actions may inevitably contribute to the growing prevalence of obesity and metabolic syndrome in the lower income groups. The prevalence of abdominal obesity is increasing at a faster velocity than in persons of higher socioeconomic status.

Conclusion

The clinical expression of the metabolic syndrome varies among ethnic groups. Hispanics, in particular the Mexican population, have high metabolic syndrome prevalence. Unfortunately there is still great uncertainty regarding which metabolic components are most useful in this group. In addition, criteria thresholds are still inadequate for estimation of disease risk. In Mexico, the value of the metabolic syndrome concept may reside in its ability to predict type 2 diabetes. Prospective studies are urgently needed to clarify these points.

Recent genetic findings hold great promise for the Mestizo-Mexican population; such work is needed in other ethnic groups. Finally, the environmental factors mentioned above must be tackled by developing new Governmental public health strategies. Emphasis must be placed on preventing and treating the peculiarities of the metabolic syndrome in the Mexican population (central obesity, atherogenic dyslipidemia and diabetes mellitus type 2).

References

[1] Meigs JB. Epidemiology of the metabolic syndrome. *Am. J. Manag. Care* 2002; 8: S283-S292.

[2] Gotto Jr AM, Blackburn GL, Dailey GE III. The metabolic syndrome: a call to action. *Coronary Art Dis.* 2006; 17: 77-80.

[3] Ford ES. The metabolic syndrome and mortality from cardiovascular disease and all-causes: findings from the National health and nutrition examination survey II mortality study. *Atherosclerosis* 2004; 173: 309-314.

[4] Banerjee D and Misra A. Do using ethnic specific criteria improve the usefulness of the term metabolic syndrome? Controversies and suggestions. *Int. J. Obesity* 2007; 31: 1340-1349.

[5] Caballero AE. Diabetes in the Hispanic or Latino population: genes, environment, culture, and more. *Current Diabetes Reports* 2005; 5: 217-225.

[6] US census Bureau. Hispanic and Asian Americans increasing faster than overall population [press release]. 2004. 14 June. http:// www.census.gov/ Press-Release/ www.releases/archives/ race/ 001839.html.

[7] Alberti KG, Zimmet PZ. Definition, diagnosis and classification of diabetes mellitus and its complications. 1. Diagnosis and classification of diabetes mellitus provisional reportof a WHO consultation. *Diabet Med.* 1998; 15: 539-553.

[8] Balkau B and Charles MA. Comment on the provisional report from the WHO consultation. European Group for the study of Insulin Resistance (EGIR). *Diabet Med.* 1999; 16: 442-443.

[9] Executive Panel on detection, evaluation, and treatment of high blood cholesterol in adults. Executive Summary of the third report of the National Cholesterol Education Program (NCEP) Expert Panel on the detection, evaluation, and treatment of high blood cholesterol in adults (Adult Treatment Panel III). *JAMA* 2001; 285: 2486-2497.

[10] Einhorn D, Reaven Gm, Cobin RH et al. American College of Endocrinology position statement on the insulin resistance syndrome. *Endocr. Pract.* 2003; 9: 237-252.

[11] Bloomgarden ZT. Definitions of the insulin resistance syndrome: The 1st World Congress on the Insulin Resistance Syndrome. *Diabetes Care* 2004; 27: 824-830.

[12] Misra A, Wasir JS and Vikram NJ. Waist circumference criteria for the diagnosis of abdominal obesity are not applicable uniformly to all populations and ethnic groups. *Nutrition* 2005; 21: 969-976.

[13] Li C and Ford ES. Definitions of the metabolic syndrome: What's new and what predicts risk? Metabolic Syndrome and related disorders 2006; 4: 237-251.

[14] Grundy SM, Cleeman JI, Daniels SR et al. Diagnosis and management of the metabolic syndrome. American Heart Association/ National Heart, Lung and Blood Institute scientific statement. *Circulation* 2005; 112: 2735-2752.

[15] Meigs JB, Wilson PWF, Nathan DM et al. Prevalence and characteristics of the metabolic syndrome in the San Antonio Heart and Framingham Offspring Studies. *Diabetes* 2003; 52: 2160-2167.

[16] Khoo CM, Liew CF, Chew SK et al. The impact of obesity as a prerequisite for the diagnosis of metabolic syndrome. *Obesity* 2007; 15: 262-269.

[17] Day C. Metabolic Syndrome, or What you will: definitions and epidemiology. *Diabetes Vasc. Dis. Res.* 2007; 4: 32-38.

[18] Smith SC Jr, Clark LT, Cooper RS et al. Discovering the full spectrum of cardiovascular disease minority health summit 2003. Report of the obesity, metabolic syndrome and hypertension writing group. *Circulation* 2005; 111: e134-e139.

[19] Razak F, Anand S, Vuksan D et al. Ethnic relationships between obesity and glucose-metabolic abnormalities: a cross-sectional population based study. *Int. J. Obesity* 2005; 29: 656-667.

[20] World Health Organization. The Asia-Pacific perspective: redefining obesity and its treatment: Health Communications, Australia, 2000, 1-56 [Reference can be found in http://www.idi.org..au/downloads/obesity-report.pdf]

[21] WHO Expert Consultation. Appropriate body-mass index for Asian populations and its implication for policy and intervention strategies. *Lancet* 2004; 363: 157-163.

[22] Olaiz-Fernández G, Rivera-Dommarco J, Shamah-Levy T. Encuesta Nacional de Salud y Nutrición 2006. Cuernavaca, México: Instituto Nacional de Salud Pública, 2006

[23] Khattar RS Swales JD, Senior R et al. Racial variation in cardiovascular morbidity and mortality in essential hypertension. *Heart* 2000; 83: 267-271.

[24] Tai ES, Lau TN, Ho SC et al. Body fat distribution and cardiovascular risk in normal weight women. Associations with insulin resistance, lipids and leptin. *Int. J. Obes. Relat. Metab. Disord.* 2000; 24: 751-777

[25] Dickinson S, Colagiuri S, Faramus E et al. Postprandial hyperglycemia and insulin sensitivity differ among lean young adults of different ethnicities. *J. Nutr.* 2002; 132: 2574-2579.

[26] Lee J, MA S, Heng D et al. Should central obesity be an optional or essential component of the metabolic syndrome? Ischemic heart disease risk in the Singapore Cardiovascular Cohort Study. *Diabetes Care* 2007; 30: 343-347

[27] Yoon YS, Lee ES, Park C et al. The new definition of metabolic syndrome by the international diabetes federation is less likely to identify metabolically abnormal but non-obese individuals than the definition by the revised national cholesterol program: the Korea NHANES study. *Int. J. Obes.* 2007; 31: 528-34

[28] Kahn R, Buse J, Ferrannini E et al. The metabolic syndrome, time for a critical appraisal: joint statement from the ADA and the European Association for the Study of Diabetes. *Diabetes Care* 2005; 28: 2289-2304.

[29] Aguilar-Salinas CA, Rojas R, Gonzalez-Villapando C et al. Design and validation of a population based definition of the metabolic syndrome. *Diabetes Care* 2006; 29: 2420-2426.

[30] Wijndaele K, Beunen G, Duvigneaud N et al. A continuous metabolic syndrome risk score. *Diabetes Care* 2006, 29; 2329.

[31] Ford Es, Giles WH and Dietz WH. Prevalence of the metabolic syndrome among US adults. *JAMA* 2002; 287: 356-359.

[32] Ford ES, Giles WH and Mokdad AH. Increasing prevalence of the metabolic syndrome among US adults. *Diabetes Care* 2004; 27: 2444-2449.

[33] Ford ES. Prevalence of the metabolic syndrome defined by the international diabetes federation among adults in the US. *Diabetes Care* 2005; 28: 2745-2749.

[34] Cook S, Weitzman M, Auinger P et al. Prevalence of the metabolic syndrome. Findings from the third National Health and Nutrition Examination Survey, 1988-1994. *Arch Pediatr Adolesc. Med.* 2003; 157: 821-827.

[35] Duncan GE, Li SM and Zhou XH. Prevalence and trends of a metabolic syndrome phenotype among US Adolescents, 1999-2000. *Diabetes Care* 2004; 27: 2438-2443.

[36] Mugo M and Sowers JR. Metabolic syndrome: Implications of race and ethnicity. *Ethnicity and Disease* 2004; 14: s2-26-s2-31.

[37] Kolovou G, Anagnostopoulou KK, Salpea KD et al. The prevalence of metabolic syndrome in various populations. *Am. J. Med. Sci.* 2007; 333: 362-371.

[38] McNeill AM, Rosamond WD, Girman CJ et al. The metabolic syndrome and 11- year risk of incident cardiovascular disease in the atherosclerosis risk in communities study. *Diabetes Care* 2005; 28: 385-390.

[39] Deepa M, Farooq S, Deepa R et al. Prevalence and significance of generalized and central body obesity in an urban Asian Indian population in Chennai, India (CURES: 47). *Eur. J. Clin. Nutr. 2007* Oct 10 [Epub ahead of printing]

[40] Tillin T, Forouhi N, Johnston DG et al. Metabolic syndrome and coronary heart disease in South Asians, African-Caribbeans and white Europeans: a UK population-based cross-sectional study. *Diabetologia* 2005; 48: 649-656.

[41] Tan CE, Ma S, Wai D et al. Can we apply the National Cholesterol Education Program Adult treatment panel definition of the metabolic syndrome to Asians? *Diabetes Care* 2004; 27: 1182-1186.

[42] Yang W, Reynolds K, Gu D et al. A comparison of two proposed definitions for metabolic syndrome in the Chinese adult population. *Am. J. Med. Sci.* 2007; 334: 184-189.

[43] Resnick HE. Metabolic Syndrome in American Indians. *Diabetes Care* 2002; 25: 1246-47.

[44] Guzman B. The Hispanic population: Census 2000 brief. Washington DC: US Census Bureau 2001.

[45] Murray CJ, Lopez AD. The global burden of disease: a comprehensive assessment of mortality and disability from diseases, injuries and risk factors in 19990 and projected to 2020. Cambridge MA: Harvard University Press, 1996

[46] Yusuf S, Reddy S, Ounpuu S et al. Global Burden of Cardiovascular Diseases. Part II: Variations in cardiovascular disease by specific ethnic groups and geographic regions and prevention strategies. *Circulation* 2001; 104: 2855-2864.

[47] Encuesta Nacional de Enfermedades Crónicas (ENEC). México. Epidemiología. Secretaria de Salud, 1993

[48] Swenson CJ, Trepka MJ, Rewers MJ et al. Cardiovascular disease mortality in Hispanics and Non-Hispanic Whites. *Am. J. Epidem.* 2002; 156: 919-928.

[49] Palaniappan L, Carnethon MR, Wang Y et al. Predictors of Incident metabolic syndrome in adults: the Insulin Resistance Atherosclerosis Study. *Diabetes Care* 2004; 27: 788-793.

[50] Lerman-Garber I, Villa AR, Caballero E. Diabetes and Cardiovascular disease. Is there a true Hispanic paradox? *Rev. Inv. Clin.* 2004; 56: 282-296.

[51] Goff DC, Nichaman MZ, Chan W et al. Greater Incidence of hospitalizad myocardial infarction among Mexican Americans than Non-Hispanic Whites. *Circulation* 1997; 95: 1433-1440.

[52] Hunt KJ, Resendez RG, Williams K et al. All- Cause and Cardiovascular mortality among Mexican- American and Non-Hispanic White older participants in the San Antonio Heart Study- Evidence against the "Hispanic Paradox". *Am. J. Epidemiol.* 2003; 158: 1048-1057.

[53] Aguilar-Salinas CA, Rojas R, Gomez-Perez FJ et al. High Prevalence of Metabolic Síndrome in México. *Arch Medical Research* 2004; 35: 76-81.

[54] Olaiz G, Rojas R, Barquera S. Encuesta Nacional de Salud 2000.Tomo 2. La salud de adultos. Cuernavaca, Morelos, México. Instituto Nacional de Salud Pública, 2003.

[55] Lorenzo C, Williams K, Gonzalez-Villapando C et al. The prevalence of the metabolic syndrome did not increase in México City between 1990-1992 and 1997-1999 despite more central obesity. *Diabetes Care* 2005; 28: 2480-2485.
[56] Lorenzo C, Serrano- Ríos M, Martínez- Larrad MT et al. Geographic variations in the International Diabetes Federation and the National Cholesterol Education Program-Adult Treatment Panel III definitions of the metabolic syndrome in nondiabetic subjects. *Diabetes Care* 2006; 29: 685-691.
[57] Florez H, Silva E, Fernandez V. Prevalence and risk factors associated with the the metabolic syndrome and dyslipidemia in White, Black, Amerindian and mixed Hispanics in Zulia State, Venezuela. *Diabetes Res. Clin. Pract.* 2005; 69: 63-77.
[58] Medina-Lezama J, Zea-Diaz H, Morey-Vargas OL et al. Prevalence of the metabolic syndrome in Peruvian Andean Hispanics: The PREVENCION study. *Diabetes Res. Clin. Pract.* 2007; 78: 270-281.
[59] Lorenzo C, Serrano-Rios M, Martinez-Larrad MT et al. Was the historic contribution of Spain to the Mexican gene pool partially responsible for the higher prevalence of type 2 diabetes in Mexican-origin populations? *Diabetes Care* 2001, 24; 2059-2064
[60] Ludwig DS, Ebbeling, Pereira et al. A physiological basis for disparities in diabetes and heart disease risk among racial and ethnic groups. *J. Nutr.* 2002; 132: 2492-2493.
[61] Landefeld CD, Wagenknecht LE, Rotter JI et al. Linkage of the metabolic syndrome to 1q23-q31 in Hispanic families. *Diabetes* 2004; 53:1170-1174.
[62] Semple RK, Chatterjee VK and O'Rahilly S. PPAR gamma and human metabolic disease. *J. Clin. Invest.* 2006; 116:581-589.
[63] Villarreal-Molina M, Arellano-Campos O, Flores-Dorantes M et al. Association of the ATP-binding cassette transporter A1 R230C Variant with Early-Onset Type 2 Diabetes in the Mexican Population. *Diabetes Care* 2007. In press.
[64] Phillips DI Birth weight and the future development of diabetes. A review of the evidence. *Diabetes Care* 1998;21 (suppl): B150- B155.
[65] Dabelea D, Pettit DJ, Hanson RL et al. Birthweight, type 2 diabetes and insulin resistance in Pima Indian children and young adults. *Diabetes Care* 1999; 22: 944-950.
[66] Gillman MW, Rifas-Shiman, Camargo CA et al. Risk of overweight among adolescents who were breastfed as infants. *JAMA* 2001; 285:2461-2467.
[67] Rivera JA, Barquera S, Campinaro F et al. Epidemiological and nutritional transition in Mexico: rapid increase of non communicable chronic diseases and obesity. *Public Health Nutr.* 2002; 5:113-122.
[68] Lanas F, Avezum A, Bautista LE et al. Risk factors for acute myocardial infarction in Latin America. The INTERHEART Latin American Study. *Circulation* 2007; 115: 1067-1074.

In: Topics in Prevalent Diseases
Editors: N. C. Chavez-Tapia and M. Uribe
ISBN 978-1-60456-959-9

Chapter 8

Prevalence of Diabetes: An International Perspective

Hamid R. Baradaran and Mohammad E. Khamseh
Institute of Endocrinology and Metabolism,
Iran University of Medical Sciences, Tehran, Iran

Epidemiology of Diabetes in South East Asia

This chapter reviews the frequency of diabetes in developing nations, and outlines some of the factors which may contribute to the cause.

Geographically, South East Asia consists of Myanmar, Thailand, Cambodia, Laos, Vietnam, the Philippines, Indonesia, Malaysia, Singapore, Brunei, the nations that surround the South China Sea and the nations in the Indian subcontinent.

A review of the literature available in 1987 showed the estimated prevalence of diabetes in the South East Asian region to be about 2-5% [1;2]. Earlier recorded studies in Malaysia, Singapore and Indonesia showed similar low estimates for Malays and Indonesians (about 1-2% for Malays in Malaysia in the 1960s, 1.4% for Malays in Singapore in 1945 and 1.5% in Indonesians in 1976). These low estimates may, however, be methodological due to the small number of subjects tested and the use of urine testing for diagnosis.

Cheah and Thai reported increasing prevalence of Type 2 diabetes in Singapore, with the overall prevalence rising from 1.99% in 1975 to 4.7% in 1984, with a further increase to 8.6% by 1992 [2]. The rise in prevalence occurred in Chinese (4% in 1984 to 8% in 1992), Malays (7.6% in 1984 to 9.3% in 1992), with the most predominant change being in the Indians, who had a 44% rise (from 8.9% in 1984 to 12.8% in 1992). The changes were attributed to rising affluence and changes in lifestyle, for example, increasing obesity and rural-urban migration [1]. However in the 1998 National Health Survey which was conducted in Singapore, the prevalence of diabetes mellitus was highest in Indians (12.9%), followed by Malays (9.3%) and Chinese (8.1%) [18]. This may indicate a genetic predisposition among the Indians, in addition to effect of migration, as a high prevalence of diabetes mellitus was found among migrant Asian Indians in many countries, such as South Africa (13%), Fiji (14%), Mauritius (17%), Canada (prevalence among South Asians was 10%, compared with 5% in Chinese and 6% in Europeans), and the UK [3].

The Indian Council of Medical Research (ICMR) reported the first reliable studies on the prevalence of diabetes in India in the early seventies. This study reported a prevalence of 2.3% in urban and 1.5% in rural areas. Indian migrants settled in different parts of the world have been shown to have a high prevalence of Type 2 diabetes [4] which was believed to be due to greater affluence and a more sedentary lifestyle compared to the resident Indian population. However, the local host population living in an identical environment in these countries had a lower prevalence of diabetes. Rising prevalence of Type 2 diabetes has been noted in Indians since 1986. Studies by Verma et al. in 1986 [4], using a questionnaire method, reported a prevalence of 3.1% in an affluent area in Darya Ganji, New Delhi. Over the same period, Ramachandran et al., in a series of cross-sectional surveys in Southern India, noted a rising trend in the prevalence of Type 2 diabetes. In 1983, the prevalence of Type 2 diabetes in adults was 5% in an urban township and it rose to 8.2% in 1988 [5]. In a more recent survey in the same urban area, the prevalence had increased to 12%, [6].

The Diabetic Association of Thailand conducted the first nationwide survey of diabetes mellitus in Thailand in 1971. Among 322,953 people screened, the prevalence of diabetes was estimated to be 2.5% [7]. Several other studies showed an increasing prevalence of diabetes [8]. Other surveys in Thailand revealed that prevalence of diabetes increased from 2.5% in 1978 to 3.3% in 1983 and 4.6% in 1986. When the prevalence of diabetes in the lower socio-economic community was studied in 1990 [9] at Klong Toey port area in Bangkok, the prevalence was 4.5% and 5.9% among slum residents and apartment house residents aged 30 years or over respectively [9].

Diabetes in the Middle East

Despite the wealth of epidemiological and clinical data published globally on diabetes, there has been a relative lack of accurate information on the exact magnitude of the problem in the Eastern Mediterranean region. Important epidemiological surveys have been reported from Bahrain, Egypt, Iran, Jordan, Oman, Pakistan and Saudi Arabia. They employed a comparable methodology and diagnostic criteria and consistently found that diabetes in these populations was at least twice as prevalent as in Europe and North America [10-13].

One of the earlier epidemiological studies in the region was performed in 1976 and 1980 on rural and urban samples of the adult Tunisian population aged 20 years and over). The age-standardized prevalence was found to be 4.6% in males and 3.5% in females in the urban sample, as compared with 2.3% and 0.6% in rural males and females respectively. A later study in an urban population sample in Tunisia found that the prevalence in subjects aged 30 years and over was 9.2% in males and 9.1% in females.

A study of a small village population aged 15 years and above in the south of Iraq found an overall prevalence of 4.8% [11]. In a survey of a rural population aged 15 years and above in Saudi Arabia, diabetes had a prevalence of 5.9% in females and 2.9% in males, with an overall prevalence of 4.3% among all ages and of 6.6% among subjects 15 years or older.

The same investigators reported an overall prevalence of diabetes of 5% in an urban sample; and 7.8% in persons aged 15 years and over [12].

In the Iranian Health Survey was found that 7.7% of adults aged 25–64 years, or 2 million adults, have diabetes, among whom one-half are undiagnosed. An additional 16.8%, or 4.4 million, of Iranian adults have impaired fasting glucose [13].

A report from Egypt derived from several surveys using WHO criteria and performed in various areas in the country [10] found a national prevalence of 4.3%. Based on available studies, a recent WHO report estimated that the total number of people with diabetes in the Middle East was 22 million in the year 2000. If current trends in population growth and urbanization continue, there will be 53 million adults with diabetes living in the Middle East in the year 2025, the majority in the middle age range. Between 1995 and 2025, the prevalence will increase by 30%, from 6.3% to 8.2%. There will be a considerable excess of diabetes in urban areas, and similar number of males and females with diabetes. Pakistan and Egypt will be amongst the ten countries with the greatest number of adults with diabetes in the world [14].

Diabetes in Africa

Africa is the second largest continent, with an estimated population of 642 million in about 50 countries, 3000 distinct ethnic groups and over 1000 languages. Despite the explosion of epidemiology data from other continents, data on the impact of diabetes in Africa using standardised (WHO) criteria are scarce. After the introduction of WHO criteria [15-16] there have been several reports of prevalence of diabetes from West Africa [17-19], East Africa [20] North Africa [21-23] and South Africa (24) .

Prevalence rates range from an absence of diabetes mellitus in Togo to higher and moderate rates in Cape Town in South Africa (8%) and Egypt in North Africa (9.3%). In sub-Saharan Africa, the prevalence of diabetes is low in both rural and urban communities in countries in West Africa and in Tanzania in East Africa. By contrast, moderate rates (5-8%) have been reported from South Africa, in a semi-urban community in the Orange Free State (OFS) (4.8%) and in urban groups in OFS (6%), Durban (Zulu) (5.3%) and Cape Town (Xhosa) (8.0%) [25].

Studies from North Africa indicate moderate prevalence rates in Sudan and Tunisia (3.4-8.3%). In an Egyptian study, overall prevalence was 9.3% and high rates (13.5%, 20%) were reported in urban populations in Cairo. Ethnic differences were examined in Tanzania and South Africa. In both countries, diabetes prevalence was lower in the indigenous African population than in the migrant Asian group (African vs. Asian; 5.3% vs. 13% in South Africa, 1.1% vs. 9.1% in Tanzania) [24-26].

From the evidence to date, it would appear that, in sub-Saharan Africa, diabetes prevalence is low in both urban and rural communities. However, in South Africa and North Africa, moderate and high rates are found and do not differ significantly from rates found in developed countries; in fact, urban Egyptians show a high prevalence. Moreover, there appears to be a difference between urban and rural prevalence.

Table 1. Epidemiological data from Latin America

Country	Prevalence rates (Age adjusted %)
Mexico	14.9
Jamaica	12.2
Cuba	11.8
Colombia	8.2
Brazil	7.6
Argentina	7.6
Chile	7.0

Adapted from Pan America Health Organization (www.paho.org).

Diabetes in Latin America

The population of Latin America is a heterogeneous group, made up of the descendants of Hispanics, Portuguese and other European Caucasians, Africans, American Indians and Japanese. Such populations reflect not only great racial and genetic heterogeneity but also socio-economic and cultural diversity. Over the last two decades populations around the world have experienced large increases in the prevalence of diabetes mellitus and of one of its most important risk factors, obesity. Latin America and the Caribbean will experience even more dramatic changes. An extensive review of the literature on diabetes and obesity trends in the region is presented. Recent data collected in seven countries are used to provide new population-based estimates of diabetes prevalence among elderly people. Results show that diabetes prevalence is higher in Barbados and Mexico. Argentina, Uruguay and Chile have the lowest rates, while Brazil and Cuba have intermediate levels. In Mexico, prevalence rates are higher in urban settings than in rural ones. Self-reported rates for Barbadians, Mexicans and Brazilians are higher than the self-reported rates found in 2001 in the United States [27]. The table 1 summarizes the available data on Type 2 diabetes prevalence in Latin American countries.

The incidence of type 1 diabetes in Latin America ranges from 0.4 to 8.3 cases per 100 000 children under 15 years of age, and the prevalence of type 2 diabetes ranges from 1.2% to 8%, with higher prevalence rates in urban areas. The frequency of diabetes in Latin America is expected to increase by 38% over the next 10 years, compared with an estimated 14% increase in the total population. The total number of cases of diabetes is expected to more than double and to exceed the number of cases in the US, Canada, and Europe by 2025. Factors underlying this increase include aging and increased life expectancy of the population, increased urbanization, and lifestyle changes among Native American populations [28].

United States

Ethnic differences in prevalence of type 2 diabetes are well documented. In 2004, the prevalence of diagnosed diabetes in the U.S. was higher for blacks and Hispanics than for whites across all age-groups [29]. For women aged 45–64 years, the prevalence was 7.8% among whites, 13.5% among Hispanics, and 15.4% among blacks. From 1980 through 2004, the age-adjusted prevalence increased by 65% among white women and 37% among black men. A random sample of 5% of Medicare fee-for-service beneficiaries 65 years of age showed the prevalence of type 2 diabetes to be the highest among Hispanics, the lowest among whites, and intermediate for blacks and Asians. The greatest increase in diabetes prevalence was observed among Asians (68%) during the 7-year period from 1997 to 2004. In a recent population-based national U.S. telephone survey, the prevalence of diabetes was significantly higher among Asian Americans than among non- Hispanic whites, after accounting for a lower BMI among Asians [29-33].

Complications of Diabetes

This section provides a review of the most relevant studies on the complications of diabetes.

Retinopathy

Prevalence rates of patients with diabetes retinopathy are available from many studies. Although rates of diabetic retinopathy vary by time and geographical location, nearly everyone with diabetes will develop diabetic retinopathy within 20 years of diagnosis. The prevalence of diabetic retinopathy in people with diabetes of a duration of less than five years varied from 0% in Detroit [34] and 2% in Portuguese [35] to 18% in Italians [36], 22% in Nauruans, 23% in African, 22% in non-Hispanic whites in the US[37] and Spanish[38], and 35% in Taiwanese [39].

Nephropathy

In diabetes, small blood vessels in the kidneys become abnormal, and proteins can leak out, first in small amounts (microalbuminuria) and then in larger amounts (proteinuria). Persistent proteinuria is taken to define overt nephropathy. Diabetic nephropathy is a serious complication of diabetes that can lead to end-stage renal failure (ESRF). Diabetic nephropathy develops in about 30% of patients with Type 1 diabetes mellitus.

The cumulative risk of nephropathy after 10 years in those with Type 2 diabetes varies with from 25% in individuals of European origin to 50% in other ethnic groups such as African-Caribbean and Asian Indians. As Type 2 diabetes is more common than Type 1 diabetes, the number of patients with Type 2 diabetes requiring renal replacement therapy (dialysis or transplantation) equals or exceeds that of Type 1 patients with diabetes. In Europe, diabetes is the only increasing cause of end-stage renal failure, and patients with diabetes represent about 16% of all new patients entering renal replacement therapy programs [40-42].

Coronary Heart Disease

Several recent North American studies have reported the prevalence of coronary heart disease (CHD) in adults with diabetes [43]. CHD prevalence rates for people with and without abnormal glucose tolerance varied, probably reflecting differences in age, ethnicity and body size [44-45]. Within populations of American , European, Mexican and Japanese ancestry, patients with diabetes nearly always had significantly more clinically manifest CHD and more silent ischemia (as defined by resting electrocardiogram) than those with normal glucose tolerance.

The Strong Heart Study provides age-adjusted prevalence rates for 13 American Indian communities in Arizona, Oklahoma and the Dakotas [46]. The prevalence of CHD defined by history and resting electrocardiogram was higher in patients with diabetes than non-diabetes in all groups and in both sexes but there is a significant unexplained difference in the prevalence of CHD by geographical area [46]. In east Finland, the frequency of symptomatic CHD and ischemic ECG abnormalities was remarkably similar among individuals with known diabetes or newly-recognized diabetes identified by oral glucose tolerance test (OGTT) screening, while among the elderly Kuopio subjects, more CHD was present in persons with known diabetes than with newly-diagnosed diabetes [47].

Studies of the prevalence of diabetes or CHD in developing countries are rare. A clinical diagnosis of CHD is less commonly made and most of the CHD prevalence data is derived from surveys of electrocardiographic abnormalities. Li and colleagues [48] have reported the low prevalence of major Q wave and ST-T wave abnormalities in 15 populations from nine countries, predominantly Asian, Melanesian, Polynesian, or Micronesian populations. Data is not shown by diabetes status, but many of these populations have high rates of diabetes.

Stroke

Diabetes is a potent risk factor for stroke, as reviewed elsewhere [49]. Most strokes occur in the elderly and are non-hemorrhagic infarctions; this is also true in patients with diabetes. As is the case CHD, diabetes is commonly not diagnosed in older adults until after the stroke. The two largest prospective studies of stroke and diabetes were conducted in the United States and describe individuals with and without clinically-recognized diabetes. The Multiple Risk Factor Intervention Trial (MRFIT) [50] determined the 12-year stroke mortality for 5163 men aged 35-57 years who reported taking medication for diabetes, and 324,815 men without a history of diabetes. The risk of fatal non-hemorrhagic stroke was increased 3.8-fold among those with diabetes, independent of age, race, income, blood pressure, cigarette smoking and other CHD risk factors.

In the Whitehall Study [51] of London civil servants, middle-aged men with a history of diabetes had a 2-fold increased risk of stroke. A seven-year follow-up of two middle aged cohorts from Finland found that, compared to non-diabetes patients, men and women with clinically diagnosed diabetes had a 3- and 5-fold higher risk of stroke, respectively [52]. During an eight-year prospective population-based study carried out as part of the MONICA project in Northern Sweden [53], the impact of diabetes on the risk of incident stroke (fatal or non-fatal) was found to be 4.1-fold in men and 5.8-fold in women. The relative risk for stroke mortality was 4.4 and 5.1, respectively.

Only a few studies of the diabetes-stroke association have been conducted in populations other than Caucasians of northern European ancestry. Early reports found no significant excess risk of stroke in Japanese men with diabetes living in Japan [54] or Hawaii [55] but an excess risk of stroke was found after a longer follow-up of the Japanese men in the Honolulu cohort [56], while African Americans have more diabetes and more strokes than white Americans. Nevertheless, follow-up of a United States national survey found that a medical history of diabetes increased the risk of stroke approximately 2.5-fold in both African American and Caucasian, and the increased risk associated with diabetes was nearly identical in men and women [57].

Lower Extremity Arterial Disease

Epidemiological studies of diabetes and lower extremity arterial disease (LEAD) will be reviewed in this section.

Amputations

The most serious complication of lower LEAD is limb amputation. In one community-based study, adults with diabetes had an up to 70-fold increased risk of gangrene and amputation [58]. A retrospective study of amputation in Kuopio, Eastern Finland, found a 10-fold excess risk of lower extremity amputation in men with diabetes and a 14-fold excess risk in women with diabetes [59]. In a US study of hospital discharge data from six states, the relative risk of lower extremity amputation in patients with diabetes was approximately 15 times the rate in nondiabetes patients, with 45% of all amputations occurring in patients with diabetes [60].

A few community-based incidence studies have been reported. A study from England reported that the amputation rate in older patients with diabetes was 8 per 1000 patient-years [61]. In Finland, the seven-year amputation rate in middle-aged patients with Type 2 diabetes was 6.6% in men, and 5.3% in women [62]. In Wisconsin, the four-year amputation rate was 2.2% in known patients with diabetes, and rates were the same in persons with onset of diabetes before or after age 30. Data about amputation rates in patients with diabetes is almost entirely from North America or Europe. The wide variations in overall amputation rates reported around the world may reflect geographical differences in diabetes prevalence, trauma, or the availability of foot care. Morris and his colleagues reported that patients with diabetes in Tayside, Scotland, had a 12.3-fold risk of an amputation compared with non-diabetes residents [63].

Foot Ulcers

A foot sore or ulcer usually precedes the gangrene that leads to amputation. The prevalence of past or current foot ulcers varies in population-based studies of patients with diabetes. A history of 'ever having had a foot ulcer' was found in approximately 5% of patients with diabetes in a United Kingdom study [64], 10% in a Swedish study, and 15% in a study from southern Wisconsin [65]. In an English patient registry study, the prevalence of past or present foot ulcer in patients with diabetes was 7.4% compared to 2.9% in age and sex matched non-diabetes patients [66].

Claudication

Intermittent claudication, usually defined as exercise-induced leg pain not present at rest, is strong evidence of LEAD. The largest study using standardized criteria for diabetes and claudication (a Finnish population-based study of 5738 men and 5224 women) found the prevalence of intermittent claudication to be 3.4 times higher in men with diabetes and 5.7 times higher in women with diabetes than in non-diabetes patients of the same sex [65].

References

[1] Chua I, Khalid B. A survey of diabetes mellitus and its complications in the general hospital, Kuala Lumpur. *J. ASEAN Fed. Endoc. Soc.* 1987; 6:74-81.

[2] Cheah J, Thai A. Epidemiology of non insulin dependent diabetes mellitus (NIDDM) in ASEAN. 7th Congress of the ASEAN Federation of Endocrine Societies A1[S6], 58. 1993.

[3] C Y Hong, K S Chia, K Hughes, S L Ling. Ethnic differences among Chinese, Malay and Indian patients with type 2 diabetes mellitus in Singapore. *Singapore Med. J.* 2004 Vol 45(4):154-160

[4] Verma N, Mehta S, Madhu S, Keen H. Prevalence of known diabetes in an urban Indian environment: the Daryaganj Diabetes Survey. *Br. Med. J.* 1986; 293:423-424.

[5] Ramachandran A, Snehalatha C, Daisy D. Prevalence of glucose intolerance in Asian Indians: urban-rural difference and significance of upper body adiposity. *Diabetes Care* 1992; 15:1348-1355.

[6] Ramachandran A, Snehalatha C, Latha E, Vijay V, Viswanathan H. rising prevalence of NIDDM in urban population in India. *Diabetologia* 1997; 40:232-237.

[7] Tandhanand S, Vannasaeng S. Diabetes Mellitus in Thiland. In: Krall L, editor. World Book of Diabetes in Practice. Amsterdam: Elsevier, 1986: 252-257.

[8] Vichayanrat A. Diabetes mellitus and nutrition in Thailand. The 2nd Asian International Workshop on Nutrition and Sciences , 36-43. 1993. Fukuoka, Japan.

[9] Bunnag S, Sitthi-Amorn C, Chandraprasert S. The prevalence of obesity, risk factors and associated diseases in Klong Toey slum and Klong Toey government apartment house. *Diabetes Res. Clin. Pract.* 1990; 10(Suppl):81-87.

[10] Arab M. Diabetes mellitus in Egypt. World Hlth Statist Quart 1992; 45:334-337.

[11] Al-Kasab F, Alkafajei A, Medbigh S. The prevalence of diabetes mellitus in a rural community in Iraq. *Int. J. Epidemiol.* 1979; 8:69-72.

[12] Fatani H, et a. Prevalence of diabetes mellitus in rural Saudi Arabia. *Diabetes Care* 1987; 10:180-183.

[13] Esteghamati A, Gouya MM, Abbasi M, Delavari A, Alikhani S, Alaedini F, Safaie A, Forouzanfar M, Gregg EW. Prevalence of diabetes and impaired fasting glucose in the adult population of Iran: National Survey of Risk Factors for Non-Communicable Diseases of Iran. *Diabetes Care* 2008 Jan;31(1):96-8.

[14] King H, Aubert R, Herman W. Global burden of diabetes, 1995-2025. Prevalence, numerical estimates and projections. *Diabetes Care* 1998; 21:1414-1431.

[15] World Health Organization. WHO Expert Committee on Diabetes Mellitus. Second Report. 626. 1980. Geneva, *WHO.* Technical Report.

[16] WHO. Diabetes Mellitus: Report of a WHO Study group. 727. 1985. Geneva, *WHO.* WHO Technical Report Series. 40

[17] Cooper R, Rotimi C, Kaufman J, Owoaje E, Fraser H, Forrester T et al. Prevalence of NIDDM among populations of the African diaspora. *Diabetes Care* 1997; 20:343-348.

[18] Ohwovoriole A, Kuti J, Kabiawu S. Casual blood glucose levels and prevalence of undiscovered diabetes mellitus in Lagos Metropolis Nigerians. *Res. Clin. Pract.* 1988; 4:153-158.

[19] Fisch A, Pichard E, Prazuck T, Leblance H, Sidibe Y, Brucker G. Prevalence and risk factors of diabetes mellitus in the rural regions of Mali (West Africa): a practical approach. *Diabetologia* 1987; 30:859-862.

[20] McLarty D, Swai A, Kitange H, Masuki G, Mtinangi B, Kilima P et al. Prevalence of diabetes and impaired glucose tolerance in rural Tanzania. *Lancet* 1989; 1:871-875.

[21] Papoz L, Ben Khalifa F, Eshwege E, Ben Ayed H. Diabetes mellitus in Tunisia: descriptions in urban and rural populations. *Int. J. Epidemiol.* 1988; 17:419-422.

[22] Herman W, Ali M, Aubert R, Engelgau M, Kenny S, Gunter E et al. Diabetes mellitus in Egypt: risk factors and prevalence. *Diabetic Medicine* 1995; 12:1126- 1131.

[23] Elbagir M, Elton M, Elmahdi E, Kadam I, Berne C. A population-based study of the prevalence of diabetes and impaired glucose tolerance in adults in northern Sudan. *Diabetes Care* 1996; 19:1126-1128.

[24] Omar M, Seedat M, Motala A, Dyer R, Becker P. The prevalence of diabetes mellitus and impaired glucose tolerance in a group of urban South African Blacks. *S Afr. Med. J.* 1993; 83:641-643.

[25] Omar M, Seedat M, Dyer R, Motala A, Knight L, Becker P. South African Indians show a high prevalence of NIDDM and bimodality in plasma glucose distribution patterns. *Diabetes Care* 1994; 17:70-73.

[26] Ramaiya K, Kodali V, Alberti K. Epidemiology of diabetes in Asians of the Indian subcontinents. *Diabetes Metab. Rev.* 1990; 6:125-146.

[27] Andrade, F. (2006, Aug) "Trends on Diabetes and Obesity Prevalence in Latin America and the Caribbean: A Review of the Literature and New Estimates" Paper presented at the annual meeting of the American Sociological Association, Montreal Convention

Center, Montreal, Quebec, Canada http://www.allacademic.com/meta/p104749_ index.html

[28] Pablo Aschner. Diabtes ternd in Latin America. Diabetes/Metabolism Research and Reviews.Volume 18, Issue S3 , Pages S27 - S31

[29] The National Center for Chronic Disease Prevention and Health Promotion: Age-specific prevalence of diagnosed diabetes, by race/ethnicity and sex, United States 2004. Available at http://www.cdc.gov/diabetes/statistics/prev/natioanl/fig2004.htm.

[30] Bolen JC, Rhodes L, Powell-Griner EE, Bland SD, Holtzman D: State-specific prevalence of selected health behaviors, by race and ethnicity: Behavioral Risk Factor Surveillance System, 1997. MMWR CDC Surveill Summ49:1–60, 2000

[31] Harris MI, Flegal KM, Cowie CC, Eberhardt MS, Goldstein DE, Little RR, Wiedmeyer HM, Byrd-Holt DD: Prevalence of diabetes, impaired fasting glucose, and impaired glucose tolerance in U.S. adults: the Third National Health and Nutrition Examination Survey, 1988–1994. *Diabetes Care* 21:518–524, 1998

[32] Brancati FL, Kao WH, Folsom AR, Watson RL, Szklo M: Incident type 2 diabetes mellitus in African American and white adults: the Atherosclerosis Risk in Communities Study. *JAMA* 283:2253–2259, 2000

[33] McBean AM, Li S, Gilbertson DT, Collins AJ: Differences in diabetes prevalence, incidence, and mortality among the elderly of four racial/ethnic groups: whites, blacks, Hispanics, and Asians. *Diabetes Care* 27:2317–2324, 2004

[34] Frank R, Hoffman W, Podgor M, et al. Retinopathy in juvenile-onset diabetes of short duration. *Ophthalmology* 1980; 2:196-201.

[35] Pinto-Figueiredo L, Moita J, Vinagre V, et a. Diabetic retiopathy in a population of 1302 insulin dependent diabetics (IDDM) diagnosed before 30 years of age. *Int. Ophthalmol.* 1992; 16:429-437.

[36] Garancini P, Micossi P, Valsania P, et a. Prevalence of retinopathy in diabetic subjects from out-patient clinics in Lombardy (Italy), and associated risk factors. A multicentre epidemiologic study. *Diabetes Res. Clin. Pract.* 1989; 6:129-138.

[37] Hamman R, Franklin G, Mayer E, et a. Microvascular complications of NIDDM in Hispanics and non-Hispanic whites. San Luis Valley Diabetes Study. *Diabetes Care* 1991; 14:655-664. 41

[38] Fernandez-Vigo J, Sanchez Macho J, Diaz Rey A, lBarros J, Tome M, Bueno J. The prevalence of diabetic retinopathy in northwest Spain. An epidemiological study of diabetic retinopathy in Galicia. I. *Acta Phthalmol.* 1993; 71:22-26.

[39] Chen M, Kao C, Chang C, et al. Prevalence and risk factors of diabetic retinopathy among noninsulin-dependent diabetic subjects. *Am. J. Ophthalmol.* 1992; 114:723-730.

[40] Viberti GC, Marshal S, Beech R, et al. Report on renal disease in diabetes. *Diabetic Med.* 1996; 13:S6-12.

[41] Groggel GC. Diabetic nephropathy. *Arch Fam. Med.* 1996; 5:513-520.

[42] Perneger TV, Brancati FL, Whelton PK, Klag MJ. End-stage renal disease attributable to diabetes mellitus. *Ann. Intern. Med.* 1994; 121:912-918.

[43] Scheidt-Nave C, Barrett-Connor E, Wingard D. Resting electrocardiographic abnormalities suggestive of asymptomatic ischemic heart disease associated with non-

insulin-dependent diabetes mellitus in a defined population. *Circulation* 1990; 81:899-906.

[44] Rewers M, Shetterly S, Baxter J, Marshal J, Hamman R. Prevalence of coronary heart disease in subjects with normal and impaired glucose tolerance and non-insulin dependent diabetes mellitus in a biethnic Colorado population. The San Luis Valley Diabetes Study. *Am. J. Epidemiol.* 1992; 12:1321-1330.

[45] Mitchell B, Hazuda H, Haffner S, Patterson J, Stern M. Myocardial infraction in Mexican-American and Non-Hispanic Whites: The San Antonio Heart Study. *Circulation* 1991; 83:54-51.

[46] Howard B, Lee E, Cowan L, Fabsitz R, Howard W, Oopik A et al. Coronary heart disease prevalence and its relation to risk factors in American Indians. The Strong heart Study. *Am. J. Epidemiol.* 1995; 142:254-268.

[47] Mykkanen L, Laakso M, Pyorala K. Asymptomatic hyperglycemia and atherosclerotic vascular disease. *Diabetes Care* 1992; 15:1020-1030.

[48] Li N, Tuomilehto J, Dowse G, Virtala E, Zimmet P. Prevalence of coronary heart disease initiated by electrocardiogarm abnormalities and risk factors in developing countries. *J. Clin. Epidemiol.* 1994; 47:599-611.

[49] Bell S. Stroke in the diabetic patient. *Diabetes Care* 1994; 14:213-219.

[50] Neaton J, Wentworth D, Cutler J, Stamler J, Kuller L. Risk factors for death from different types of stroke. Multiple Risk Factor Intervention Trial Research Group. *Ann. Epidemiol.* 1993; 3:493-499.

[51] Fuller J, Shipley M, Rose G, Jarrett R, Keen H. Mortality from coronary heart disease and stroke in relation to the degree of glycaemia: the Whitehall study. *Br. Med. J.* 1983; 287:867-870.

[52] Lehto S, Ronnemaa T, Pyorala K, Laakso M. Predictors of stroke in middleaged patients with non-insulin-dependent diabetes. *Stroke* 1996; 27:63-68.

[53] Stegmayr B, Asplund K. Diabetes mellitus as a risk factor for death from stroke. *Diabetologia* 1995; 38:1061-1068.

[54] Sasaki A, Vehara M, Horiuchi N, Hasagawa K. A long-term follow-up study of Japanese diabetic patients: mortality and causes of death. *Diabetologia* 1983; 25:309-312.

[55] Yano K, Kagan A, McGee D, Rhoads G. Glucose intolerance and nine-year mortality in Japanese men in Hawaii. *Ame. J. Med.* 1982; 72:71-80.

[56] Abbott R, Donahue R, MacMahon S, Reed D, Yano K. Diabetes and the risk of stroke. The Honolulu Heart Program. *J. Am. Med. Assoc.* 1987; 257:949-952.

[57] Kittner S, White L, Losonczy K, Wolf P, Hebel J. Black-White differences in stroke incidence in a national sample. The contribution of hypertension and diabetes mellitus. *J. Am. Med. Assoc.* 1990; 264:1267-1270.

[58] Waugh N. Amputations in diabetic patients: a review of rates, relative risks and resource use. *Comm. Med.* 1988; 19:279-288.

[59] Siitonen O, Niskanen L, Laakso M, Siitonen J, Pyorala K. Lower-extremity amputations in diabetic and nondiabetic patients. A population-based study in eastern Finland. *Diabetes Care* 1993; 16:16-20.

[60] Most R, Sinnock P. The epidemiology of lower extremity amputations in diabetic individuals. *Diabetes Care* 1983; 6:87-91.

[61] Morris A, McAlpine R, Steinke D, Boyle D, Ebrahim A, Vasudev N et al. Diabetes and Lower-Limb Amputations in the Community: A retrospective cohort study. *Diabetes Care* 1998; 21(5):738-743.

[62] Kumar S, Ashe H, Parnell N, Fernando D, Tsigos C, Young R et al. The epidemiology of foot ulceration and its correlates in Type 2 diabetic patients: a population-based study. *Diabetic Medicine* 1994; 11:480-484.

[63] Klein R, Klein B, Moss S. Relation of glycaemic control to diabetic microvascular complications in diabetes mellitus. *Ann. Intern. Med.* 1996; 124:90- 96.

[64] Walters D, Gatling W, Mullee M, Hill R. The prevalence, detection, and epidemiological correlates of peripheral vascular disease: a comparison of diabetic and non-diabetic subjects in an English community. *Diabetic Medicine* 1992; 9:710-715.

[65] Reunanen A, Takkunen H, Aromaa A. Prevalence of intermittent claudication and its effect on mortality. *Acta Med. Scand.* 1982; 211:249-256.

[66] Marshall J, Hamman R, Baxter J, Mayer E, Fulton D, Orleans M et al. Ethnic differences in risk factors associated with prevalence of non-insulin-dependent diabetes mellitus. *Am. J. Epidemiol.* 1993; 137:706-718.

In: Topics in Prevalent Diseases
Editors: N. C. Chavez-Tapia and M. Uribe
ISBN 978-1-60456-959-9

Chapter 9

Hypercholesterolemia in Minorities

Carlos J. Rodriguez*[1] *and Juan C. Brenes
Columbia University Medical Center, College of Physicians and Surgeons / Mailman School of Public Health, Division of Cardiology, Columbia University, New York, New York, USA

Introduction

The United States of America (USA) has undergone significant demographic and ethnic changes over the past 50 years. The growth of the population along with an increasing age has caused a direct impact in the epidemiology of cardiovascular disease (CVD). Despite a decrease in mortality rates, CVD remains still as the most common cause of death in this country.[1]

It is not surprising that CVD, being influenced by varied and complex conditions, remains at the top of the list of causes of death in the industrialized world. The genetic, environmental [educational level and socioeconomic status (SES)] and lifestyle (diet) patterns of a population have a direct effect on the prevalence of risk factors for CVD, which are concurrently related to race, ethnicity and sex. The USA along with many other developed countries is faced today with an increasingly diversified population, with many different ethnicities and behavioral patterns.

Today, CVD has become the leading cause of death among minority populations in the USA. Unfortunately, marked disparities exist in the prevalence, morbidity, and mortality associated with CVD and the major risk factors between minority and majority groups.[2] The elimination of such differences is one of the main goals of a national public agenda.[3] Among minority groups, Hispanics are the fastest growing, representing 13.3% of the US population, followed by African-Americans (13%).[4] Furthermore, Hispanic-Americans are a heterogeneous group, with Mexican-Americans constituting approximately 64% of its

622 W. 168th Street, PH 3-342, New York, NY 10032.

population.[5] Native-Americans represent another minority group whose CVD prevalence has increased in the last decade.

Over three decades ago a statistical association was made between total serum cholesterol and the incidence of CVD.[6] Hyperlipidemia remains among the leading risk factors for developing atherothrombotic disease.[7] Furthermore, hyperlipidemia has become one of the most easily modifiable and treatable risk factors. An understanding of the differences in the indicators of hyperlipidemia among different population minority groups is among the steps that need to be taken towards a better prevention and treatment of CVD.

Epidemiology of Hyperlipidemia in Minority Populations

Several studies have evaluated hypercholesterolemia as a CVD risk factor by race and ethnicity. In most of these, there has not been one minority group to be consistently associated with a higher or lower prevalence of hyperlipidemia.[8] However, prevalence and treatment patterns of dyslipidemia among minorities are not as well known as their majority counterparts due to relative under representation of minorities in epidemiologic studies and clinical trials. Furthermore, hyperlipidemia is likely influenced by other variables such as obesity, diabetes, and SES in relation to diet and sedentarism which are themselves associated with race and ethnicity. In the past we have been comfortable extrapolating data from majority groups in large lipid clinical trials however this strategy may not fully apply to the problem of hyperlipidemia in minority groups.

African-Americans have a higher rate of CVD morbidity and mortality than do Caucasians, yet they are often underdiagnosed and undertreated.[1, 9, 10] The average life expectancy of African Americans in the USA is approximately 69 years, vs. the 76 years for the general population. CVD largely contributes to this disparity. Although African-Americans have a greater incidence of hypertension, the rates of coronary heart disease (CHD) among African-American men are no higher than those among non-Hispanic Caucasian men.[1] This may be in part because African-American men have 20% higher levels of high-density lipoprotein cholesterol (HDL-c) when compared to non-Hispanic Caucasian men,[11] along with lower values of low-density lipoprotein cholesterol (LDL-c) and apolipoprotein B (apoB)[12] and triglyceride levels. However, African-Americans also have higher levels of lipoprotein(a) [Lp(a)] as compared with the level in non-Hispanic Caucasians.[13]

The Third National Health and Nutrition Examination Survey (NHANES 1998-1994) is one of the largest epidemiologic studies in minority women, namely African-Americans and Mexican-Americans.[5] The population included 1762 African-American, 1481 Mexican-American, and 2023 non-Hispanic Caucasian women. They found that after adjusting for SES, African-American women had lower non-high-density lipoprotein cholesterol (non HDL-c) levels than non-Hispanic Caucasians women. However, women with the lowest SES from each of the three ethnic groups had significantly higher levels of non HDL-c compared with the ones on a higher SES. Others have found that African American men have a higher HDL-c levels and similar levels of total cholesterol as compared with non-Hispanic

Caucasians men. African American men and women have higher levels of apolipoprotein A-I (apoA-1), and Lp(a) and lower levels of triglycerides as compared with non-Hispanic Caucasian men and women.[14] A similar study concluded that environmental, lifestyle, and social factors may contribute significantly in the levels of HDL-c, its fractions HDL2, HDL3, and apoA-1 among African-Americans.[10]

In the Washington Height and Inwood Community Aging Program Study (WHICAPS) a cross-sectional study of 1,118 men and women living in Northern Manhattan, race was an independent predictor of all lipid and lipoprotein levels. The prevalence of hyperlipidemia was higher among non-Hispanic Caucasians and Hispanics compared to African-Americans. Low HDL-c (men < 40 mg/dl; women < 50 mg/dl) and high triglycerides (TG > 150 mg/dl) were more common in Hispanics as compared to non-Hispanic Caucasians. Elevated LDL-c (≥ 130 mg/dl) was more prevalent in non-Hispanic Caucasians than in Hispanics. Hispanics had lower mean HDL-c and higher mean triglyceride levels. African-Americans had higher mean HDL-c with a greater percentage having HDL-c levels >55mg/Dl compared to Hispanics or non-Hispanic Caucasians. Triglycerides levels were also lower among African-Americans.[15] Other studies have found that non-Hispanic Caucasians have a higher mean serum cholesterol values than Hispanics,[16, 17] and suggested that the independent effect of Hispanic ethnicity on HDL-c is minimal.[18]

More recently, data from a large cohort involving over 3000 individuals showed that dyslipidemia significantly varied among race-ethnic groups. The Northern Manhattan Study (NOMAS) is a community-based epidemiological study consisting of a randomly sampled cohort of 3298 participants, of whom 54% are Hispanic, 21% non-Hispanic Caucasians, and 25% African-American (47% women; mean age 69 ± 10 years). Almost 16% of African-Americans, 17.8% of non-Hispanic Caucasians and 16.2% of Hispanics had total cholesterol > 240mg/dl (P=0.52). Moreover 42.3% of African-Americans, 50.5% of non-Hispanic Caucasians and 47.5% of Hispanics had LDL-c >130mg/dl; (P=0.01). Hispanics had greater prevalence of low HDL-c (40.8%) than did non-Hispanic Caucasians (28.8%) or African-Americans (23.2%); (P=<0.0001). Hispanics had greater prevalence of high triglyceridemia (35.2%) than did non-Hispanic Caucasians (28.1%) or African-Americans (17.5%); (P=<0.0001) Figure 1[19].

Increasing the awareness in the general public that elevated cholesterol levels constitutes a risk for developing CVD is one step towards its treatment. One way of doing this is by screening for hypercholesterolemia. According to the National Cholesterol Education Program (NCEP), all adults over 20 years of age should be screened for elevated cholesterol levels at least once every 5 years.[7] The screening prevalence among Hispanics is among the lowest in the country (55%), compared to non Hispanic Caucasians (73%).[20]

Furthermore, there are important ethnic differences regarding awareness and treatment of hypercholesterolemia. Only 34% of Hispanics were found be aware of having elevated total cholesterol (> 200 mg/dl), 57% had it checked, and only 13% were receiving treatment, compared to 51%, 71%, and 24% respectively of the non-Hispanic Caucasians population.[21] NOMAS found treatment of hypercholesterolemia was particularly low among Hispanics with only 13.7% (P < 0.01) of Hispanics with LDL-c >130 and 17% (P < 0.01) with total cholesterol >240mg/dl receiving lipid lowering therapy.[19]

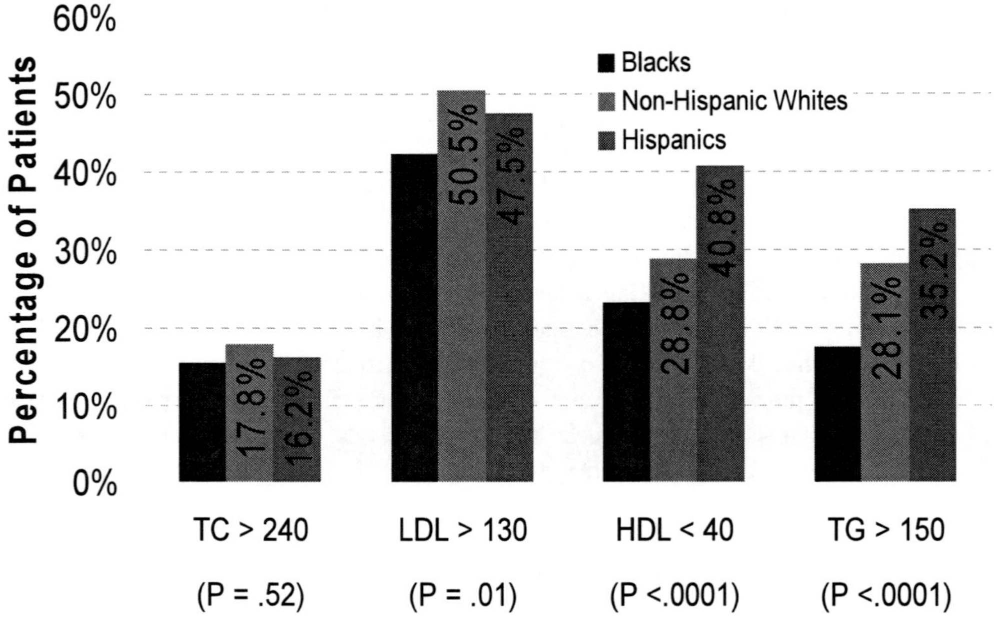

Figure 1. Prevalence of dyslipidemia type by race-ethnicity. Significant race-ethnic differences are noted for each dyslipidemia type.

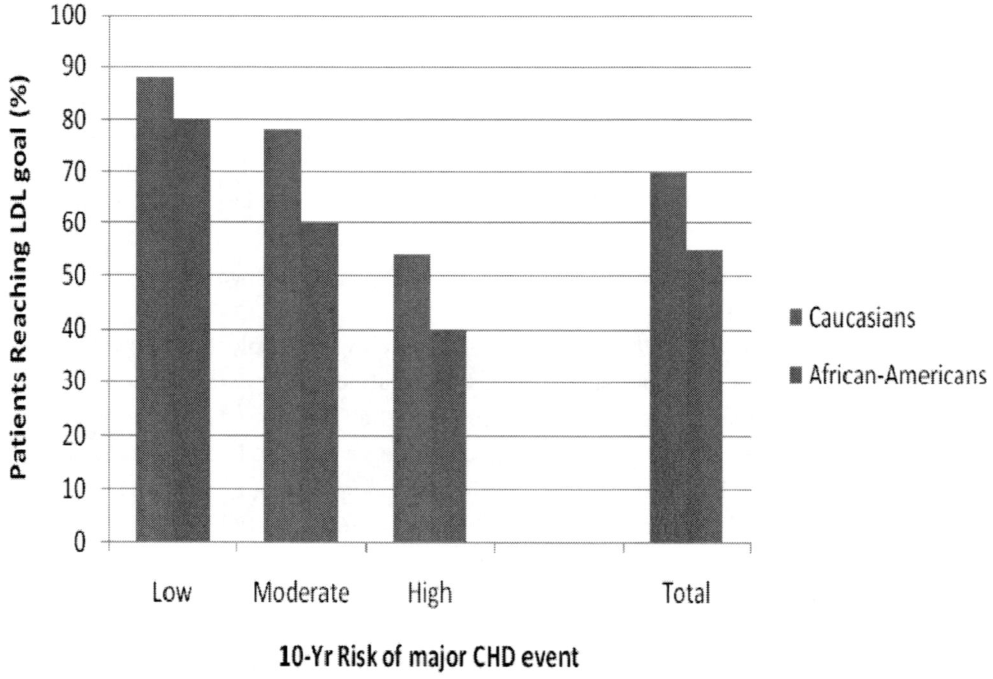

Figure 2. National Cholesterol Education Program Adult Treatment Panel III LDL cholesterol goal achievement by risk category in non-Hispanic white and African-American patients.

The National Cholesterol Education Program Evaluation Project Utilizing Novel E-Technology (NEPTUNE) II survey evaluated provider compliance with the current version of the NCEP guidelines. The study included almost 400 physicians who submitted data related to cholesterol management in 4885 outpatients. They showed that African Americans were significantly less likely to achieve goals of therapy when compared with Caucasian patients (54% vs. 69%, respectively; $P < .0001$).[22] This disparity was worse for those at higher risk (Figure 2). A greater proportion of African Americans had high risk for CHD, but they were significantly less likely than Caucasians to reach LDL-c goals. Further analysis confirmed that African-American race was a strong predictor of inadequate treatment in a variety of population subgroups. Whether these differences are related to therapeutic inertia or patient compliance or a combination of both remains unclear. However, this report did suggest that more patients are currently receiving the standard of care than did so in the past. In an older report, only 39% of Caucasians and 29% of African Americans had reached LDL-c goals.[23] However, despite the progress, disparities have persisted and there remains much room for improvement.

Table. Comparison of non-Caucasian participation in major Lipid Clinical Trials

Study	Total Patients	Non- Caucasian Participants
WOSCOPS	6595	-----
AFCAPS / TexCAPS	6605	561
LIPID	9014	-----
CARE	4159	308
4S	4444	-----
VA-HIT	2531	265

The Strong Heart Study has provided us with rates of dyslipidemia (defined as total cholesterol $\geq$ 200mg/dl) among Native Americans of 34-38%, which are higher than the general US population.[24] A recent retrospective study involving 2095 Native Americans with history of coronary artery disease evaluated the use of 3-hydroxy-3-methylglutaryl coenzyme A reductase inhibitors (statins). Almost 60% of the patients did not have a statin prescription dispensed a year after being diagnosed with coronary artery disease. [25] In this same study, Native Americans who were 80 years or older and women were less likely to receive statins. Although statins are underutilized in this population,[25] the clinical management of dyslipidemia in this population through a comprehensive CVD risk reduction program including a trained dietician in a multidisciplinary health team significantly reduced CVD risk while minimizing the need for pharmacotherapeutic interventions.

Are Lipid-lowering Drugs Effective in Minorities?

The statins remain the cornerstone of therapy and they significantly lower total cholesterol, LDL-c, triglycerides and to a lesser extent can increase HDL-c. Lowering the LDL-c to less than 100 mg/dl (optimal goal of < 70mg/dl) is the target for patients with high risk for CHD (10-year risk > 20%), prior myocardial infarction, peripheral vascular disease or diabetes. These 10-year risk scores are primarily based on a Caucasian population. African-Americans and other minority populations likely have a higher absolute risk for any given Framingham risk score thus their CHD risk is underestimated by this scoring system. As previously mentioned, minority patients have been traditionally under-represented in lipid lowering and cardiovascular trials. This is one of the problems encountered when assessing the pharmacologic effects of statins in this minority group. The efficacy of lipid lowering agents in minority populations has been extrapolated from data in non-Hispanic Caucasian populations however these extrapolations may not be appropriate (Table).

One of the few Hispanic-only trials available, is The STudy Assessing RosuvaStatin in HIspanic Population (STARSHIP).[26] This study was undertaken to provide data on the effects of rosuvastatin and atorvastatin in an exclusively Hispanic population of hypercholesterolemic patients, 696 Hispanic patients at a medium to high risk for CHD, in 86 centers across the US were randomized to treatment with 10 or 20mg of rosuvastatin or 10 or 20 mg of atorvastatin. As expected, a significant higher proportion of patients under the rosuvastatin therapy achieved goal LDL-c levels as compared to atorvastatin (45% reduction at 6 weeks). The authors state that this effect is a similar finding when compared to large non-Hispanic trials of rosuvastatin.

In the EASE study a large (3030 patients) double-blind, randomized trial that evaluated the effectiveness of adding ezetimibe on the lipid profile, in patients already taking a statin.[27] Hispanics conformed 5% of the study population and 9% were African-Americans. There was a statistically significant reduction in LDL-c to ATP-III goal levels in the three different ethnic groups. This response rate was less for Hispanics than for the other groups, but was not statistically significant.

The African-American Rosuvastatin Investigation of Efficacy and Safety (ARIES) trial followed up 774 patients on open-label treatment with one of two statins. On randomization, patients were provided a 6-week supply of rosuvastatin or atorvastatin. Patients received either 10 mg or 20 mg of the statin; the respective doses of rosuvastatin lowered LDL-c by 37% and 46%, and atorvastatin lowered LDL-c by 32% and 39%. Rosuvastatin lowered non HDL-c by 34% and 42%, as did atorvastatin by 30% and 36%. The 10-mg and 20-mg doses of rosuvastatin raised HDL-c 7% and 6%, and the same doses of atorvastatin raised HDL-c 6% and 4%. The milligram-equivalent doses of rosuvastatin were more efficacious than atorvastatin. Despite the fact that both statins significantly decreased LDL-c levels, the authors noted that the LDL-c reductions in ARIES seem lackluster in comparison to similar trials of mostly Caucasian populations.[28]

The rates of goal achievement and LDL-c lowering are less than expected based on response in Caucasians. It is important to determine if this is true and if so, to find a biological basis. Simon and colleagues make an excellent attempt at this important question in the Cholesterol and Pharmacogenetics (CAP) study.[29] The study started with a placebo run-in phase to exclude subjects who did not maintain a 90% or greater adherence rate with a nightly medication. The study included 300 African Americans and 600 Caucasians who took 40 mg of simvastatin for 6 weeks. During that time, investigators performed pill counts every 2 weeks to assure adherence of 90% or better. After correction for multiple confounding variables, African Americans had a weaker response to the statin compared with

Caucasians. The decrease in LDL-c was 3 mg/dL less than that achieved by Caucasians, and the rise in HDL-c was 1 mg/dL less. The decrease in apo-B for African-Americans was 3 mg/dL less than that in Caucasians. This meticulous study confirms a biological racial disparity in LDL-c response to simvastatin that is similar to that suggested by other trials of rosuvastatin and ezetimibe.

Do We Have a Biological Explanation for Racial Disparity in LDL-c Response?

LDL-c may not be the most accurate marker of dyslipidemia among minority groups. LDL particles contain most of the cholesterol in plasma but LDL particles differ in composition. Small dense LDL species are more atherogenic than larger LDL particles thus LDL-c levels alone do not reflect total atherogenic risk. Each LDL particle regardless of size contains one molecule of apoB. Unlike LDL levels, plasma apoB levels reflect the total number of pro-atherogenic particles. Furthermore, apolipoprotein A-I (apo A-I) is more important than HDL-c content for biochemical pathways that render HDL-c antiatherogenic. A series of large, prospective epidemiological studies has shown that apoB is superior to LDL-c as a predictor of the risk of vascular disease and that the apo B:apo A-I ratio was associated with future CVD events independent of traditional lipid values.[30, 31] ApoB or the apo B:apo A-I ratio may provide a better approach than LDL-c in characterizing dyslipidemia and response to therapy among minorities particularly Hispanics and African-Americanss that in general have more of mixed dyslipidemia and lower prevalence of elevated LDL-c. Although this has been looked at in majority populations[32] it remains to be extensively studied among minorities.

Lipoprotein(a) [Lp(a)] has been found in epidemiologic studies to be associated with CHD, and in some studies this association was stronger in Caucasians compared with African Americans. [33] An expert panel of the NIH advised that Lp(a) above 75 nmol/L should be considered as a CHD risk factor for Caucasians, but a cutoff for African-Americans has not been determined.[34] This is an important point because among healthy people, African Americans have Lp(a) levels twice that of Caucasians[35] and not enough is known about Lp(a) levels in other minority groups.

Lp(a) not typically lowered by statins but is included in the measurement of LDL-c. Most lipid-lowering studies do not measure LDL-c directly. Instead, they calculate LDL-c using the Friedwald equation. On average, the calculated LDL-c overestimates the directly measured LDL-c by 4% or more in people in the lowest tertile of Lp(a), compared with 20% or more in those in the highest tertile. The NCEP has long advised that the LDL-c calculation is prone to greater error from Lp(a) in higher-risk patients,[36] and they reaffirmed this in recent guidelines.[37] When Lp(a) is high, this leads to a systematic approximation bias that may lead to erroneous scientific and clinical consequences in African-Americans. First it leads to a systematic overestimation of LDL-c in African-Americans. Second, high Lp(a) leads to the illusion that LDL-c is less responsive to statins. This is because a portion of the approximated LDL-c is not LDL-c at all and is therefore not responsive to statins. A patient with high Lp(a) may seem to have an LDL-c that changes little despite statin treatment, when true LDL-c may be responding well. This can be frustrating for both physicians and patients, and African-Americans are much more likely to encounter this unfortunate clinical problem. This may affect other minority groups but not enough is known about Lp(a) in other minority groups. Clinicians can avoid this by simply checking Lp(a) in those with high LDL-c, especially African-Americans. Though the clinical solution is straightforward, currently some insurance companies will not reimburse for measurement of Lp(a).

Can Biological Differences Explain the Racial Disparity in LDL-c Goal Achievement?

Although biological differences likely do exist among different race-ethnic groups, biological reasons are probably not the major culprit in the consistent undertreatment and poor control of lipids among minority populations. The magnitude of racial disparities coupled with a wide variety of failed general prevention benchmarks suggest that a tendency for dyslipidemia among minority groups was strongly influenced by lower access to health care.

Massing and colleagues[38] recently performed a large study of CVD patients which confirmed that African-Americans are less likely to have their cholesterol measured, let alone treated and controlled. To explain this finding, they noted evidence that continuity of care and time with physicians were more limited in African-Americans with chronic medical conditions. Massing also cited evidence that Caucasians may be more trusting of their physicians than African-Americans, who felt physician encounters were less participatory (though this improved with African-American physicians). Moreover, 16% of older African Americans had to forego filling a prescription because they could not afford it—more than twice the rate in Caucasians. Other possible factors for the relative undertreatment of African-Americans, include less knowledge about cholesterol, lower adherence rates, inadequate monitoring by physicians, and weaker physician oversight.

More recently, Trivedi and colleagues[39] examined data from almost 2 million observations to determine whether quality of care improved between 1997 and 2003. Indicators for diabetes and cardiovascular care included testing and control of LDL-c. Both of these were improved substantially. Unfortunately, African-Americans with CHD continued to lag behind Caucasians in control of LDL-c. For example, the percentage of Caucasian diabetic patients with controlled LDL-c increased from 36% to 75%, and the percentage of African Americans increased from 23% to 66%, narrowing the disparity from 13% to 9%. The investigators studied whether patients admitted for an myocardial infarction or revascularization procedure had achieved an LDL-c below 130 mg/dL. Caucasian patients with CHD were more likely to achieve this goal, improving from 47% to 68% success by 2002. African-Americans also improved from 33% to 51% success, but the disparity between the groups persisted; 14% to 17% fewer high-risk African-Americans than Caucasians achieved LDL-c below 130 mg/dL, revealing that the disparity had not changed significantly over time (Figure 3).

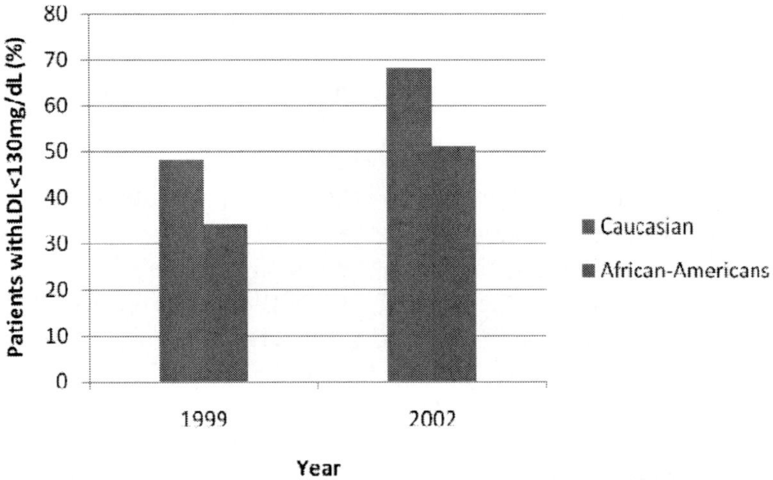

Figure 3. Overall improvements in the quality of care for both African-American and non-Hispanic whites from 1999 to 2002 with no narrowing of the disparity between races in the control of LDL cholesterol below a level of 130 mg per deciliter after myocardial infarction (MI) or a coronary revascularization procedure ($P<0.001$).

Summary

Minority populations represent a significant percentage of the US population. Important health disparities exist regarding hyperlipidemia, influenced by socioeconomic, lifestyle, and possibly biological and genetic variables. Some inappropriate bias has existed among the health care system. Minority groups have been classically under-represented in major lipid clinical trials and minority patient-physician encounter needs further improvement. Progress has been made in the awareness and treatment of hyperlipidemia as a risk factor for CVD among minority groups. However, important gaps are still present between the different ethnic groups that translate into different cardiovascular mortality and morbidity rates.

References

[1] Rosamond W, Flegal K, Friday G, Furie K, Go A, Greenlund K, et al. Heart disease and stroke statistics--2007 update: a report from the American Heart Association Statistics Committee and Stroke Statistics Subcommittee. *Circulation* 2007 Feb 6; 115(5):e69-171.

[2] Mensah GA, Mokdad AH, Ford ES, Greenlund KJ, Croft JB. State of disparities in cardiovascular health in the United States. *Circulation* 2005 Mar 15;111(10):1233-41.

[3] Mokdad AH, Marks JS, Stroup DF, Gerberding JL. Actual causes of death in the United States, 2000. *Jama* 2004 Mar 10;291(10):1238-45.

[4] Chowdhury PP, Balluz L, Okoro C, Strine T. Leading health indicators: a comparison of Hispanics with non-Hispanic whites and non-Hispanic blacks, United States 2003. *Ethnicity and disease* 2006 Spring;16(2):534-41.

[5] Winkleby MA, Kraemer HC, Ahn DK, Varady AN. Ethnic and socioeconomic differences in cardiovascular disease risk factors: findings for women from the Third National Health and Nutrition Examination Survey, 1988-1994. *Jama* 1998 Jul 22-29;280(4):356-62.
[6] Kannel WB, Castelli WP, Gordon T, McNamara PM. Serum cholesterol, lipoproteins, and the risk of coronary heart disease. The Framingham study. *Annals of internal medicine* 1971 Jan;74(1):1-12.
[7] Third Report of the National Cholesterol Education Program (NCEP) Expert Panel on Detection, Evaluation, and Treatment of High Blood Cholesterol in Adults (Adult Treatment Panel III) final report. *Circulation* 2002 Dec 17;106(25):3143-421.
[8] Kurian AK, Cardarelli KM. Racial and ethnic differences in cardiovascular disease risk factors: a systematic review. *Ethnicity and disease* 2007 Winter;17(1):143-52.
[9] Williams RA, Flack JM, Gavin JR, 3rd, Schneider WR, Hennekens CH. Guidelines for management of high-risk African Americans with multiple cardiovascular risk factors: recommendations of an expert consensus panel. *Ethnicity and disease* 2007 Spring;17(2):214-20.
[10] Metcalf PA, Sharrett AR, Folsom AR, Duncan BB, Patsch W, Hutchinson RG, et al. African American-white differences in lipids, lipoproteins, and apolipoproteins, by educational attainment, among middle-aged adults: the Atherosclerosis Risk in Communities Study. *American journal of epidemiology* 1998 Oct 15;148(8):750-60.
[11] Glueck CJ, Gartside P, Laskarzewski PM, Khoury P, Tyroler HA. High-density lipoprotein cholesterol in blacks and whites: potential ramifications for coronary heart disease. *American heart journal* 1984 Sep;108(3 Pt 2):815-26.
[12] Okosun IS, Choi S, Hash R, Dever GE. Apolipoprotein B, ratio of total cholesterol to HDL-C, and blood pressure in abdominally obese white and black American women. *Journal of human hypertension* 2001 May;15(5):299-305.
[13] Schreiner PJ, Morrisett JD, Sharrett AR, Patsch W, Tyroler HA, Wu K, et al. Lipoprotein[a] as a risk factor for preclinical atherosclerosis. *Arterioscler. Thromb.* 1993 Jun;13(6):826-33.
[14] Harris-Hooker S, Sanford GL. Lipids, lipoproteins and coronary heart disease in minority populations. *Atherosclerosis* 1994 Aug;108 Suppl:S83-104.
[15] Rodriguez C, Pablos-Mendez A, Palmas W, Lantigua R, Mayeux R, Berglund L. Comparison of modifiable determinants of lipids and lipoprotein levels among African-Americans, Hispanics, and Non-Hispanic Caucasians > or =65 years of age living in New York City. *The American journal of cardiology* 2002 Jan 15;89(2):178-83.
[16] Finkelstein EA, Khavjou OA, Mobley LR, Haney DM, Will JC. Racial/ethnic disparities in coronary heart disease risk factors among WISEWOMAN enrollees. *Journal of women's health* (2002). 2004 Jun;13(5):503-18.
[17] Wei M, Mitchell BD, Haffner SM, Stern MP. Effects of cigarette smoking, diabetes, high cholesterol, and hypertension on all-cause mortality and cardiovascular disease mortality in Mexican Americans. The San Antonio Heart Study. *American journal of epidemiology* 1996 Dec 1; 144(11):1058-65.
[18] Fulton-Kehoe DL, Eckel RH, Shetterly SM, Hamman RF. Determinants of total high density lipoprotein cholesterol and high density lipoprotein subfraction levels among

Hispanic and non-Hispanic white persons with normal glucose tolerance: the San Luis Valley Diabetes Study. *Journal of clinical epidemiology* 1992 Nov;45(11):1191-200.

[19] Rodriguez C, Jin Z, Boden-Abala B, Homma S, DiTullio MR, Sacco RL. Prevalence and Treatment Data on Dyslipidemia among Hispanics in the Northern Manhattan Study. *Circulation* 2006:e379.

[20] Brown DW, Giles WH, Greenlund KJ, Croft JB. Disparities in cholesterol screening: falling short of a national health objective. *Preventive medicine* 2001 Dec;33(6):517-22.

[21] Ford ES, Mokdad AH, Giles WH, Mensah GA. Serum total cholesterol concentrations and awareness, treatment, and control of hypercholesterolemia among US adults: findings from the National Health and Nutrition Examination Survey, 1999 to 2000. *Circulation* 2003 May 6;107(17):2185-9.

[22] Clark LT, Maki KC, Galant R, Maron DJ, Pearson TA, Davidson MH. Ethnic differences in achievement of cholesterol treatment goals. Results from the National Cholesterol Education Program Evaluation Project Utilizing Novel E-Technology II. *J. Gen. Intern. Med.* 2006 Apr;21(4):320-6.

[23] Pearson TA, Laurora I, Chu H, Kafonek S. The lipid treatment assessment project (L-TAP): a multicenter survey to evaluate the percentages of dyslipidemic patients receiving lipid-lowering therapy and achieving low-density lipoprotein cholesterol goals. *Archives of internal medicine* 2000 Feb 28;160(4):459-67.

[24] Howard BV, Lee ET, Cowan LD, Fabsitz RR, Howard WJ, Oopik AJ, et al. Coronary heart disease prevalence and its relation to risk factors in American Indians. The Strong Heart Study. *American journal of epidemiology* 1995 Aug 1;142(3):254-68.

[25] Cooke CE, Bresette JL, Khanna R. Statin use in American Indians and Alaska Natives with coronary artery disease. *Am. J. Health Syst. Pharm.* 2006 Sep 15;63(18):1717-22.

[26] Lloret R, Ycas J, Stein M, Haffner S. Comparison of rosuvastatin versus atorvastatin in Hispanic-Americans with hypercholesterolemia (from the STARSHIP trial). *The American journal of cardiology* 2006 Sep 15;98(6):768-73.

[27] Pearson TA, Denke MA, McBride PE, Battisti WP, Gazzara RA, Brady WE, et al. Effectiveness of ezetimibe added to ongoing statin therapy in modifying lipid profiles and low-density lipoprotein cholesterol goal attainment in patients of different races and ethnicities: a substudy of the Ezetimibe add-on to statin for effectiveness trial. *Mayo Clinic proceedings* 2006 Sep;81(9):1177-85.

[28] Ferdinand KC, Clark LT, Watson KE, Neal RC, Brown CD, Kong BW, et al. Comparison of efficacy and safety of rosuvastatin versus atorvastatin in African-American patients in a six-week trial. *The American journal of cardiology* 2006 Jan 15;97(2):229-35.

[29] Simon JA, Lin F, Hulley SB, Blanche PJ, Waters D, Shiboski S, et al. Phenotypic predictors of response to simvastatin therapy among African-Americans and Caucasians: the Cholesterol and Pharmacogenetics (CAP) Study. *The American journal of cardiology* 2006 Mar 15;97(6):843-50.

[30] Keavney B, Palmer A, Parish S, Clark S, Youngman L, Danesh J, et al. Lipid-related genes and myocardial infarction in 4685 cases and 3460 controls: discrepancies

between genotype, blood lipid concentrations, and coronary disease risk. *International journal of epidemiology* 2004 Oct;33(5):1002-13.

[31] Pischon T, Girman CJ, Sacks FM, Rifai N, Stampfer MJ, Rimm EB. Non-high-density lipoprotein cholesterol and apolipoprotein B in the prediction of coronary heart disease in men. *Circulation* 2005 Nov 29;112(22):3375-83.

[32] van der Steeg WA, Boekholdt SM, Stein EA, El-Harchaoui K, Stroes ES, Sandhu MS, et al. Role of the apolipoprotein B-apolipoprotein A-I ratio in cardiovascular risk assessment: a case-control analysis in EPIC-Norfolk. *Annals of internal medicine* 2007 May 1;146(9):640-8.

[33] Danesh J, Collins R, Peto R. Lipoprotein(a) and coronary heart disease. Meta-analysis of prospective studies. *Circulation* 2000 Sep 5;102(10):1082-5.

[34] Grundy SM, Cleeman JI, Merz CN, Brewer HB, Jr., Clark LT, Hunninghake DB, et al. Implications of recent clinical trials for the National Cholesterol Education Program Adult Treatment Panel III guidelines. *Arteriosclerosis, thrombosis, and vascular biology* 2004 Aug;24(8):e149-61.

[35] Guyton JR, Dahlen GH, Patsch W, Kautz JA, Gotto AM, Jr. Relationship of plasma lipoprotein Lp(a) levels to race and to apolipoprotein B. *Arteriosclerosis* (Dallas, Tex. 1985 May-Jun;5(3):265-72.

[36] [Li KM, Wilcken DE, Dudman NP. Effect of serum lipoprotein(a) on estimation of low-density lipoprotein cholesterol by the Friedewald formula. *Clinical chemistry* 1994 Apr;40(4):571-3.

[37] Marcovina SM, Koschinsky ML, Albers JJ, Skarlatos S. Report of the National Heart, Lung, and Blood Institute Workshop on Lipoprotein(a) and Cardiovascular Disease: recent advances and future directions. *Clinical chemistry* 2003 Nov;49(11):1785-96.

[38] Massing MW, Foley KA, Carter-Edwards L, Sueta CA, Alexander CM, Simpson RJ, Jr. Disparities in lipid management for African Americans and Caucasians with coronary artery disease: a national cross-sectional study. *BMC cardiovascular disorders* 2004 Aug 18;4:15.

[39] Trivedi AN, Zaslavsky AM, Schneider EC, Ayanian JZ. Trends in the quality of care and racial disparities in Medicare managed care. *The New England journal of medicine* 2005 Aug 18;353(7):692-700.

In: Topics in Prevalent Diseases
Editors: N. C. Chavez-Tapia and M. Uribe
ISBN 978-1-60456-959-9

Chapter 10

Involuntary Exposure to Environmental Tobacco Smoke in Vulnerable Groups

Tonatiuh Barrientos-Gutiérrez [1,2] ***and***
David Gimeno Ruiz de Porras [3,4, 5, 6]
[1] Departamento de Investigación sobre Tabaco. Centro de Investigación en Salud Poblacional, Instituto Nacional de Salud Pública, Cuernavaca, Morelos, México
[2] The University of Texas School of Public Health, Health Science Center at Houston, Division of Occupational and Environmental Health Sciences, Texas, USA
[3] The University of Texas School of Public Health, Health Science Center at Houston, Division of Occupational and Environmental Health Sciences, San Antonio Regional Campus, Texas, USA
[4] Department of Epidemiology and Public Health, University College London Medical School, London, England, United Kingdom
[5] The Institute for Work and Health, Toronto, Canada
[6] CIBER Epidemiología y Salud Pública (CIBERESP), Spain

1. Introduction

Environmental tobacco smoke (ETS), also known as secondhand smoke, is a complex mixture of compounds produced during the combustion of tobacco. More than 4000 compounds have been detected in ETS, and at least 250 of them are considered carcinogenic (e.g., arsenic, benzene, chromium, and polonium-210) or toxic (e.g., toluene, ammonium formaldehyde, hydrogen cyanide or nicotine).[1, 2] According to the US Environmental Protection Agency ETS is considered a type-A carcinogen for humans, and nicotine environmental levels as low as 0.0075 $\mu g/m^3$ are considered to produce *de minimis* risk for carcinogenic effects.[2,3] Unlike other pollutants, no safe level of exposure to ETS exists.

Half the world's children population is exposed to ETS.[4] Sixty percent of non-smoking households have detectable levels of nicotine in the environment, associated to increased levels of hair nicotine in children and non-smoking women.[5] ETS exposure is causally associated with health effects in children (i.e., sudden infant death syndrome, lower respiratory tract illness, respiratory symptoms, asthma, lower lung function, and middle ear disease) as well as in adults (i.e., cardiovascular disease, and lung cancer).[1]

Overall, 200,000 deaths among the working population are ETS related.[6] ETS-related disease and financial burden are a fundamental concern, recognized by more than 160 countries under the World Health Organization sponsored Framework Convention on Tobacco Control, which considers ETS exposure elimination as an attainable primary prevention goal to reduce disease and mortality.[7] Recent efforts to ban smoking in public places have reduced workplace ETS exposure, but certain worksites, particularly in the hospitality sector, remain major sources of ETS exposure.[8, 9]

As with many other pollutants, ETS exposure is not equally distributed across society and some groups are more affected than others. ETS is largely generated by male active smoking [10, 11] in a male dominated society[12] where non-smoking women and children are subject to involuntary exposure to ETS. At home women may lack the necessary resources or leverage to impose, negotiate, or discuss smoking restrictions to their male partners.[13] However, power imbalance in detriment of women is not limited to individual's relationships. All over the world women experience structural differences (e.g., restricted access to work, education, information, or income)[12] limiting their capability to identify risks and take actions to eliminate exposure. At work power imbalance between employees and employers facilitates involuntary ETS exposure, requiring State interventions to assure health protection.[14] Such is the case of the hospitality sector, where smoking is considered a fundamental commodity for costumers, placed over workers' health. More complex scenarios, such as women and children from ethnic minorities or working women in male-dominated markets, are not uncommon.

In this chapter we review the scientific evidence related to ETS exposure and its health effects in children, women, workers and, when available, racial/ethnic groups. Then we present potential interventions to eliminate ETS exposure and create healthier homes and workplaces.

2. Children and Adolescents

2.1. Prevalence

According to the Global Youth Tobacco Survey, 44% of 13 to 15 year old students are exposed to ETS at home, and 56% are exposed in public places.[15] Among never smokers, highest ETS exposure is reported in Europe (71.5%) and lowest in Africa (22.6%). Reports from other regions vary from 57.3% in the Western Pacific to 37% in the Eastern Mediterranean region. A similar pattern is found in public places. Here ETS exposure is more frequently reported in Europe (79.4%), less frequently in Africa (38.2%), and reportedly varying from 52.6% in the Western Pacific region to 38.8% in South-East Asia. While exposure in South-West Asia and the Western Pacific occurs more frequently at home, in Africa, Europe, the Eastern-Mediterranean, and the Americas ETS exposure occurs more frequently in public places (see Figure 1).[16] Similarly, a study conducted in households from 31 countries in Europe, Middle-East, America, and Asia found 48% of the children were exposed in public places. Up to 78% of children and non-smoking women living with smokers exhibited detectable concentrations of nicotine in hair, whereas the percentage was 59% among those not living with smokers. Hair nicotine concentrations of children living with a smoker were higher in Asia, followed by Europe/Middle-East, and Latin America.[5]

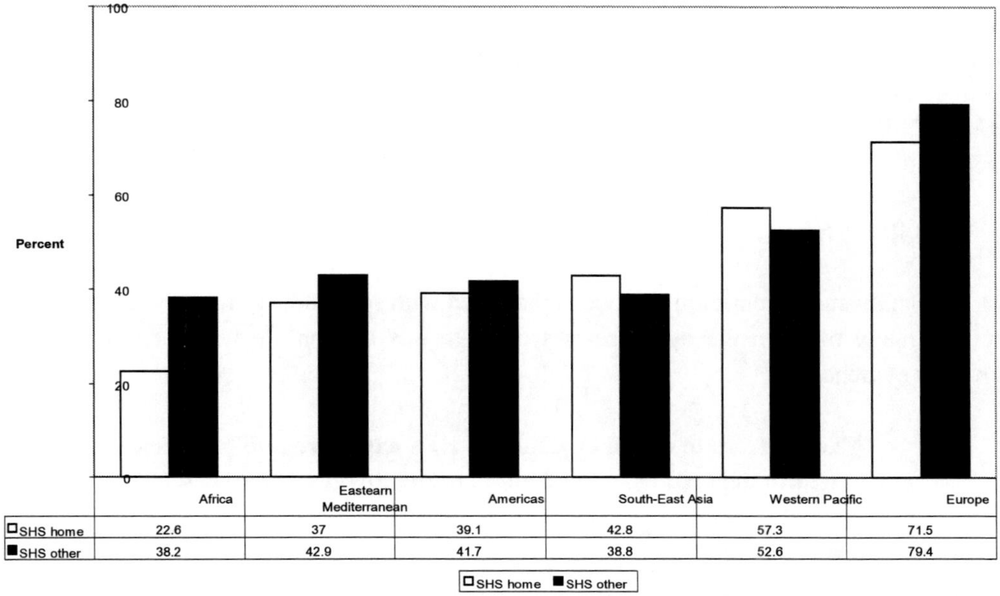

Figure 1. Prevalence of ETS exposure in never-smoker students 13 to 15 years old by WHO region according to the GYTS 2000-2007 [15]

2.2. Determinants

Parental smoking is one of the most direct predictors of ETS exposure at home and urinary cotinine in children. ETS exposure increases with every smoker living in the household,[5, 17] children's urinary cotinine is three-fold higher when one of the parents is a smoker, and six-fold higher when both parents are smokers.[18] While both parents may contribute to ETS exposure at home,[19] in some countries the influence is mainly paternal (e.g., Greece) [20] whereas in others it is maternal (e.g., Spain, Italy, and South Africa).[21-23] Despite parents being the obvious source of ETS exposure at home, other individuals (i.e., day-care providers) may also be direct contributors.[24] Parental smoking influence is reflected in differential urinary cotinine age-differences among children, with higher concentrations observed in younger children.[5,18]

Socioeconomic factors are heavily influencial on parental smoking. Particularly, increased maternal education is associated with reduced exposure.[21, 25, 26] Differences in children exposure to ETS have consistently been observed between income/education levels and race/ethnicity groups. Half of the children from families earning less than 10,000 USD per year experience ETS exposure, an abysmal difference when compared to 20% exposed children from families earning more than 50,000 USD per year.[27] Studies on parental education have shown lower ETS exposure levels as mother's education increases.[28]

In the US, African Americans, Hispanics, and Asians report lower rates of ETS exposure at home than Caucasians[28] although urinary cotinine levels among African Americans consistently double the concentration observed among Caucasians. While metabolic differences have been proposed as potential explanation for this difference, [29-31] some authors suggest cotinine differences are a true reflection of higher ETS exposure among African Americans.[32] Other factors such as time spent with smokers and distance to sources may contribute to reported differences.[5, 25] Finally, we should bear in mind that none of these factors occur in isolation, and certain groups may combine several risk factors.[33, 34]

2.3 Health Effects

ETS exposure in children has been associated with several health outcomes (see Table 1), but for many of them the evidence is scarce. In this section we will focus on those with stronger evidence.

Table 1. State of the evidence of ETS exposure and children's health according to the Report of the Surgeon General, 2006

Health indicator	Evidence
Growth and development	
Low birth weight	Suggestive
Congenital malformations	Inadequate
Cognitive development	Inadequate
Behavioral development	Inadequate
Height/growth	Inadequate
Infant death	
Sudden infant death syndrome	Sufficient
Infant death	Inadequate
Respiratory	
Lower respiratory illnesses	Sufficient
Respiratory symptoms	Sufficient
Ever having asthma	Sufficient
Wheeze illnesses	Sufficient
Lower lung function	Sufficient
Athopy	Inadequate
Asthma onset	Suggestive
Cancer	
Childhood cancer	Suggestive
Ear and throat	
Middle ear disease	Sufficient
Adenoidectomy	Inadequate

*Elaborated by the authors based on the Report of the Surgeon General, 2006.[1]

2.3.1. Low Birth Weight (LBW)

Maternal active smoking association with LBW has been known for decades, suggesting a potential role for ETS as LBW contributory factor.[35] In non-smoking women exposed to ETS by 20% increased odds of LBW at term have been reported, which has been associated with an average loss of 28 grams, although some studies rendered weight losses as large as 80 grams.[36, 37] ETS exposure, both at home and at work, has been related to weight losses up to 90 grams in newborns with mothers older than 30 years old.[38] Given limitations in the design of the reported studies, a causal relationship between ETS and LBW can not yet be confirmed.

Proposed biological pathways are the same as for active smoking, basically, reduced oxygen intake for the fetus due to increased CO and vasoconstriction produced by nicotine, thereby reducing the blood flow in the umbilical cord and the uterus. Evidence of fetal hypoxia, including increased nuclear red blood cells and levels of erythropoietin in fetal blood of ETS exposed children, supports this hypothesis.[1]

2.3.2. Sudden Infant Death Syndrome (SIDS)

Postnatal exposure to ETS has been associated with increased risk of SIDS (pooled OR=1.9)[1], even after controlling for the effect of maternal smoking during pregnancy.[39] Other studies have found an increased risk of SIDS only when the father smoked.[40]

Potential biological pathways linking ETS exposure to SIDS are not fully understood, but nicotine has been hypothesized as being at least part of the pathway. Nicotine may induce placental modifications, leading to low birth weight and brain development impairment. Nicotine may as well interfere the neuro-regulation of ventilation and heart rate occurring during sleep hypoxia, either by blocking the cholinergic system or through an increase in dopamine levels.[41] Finally, the effect of bacterial toxins could be dramatically increased when nicotine is present.[42]

2.3.3. Respiratory Problems

While some evidence points to a potential role of prenatal exposure to ETS in the development of respiratory symptoms, some evidence supports a stronger effect of postnatal exposures, particularly from maternal sources.[1, 43] For instance, odds of respiratory symptoms are higher in countries were maternal smoking is rare, also, odds of postnatal maternal smoking are stronger compared to those for smoking during pregnancy.[1]

In addition, maternal smoking appears to have a stronger impact on children's health than other people smoking. Thus, the odds of children experiencing wheeze symptoms compared to children of non-smoking parents increases by 41% if both parents smoke, 28% if the mother smokes, and 13% if the father smokes. Figures for cough are 64%, 34%, and 22% respectively, and the odds of experiencing phlegm increases 42% when both parents smoke.[1] Also, lower respiratory illness (LRI) is more strongly related to maternal smoking

[1] The OR (odds ratio) is a common and useful measure that allows the assessment of the association between an event (e.g., infant death) in a group (e.g., mothers smokers) as compared to the occurrence of the same event in another group (e.g., mothers non-smokers). For example, an OR of 2 would simply mean that infants from mothers that smoked during pregnancy had two times more risk of SIDS as compared to non-smoking mothers.

(OR=1.7) than to paternal smoking (OR=1.3) or smoking from other family members (OR=1.3).[44] Moreover, children exposed to ETS have 42% more chance of ever experiencing asthma if both parents smoke, 33% if only the mother smokes and a 7% non-significant increase if the father smokes.[1] These findings would be consistent with the role of mothers as the primary child-caregiver.[1]

Children's age seems to have a large effect on the intensity of the association between ETS exposure and respiratory symptoms. Reported cough and wheeze in ETS exposed children are more common in younger children and reduces with age.[45, 46] The influence of ETS on LRI is stronger for children 2 years old and younger (OR=1.7) than for older children (OR=1.25).[47] Odds for wheezing illness incident are 31% higher among ETS exposed children under six years old, but only 13% higher at older ages.[48] This differential finding by age has implications in the discussion of whether ETS initiates or exacerbates asthma. While age differences in incidental wheezing could be explained by a reduction in ETS exposure as children grow older, it could also reflect misclassification of the underlying pathological process. Wheezing illness in children under six years old could be related to infectious processes, such as bronchiolitis or bronchitis, and not to atopic asthma as expected in older children. The benign course of wheezing illness observed in younger children supports the idea of a transitory infectious process, contrasting with the less benign prognosis expected from atopic asthma.[48] Also, if ETS was an inductor of asthma, it should be associated with increased odds of bronchial hyperreactivity, but published evidence is limited.[49] Current evidence suggest that ETS exacerbates rather than initiates asthma, thus triggering acute asthma response but not affecting bronchial hyperresponsiveness.

Immunological and lung function impairment are the two main mechanisms proposed to explain how ETS leads to respiratory problems.[1] Nicotine potentially reduces phagocytic activity, inhibits the production of immunoglobulines (IgA and IgG2), increases the liberation of cytokines involved in atopic responses, increases IgE production, suppresses natural killer cells, and increases bacterial adherence to mucosal surfaces.[42] Uterus stress, derived from nicotine-induced hypoxia is a potential mechanism for lung hypoplasia, structural changes in fetal lung development and faster lung maturation.[1] Maternal prenatal smoking is associated with a 1% reduction in FEV1, and a 6% reduction in maximal expiratory flow at 25% of vital capacity.[50] Until the fourth year of age postnatal ETS exposure could also interfere with alveoli development and lung function.[51] Children have higher relative ventilation rates than adults, therefore increasing ETS intake under similar exposure levels.[52] Effects of postnatal exposure to ETS on pulmonary function are smaller than for prenatal exposure, still, a 0.5% reduction in FEV1 and 2% reduction in maximal expiratory flow at 25% has been observed.[50] Early life impacts on lung function and development remain over time and increase the risk of pulmonary disease later on in life.[53]

2.3.4. Cancer

One of potential roles of ETS in childhood cancer derives from known links between toxic and carcinogenic compounds in ETS and lung cancer in adults.[2] Examination of urine of ETS exposed children have found increased levels of carcinogen biomarkers (e.g., 4-aminobiphenyl hemoglobin adducts, PAH-albumin, NNAL, and NNAL-Gluc),[54, 55] and oxidative stress, a proposed pathway for cancer (i.e., increased plasma peroxide levels and oxidative stress indices, and reduced vitamin C, thiol, and total antioxidant capacity).[56, 57]

However, only weak associations between ETS exposure and some childhood cancers (i.e., brain tumors, leukemia, and lymphoma) have been observed.[58] Whereas maternal smoking during pregnancy is not considered to have a large effect on childhood cancer (OR=1.1),[1] paternal smoking has been associated with non-Hodgkin's lymphoma (RR= 2.0) and brain tumors (RR=1.2).[59] Paternal preconceptional smoking has been associated with a significant increased odds ratio of acute myeloid leukemia (OR=3.8).[60] The main biological pathway from paternal smoking to childhood cancer could be preconceptional DNA damage of sperm.[1] Nevertheless, although plausible biological pathways have been proposed, the available evidence between ETS and childhood cancer is inconclusive.

2.3.5. Middle Ear Disease (MED)

There is sufficient evidence to support a causal association between ETS exposure and certain MEDs. The likelihood of experiencing recurrent otitis media is 32% greater in children exposed to smoking of either parent and 37% higher if exposed to maternal smoking.[1] Likelihood of getting middle ear effusion is 38% higher in children exposed to ETS compared to non-exposed children.[61] For other conditions, such as acute otitis media, findings are contradictory, with some studies estimating ORs ranging from 1.0 to 1.6,[61] and other studies stating the effect of either parent smoking as non-significant (OR=0.99).[1]

3. Women

3.1. Prevalence

No global estimates of ETS exposure prevalence in adult women exist. Since active smoking prevalence is lower in women than in men (22% vs. 35% in developed countries, and 9% vs. 50% in developing countries)[62] it is possible that more women are exposed to involuntary smoking than men, particularly in developing countries. According to surveys conducted in China, 57% of the non-smoking women are exposed to ETS compared to 45% of non-smoking men.[11] In the US from 1988 to 2001, serum cotinine levels have decreased by 77% in both women (from 0.19 ng/mL to 0.04 ng/mL) and men (0.29 ng/mL to 0.07 ng/mL). However, racial/ethnicity disparities have been observed with larger reduction in Whites (79%) than in Hispanics (71%) or Blacks (67%).[1]

Data on women's ETS exposure in places other than home is scarce. One study found the prevalence of self-reported ETS exposure in other places than home was 68% in Europe, and 64% in Asia and Latin America.[5] While household exposure is probably the primary site of women's exposure, the workplace reaches a similar importance, particularly with the raising incorporation of women to the labor market. Attributable fractions of exposure derived from households or workplaces are difficult to disentangle. According to the first European Community Respiratory Health Survey (ECRHS I, 1990 to 1994) among the adult population ETS exposure was greater at the workplace (21%) than at home (18%). ECRHS II (1998) confirmed this pattern, despite a 9% reduction of exposure at home and 11% at the workplace.[63] In Switzerland ETS exposure is slightly greater at home (42%) than at the workplace (40%).[64] Finally, exposure may also occur in places other than home or workplace (e.g., in a convenience sample of non-smoking Mexican women 72% reported ETS exposure in the transportation system, 52% in public places, and 37% in restaurants).[17]

3.2. Determinants

The main source of ETS at home for women is living with a smoking partner.[1] Across countries, the number of smokers at home is highly correlated with women's hair nicotine concentrations.[5] In addition, nicotine concentrations in hair among women living with smokers are higher in Asia than in Europe or Latin America, reflecting either longer time spent at home or more intense exposure levels.

Socioeconomic factors (e.g., women's education and income) and self-efficacy are important determinants of exposure,[65] although partner's educational level has also been associated with ETS exposure.[66] Given that women do take actions to control ETS at home, the role of women's education may be particularly relevant to help them develop more effective strategies.[67] Also, racial/ethnic disparities have been reported with ETS exposure being higher among Blacks as compared to Whites,[68] but evidence is still weak.

Regarding exposure at the workplace, low socioeconomic status constitutes its main determinant.[69] Women from low socioeconomic status are more frequently exposed, experience higher levels of ETS exposure,[64] and work more often in places with no compliance with smoking bans.[14] Overall, reductions in exposure to ETS both at home and in the workplace occur at slower rates among low-socioeconomic status population.[63]

3.3. Health Effects

Table 2 summarizes the state of the evidence regarding ETS exposure and health effects in adults [1].

3.3.1. Preterm Delivery

Evidence of ETS effects on preterm delivery is limited and mixed.[1] Three out of eight studies did not find any association, whereas the rest found statistically significant differences only in some groups (e.g., women older than 30 years of age exposed at work for more than 7 hours every day, or those with evidence of high ETS exposure experiences). The biological pathway is not yet well defined, although evidence linking active smoking and preterm delivery suggests there may be a biologically plausible association with ETS.[36]

Table 2. State of the evidence on ETS exposure and adult's health. Report of the Surgeon General, 2006

Health Indicator	Evidence
Reproductive	
Preterm delivery	Suggestive
Female fertility	Inadequate
Spontaneous abortion	Inadequate
Respiratory	
Nasal irritation	Sufficient
Respiratory symptoms	Suggestive
Chronic respiratory symptoms	Suggestive
Decline in lung function in asthmatics	Suggestive
Small decrement in lung function	Suggestive
Adult-onset asthma	Suggestive
Worsening of asthma control	Suggestive
COPD	Suggestive
Morbidity in persons with COPD	Inadequate
Decline lung function healthy persons	Inadequate
Cancer	
Lung cancer	Sufficient
Breast cancer	Suggestive
Nasal sinus cavity cancer	Suggestive
Nasopharyngeal carcinoma	Inadequate
Cervical cancer	Inadequate
Cardiovascular	
Coronary heart disease	Sufficient
Stroke	Suggestive
Atherosclerosis	Suggestive

*Elaborated by the authors based on the Report of the Surgeon General, 2006.[1]

3.3.2. Respiratory Symptoms and Diseases

Exposure to ETS has been linked to nasal irritation, acute respiratory symptoms, presence of cough and dyspnea, and although weakly, phlegm and wheeze.[1]

Frequency of cough and phlegm in non-smoking women increases as a function of the number of smokers at home. In cases were women share the household with at least two smokers and use coal heating a three-fold increase in the odds of experiencing cough, phlegm and dyspnea was observed.[70] Women exposed to husband's smoking showed a 72% significant increase in odds of morning cough and morning phlegm.[71] For wheeze a 73% increased odds ratio has been observed among women exposed to partner's smoke.[72]

Exposure to ETS in adults, both female and male, have been linked to 40 to 60% increased risk of adult asthma.[1] Women exposed to ETS seem to experience more bronchial hyperactivity, requiring up to 13% more frequent use of bronchodilatator.[73] Asthma worsens in patients exposed to ETS, consequently requiring more medication, visits to the hospital, and ultimately reducing their quality of life. For chronic obstructive pulmonary disease (COPD) active smoking is the most predominant risk factor. It has been hypothesized that an important portion of the COPD observed in non-smoking population could be linked to ETS exposure. The proportion of COPD patients among non-smokers is slightly larger among women (5.1%) than men (3.7%).[74] While few studies are available to evaluate ETS association with COPD, some studies have found an association between being exposed to husband's smoke and an increased risk of COPD in never-smoking women.[75, 76]

So far most studies on ETS and respiratory health have either centered their attention to exposure at home or in the workplace; concurrent exposure at home and at work for respiratory symptoms and diseases has been rarely studied. Concurrent exposure to ETS from husbands at home and coworkers at the worksite was associated with increased odds for dyspnea, shortness of breath, wheeze, asthma diagnosis and symptoms, COPD, cough, phlegm, and rhino-conjunctivitis among non-smoking women.[77] Odds were smaller for either home or work exposure, thus highlighting the importance of studying complex exposure patterns in women.

3.3.3. Cancer

According to current meta-analytic risk estimates, there is a 22% higher likelihood of developing lung cancer among non-smoking women exposed to husband's smoke compared to non-smoking marriages.[1] Lung adenocarcinoma has been linked to the frequency and intensity of husband's smoking in a Japanese cohort of non-smoking women.[78] Up to 37% of the lung tumors in Taiwanese women are attributable to ETS exposure.[79]

Increased susceptibility of women to carcinogenesis has been proposed, but this hypothesis remains to be proved.[80] The carcinogenic potential of ETS is the most likely cause of increased DNA damage deriving in lung cancer among ETS exposed subjects.[1]

Meta-analysis evidence shows a 40% increase in the risk of breast cancer associated with the fact of ever been exposed to ETS over the lifetime.[1, 81] However, this finding remains controversial since it has been observed in premenopausal women (85% increased risk) but not for postmenopausal women.[82-84] No biological explanation for this difference is available, but no evidence linking active smoking and breast cancer has been found,[85-87] challenging the biological plausibility of an association with ETS.

Finally, limited evidence shows that non-smoking women have an 40% increased odds of nasal sinus cancer if exposed to one smoker, but a five-time increase if more than one smoker is present in the household.[88] This potential association might follow the same biological pathway for active smoking.[1]

3.3.4. Cardiovascular Disease (CVD) and Stroke

Women exposed to ETS have a 24% increased risk of CVD compared to non-exposed women,[89] and CVD mortality risk has been estimated to be 15% increased for non-smoking women exposed to ETS.[90]

Evidence for stroke is less clear. While some studies did not find a significant association,[1] women's exposure to ETS at home has been linked to a significant 24% and 66% increase in the likelihood of stroke.[91, 92] The likelihood of stroke was 28% greater for women exposed to ETS from less than 9 cigarettes per day, 32% greater for exposures to 10 to 19 cigarettes, and 62% greater for more than 20 cigarettes per day.[93]

CVD and stroke may share a biological pathway. The most likely biological pathway proposed for CVD is increased platelet aggregation.[94] Other factors (e.g., endothelial dysfunction, atherosclerosis, increased oxidative stress, decreased energy metabolism, increased insulin resistance, and increased inflammation) are still under investigation.[1, 81]

4. Workers

4.1. Prevalence

There are no global estimates of ETS exposure among workers. Furthermore, current implementation of 100% smoke-free workplaces creates large variations in short-term across countries complicating the estimation of prevalence. For instance, according to the first phase of the Third National Health and Nutrition Examination Survey (NHANES III, 1988-1991) 71% of workers are considered exposed based on serum cotinine data from workers not exposed at home. The percentage declined to 55% in phase 2 of NHANES III (1991-1994).[8] This later phase is the last one that provided estimates of exposure among workers, showing occupational variations in both frequency and intensity of exposure. Non-construction laborers (93%), waiters/waitresses (90%), textile machine operators (87%), motor vehicle operators and mechanics (84%), and cooks (80%) were the occupations more frequently exposed.[8] The ranking in terms of intensity was lead by waiters/waitresses (0.5 ng/mL), non-construction laborers (0.4 ng/mL), textile machine operators (0.3 ng/mL), and food preparators and construction traders (0.2 ng/mL).

Recent research on ETS concentrations in public places, including workplaces, has shown that, in Europe, bar and discotheques had the highest environmental nicotine concentrations (19-122 $\mu g/m^3$), followed by restaurants (0.01-18 $\mu g/m^3$), universities (0.01-19.4 $\mu g/m^3$), hospitals (0.01-17.6 $\mu g/m^3$), train stations (0.5-10 $\mu g/m^3$), airports (0.1-5 $\mu g/m^3$), and schools (0.01-2 $\mu g/m^3$). In Latin America, 93% of the public monitored places (i.e, bars and restaurants, governmental buildings, airports, schools, and hospitals) had detectable nicotine levels.[9] Bars and restaurants had the highest median concentrations (3.65 and 1.24 $\mu g/m^3$ respectively),[9] an observation also reported in China.[95]

4.2. Determinants

The main determinant of ETS exposure at work is whether or not the workplace has an enforced smoking ban on its premises. In US offices, a 8.6 $\mu g/m^3$ nicotine concentration was measured in smoking-allowed spaces, compared to 1.3 $\mu g/m^3$ in restricted-smoking areas, and 0.3 $\mu g/m^3$ in places with total ban. Figures for non-office spaces were, respectively, 2.3 µg/m3, 0.7 µg/m3, and 0.2 µg/m3.[96]

Table 3. Sources of variation in ETS-exposure concentrations in bars and restaurants

Smoking vs. Non-smoking areas		
	SMK Restaurants	*N-SMK Restaurants*
Akbar-Khanzadeh*, 2003	16.8 (0.5-121.7)	0.7 (0.1-54.4)
Ceno, 2004°	23.4 (16.5-38.8)	4.4 (<0.1-8.7)
	SMK Bars	*N-SMK Bars*
Gee, 2006*	63 (23-132)	21.1 (10-42)
Ventilation types		
Gee, 2006§	*SMK areas*	*Bar areas*
Mechanical	68.6 (19.5)	75.5 (21.6)
Extractor	93.0 (10.6)	81.0 (12.2)
Natural	67.0 (17.2)	53.1 (21.5)
Deprived vs. non-deprived location		
	Affluent food serving	*Non-affluent food serving*
Edwards, 2006‡	160.3 (59.3-424)	329.8 (54.1-1395.1)

*Vapor phase nicotine, active monitoring: Median (IQR)
°Vapor phase nicotine, active monitoring: Mean (range)
§Vapor phase nicotine, active monitoring: Mean (SE)
‡ RSP-PM2.5, active monitoring:
Median (IQR)

Social inequalities in the exposure to ETS at workplace exist by gender, race/ethnicity, and occupation. First, working without smoking regulations is reported by 20% of the women living at or under the poverty line, but only by 10% of those living 150% above the poverty line.[97] Second, absence of smoking regulations is more frequently reported by Hispanics (15%), American Indians (14%), and Asian-American (13%) than by Caucasians or African-American women (10.7% and 10.5%, respectively).[97] Third, the likelihood of exposure is four times higher for manual than for non-manual jobs in men, and three times higher in women - [98] In addition to being two times higher in hospitality workers compared to workers in other sectors.[99, 100] Workplace ETS exposure also varies by age group, with workers younger than 30 being more frequently exposed.[98, 101]

Beyond the individual, certain physical features of the work environment (See table 3), such as creating smoking and non-smoking areas [102, 103] or using natural ventilation systems,[104] reduce ETS exposure, although, none eliminates the exposure.[105] Finally, in terms of economic inequalities, more deprived establishments have higher ETS exposure levels.[106]

4.3. Health Effects

Overall, ETS exposure in the workplace is associated with the same health effects observed in exposed adults in the general population. However, considering the peculiarities of the workplace, research has evaluated whether working populations experience health effects of larger magnitudes.

4.3.1 Respiratory Function and Symptoms

Natural experiments, such as the introduction of smoking bans, provide evidence on the impact of ETS on respiratory problems. Overall, smoking bans seem to improve workers' respiratory function and diminished the number of respiratory symptoms. Data from Ireland [107] showed that barmen's lung function improved between measures taken prior to the Irish ban and one year after (e.g., FVC increased from 92% to 95%, PEF increased from 94% to 97%,) and their respiratory symptoms diminished (e.g., cough in the morning (31% to 11%), cough during the day (55% to 34%), phlegm (68% to 40%), runny nose (65% to 32%), and sore throat (47% to 21%)). In Norway,[108] cross-shift differences (i.e., before and after work shift) in lung function measures were significantly larger before the smoking ban was enforced (e.g., FVC was 81 ml vs. 52 ml; and FEV1 was 89 ml vs. 46 ml). These reductions were interpreted as reductions in the bronchial responsiveness due to reductions in ETS-components.

4.3.2. Lung Cancer

Meta-analysis data shows ETS at work is associated with increase in the likelihood of lung cancer, which is significantly greater in women (22%) compared to non-significant increases of 12% in men.[1] Intensively exposed workers, that is those working in restaurants and bars, could experience up to 50% increased risk of lung cancer compared to the general population, even after controlling for active smoking.[99]

4.3.3. Cardiovascular Disease (CVD)

Meta-analytical data shows a 21% increased risk of CVD among non-smokers exposed to workplace ETS,[109] which would yield 7 deaths from CVD for every 1000 workers, superseding the 1 for every 1000 workers threshold marked by the US Occupational Safety and Health Administration. Potential mechanisms of this association include increased heart rate at rest [110] and heart variability,[111, 112] changes in aortic and brachial blood pressure,[113] and vascular endothelial dysfunction.[114]

5. Interventions

Since ETS exposure has a single source, active smoking, the first action to be taken to eliminate ETS is to reduce active smoking in the general population. However, this is a long-term goal common to all tobacco control policies, and it is unattainable in the short term. Moreover, as any other tobacco control activity, elimination of ETS exposure will not be attained by means of a single intervention,[13, 115-117] thus requiring a comprehensive approach based in several simultaneous mechanisms: taxation, advertisement regulation, education, legislation, information generation, along with punctual interventions.[4, 7]

Media campaigns for ETS control are common, but they have limited impact.[115] Smoking bans (i.e., smoke-free legislation bills) in public places (e.g., governmental buildings, transportation centers, education facilities, and most workplaces) have proven to be more efficient. After their implementation, children's ETS exposure has been reduced in schools, hospitals, restaurants, and other public places.[118] While it seems natural to enforce public health measures in public places, enforcing measures of control in private places (e.g., home) is controversial. Still, exposure to ETS at home is, together with the workplace, where most of the ETS exposure occurs, especially for children. Thus, current regulations are for instance considering to enforce penalties for smoking in cars, since evidence shows toxicity could be higher than at home.[13] However, it may be extremely difficult to develop legislation to protect people's health at home while maintaining other constitutional rights.[4]

In view of this dilemma, recent research has focused in developing educational programs and behavioral interventions aimed to convince smokers to voluntarily reduce ETS at home. Developed countries in the Americas have successfully reduced ETS exposure rates. In the US, home ETS has declined over the last 30 years, yielding a significant reduction from 35.6% to 25.1% in exposure prevalence at home documented for the period between 1992 and 2000.[28] Similar trends have been documented in Canada, where parents' consent that smoking close to children should be avoided increased from 51% to 70% from 1992 to 1996, reflected in 80% of households with children being smoke-free in 1996.[119]

5.1. Reducing Exposure to ETS at Home

Interventions to reduce ETS smoke are relatively new and have mainly focused on getting parents to quit smoking or modify their smoking behavior by restricting smoking indoors or in the presence of children. In a recent systematic review [13] only one study showed increased quitting rates at 6 months (5.9% in the program group vs. 2.7% in controls) and lower relapse rates (45% vs. 55%, respectively); more evidence was found for programs aimed to reduce the self-reported number of cigarettes smoked, although reductions in cotinine levels were observed only in one study; and only two studies found significant reductions in indoor smoking or air nicotine without increasing quitting rates. Most of the success has been observed in self-reported outcomes, but rarely in objective outcomes.[117] Despite the relatively positive effect of the interventions aiming to obtain behavioral modifications, regulation alone may not suffice to reduce objective measurements of exposure.[120, 121]

Most interventions are delivered by health care related personnel, either in health services by nurses or doctors, or directly at home by health-promotion personnel.[13] Although people tend to be receptive to professional advice in health services, medical interventions are costly and usually of short duration. Home interventions have the advantage of potentially allowing a larger intervention in a more friendly environment.[115] It is likely that larger and more frequent interventions, such as those provided at home, could render better results but evidence is still insufficient to conclude which type is more efficient.[13, 115]

Future intervention research should consider the following challenges: the incorporation of strong theoretical frames,[13, 115] development of culturally and socially sensitive programs, improvement of understanding of home smoking negotiation by women and/or children in the household,[115] inclusion of fathers as primary targets of interventions, and evaluation of success from objectively measured outcomes since most of the prior evidence is based on self-reported results. Additionally, customized interventions are particularly needed for low-income families and ethnic minorities where fewer ETS exposure restrictions at home have been observed.[1]

5.2. Reducing Exposure to ETS in the Workplace

Interventions in the workplace are centered in the development of smoke-free policies. Practically unknown before 1986, smoke-free regulations were implemented rapidly as awareness on ETS deleterious effects increased. By 1999, 70% of the US working population labored in a smoke-free workplace. [8] Studies in the US and abroad have shown a consistent decrease in ETS exposure after implementation of smoke-free regulations. [122-126] The impact of the regulations on health indicators has been strong and consistent. Smoking bans across the world have been linked to reduced respiratory symptoms, [107, 127] improved respiratory function, [107, 108, 127] reduced hospital admission for myocardial infarction, [128] and reduced active smoking.[129]

Since there are no safe levels of exposure to ETS, the ultimate goal of any intervention must be to completely eliminate environmental ETS,[118] and such goal can only be attained with a 100% indoor-smoke ban, which is the only intervention recognized as effective by the WHO. Tobacco companies have tried to block 100% smoke-free bans suggesting "alternatives", such as ventilation or physical separation between smoking and non-smoking areas.[130] However, while increased ventilation, separation of spaces, and restrictions to smoke in certain areas may reduce ETS exposure, none of these interventions are effective to eliminate ETS exposure and related health risks.[105]

The WHO recommends the development of clear and simple legislations defining all public premises and workplaces as 100% smoke-free with universal coverage and mandatory compliance. Additionally, affirmative steps must be taken to assure the law is implemented and enforced.[105] Unfortunately, getting this type of ordinance to work for countries, states, or cities is not easy.[131-133] All parties involved in developing and enforcing the regulations must be ready to face strong and steady opposition, especially from the tobacco industry.[105] Tobacco companies are very aggressive in hampering efforts to generate 100% smoke-free environments and systematically avoid attempts to stop smoking bans, either by direct (e.g., manipulation of information) or indirect means, for instance, trough manipulation of a third party, such as the hospitality sector.[134-136]

6. Conclusions

In this chapter we have reviewed the evidence on exposure to ETS in women, children, and workers, and to a certain extent, in race/ethnicity groups. Rather than considering them as "minorities", which they are not from a numerical standpoint, we considered them as "vulnerable groups" from a power imbalance perspective. That means, depending on the social context, these groups are forcefully or involuntarily exposed to ETS, and may lack the power to impose or negotiate the elimination or avoidance of such exposure.

Despite global efforts to control it, ETS exposure is still highly prevalent among children, women, and workers. Due to its chemical properties no safe levels of ETS exist, and even the smallest exposure bears health risks.[137] In children health effects range from death to dysfunctions over the lifetime, such as those produced by respiratory impairment. In women ETS has a large toll on mortality and morbidity, reducing life quality, and producing unnecessary suffering and pain. Although workplaces around the globe are starting to impose smoking bans, a large proportion of workers are still exposed to very high concentrations of ETS, thus increasing health related-risks.

Aside from the health effects on exposed children, ETS exposure in children and adolescents plays a critical role for the reproduction of the tobacco market. Tobacco companies target adolescents and children because they represent a full new wave of potential "costumers". Either by creating biochemical dependence or through introjections of role models learnt from parents or guardians, children exposed to ETS have been observed to have higher odds of active smoking later on in life.[16] Thus, along with marketing efforts to construct behavioral models, such as "cool" or "sexy", firmly attached to smoking, ETS exposure facilitates the initiation of children and adolescents as smokers. Efforts to destroy such media myths and to build healthier role models must be conducted by the society at large, and smoking bans represent very good vehicles for it. Smoking bans not only reduce ETS exposure, they also set a public position towards smoking, and break the social normality and desirability of smoking behaviors.

Although no formal study has been conducted so far to evaluate the effect of womens' or couple's socioeconomic status on the smoking-ban negotiation process at home, data supports that as socioeconomic status increases women are more able to avoid or eliminate ETS exposure from their environments, a reflection of a more equitable distribution of power in the household. In any case, as with other tobacco control policies,[138] women's empowerment represents a milestone to successfully eliminate ETS from homes. Further research is required to understand the inner dynamics of the bargain process to successfully develop smoking bans at home.

Workers exposure to ETS not only has implications on the individual level. ETS has a direct economic impact on business and nations through increased costs from medical attention or loss of productivity.[139-141] In countries with smoking regulations most workplaces are now considered smoke-free. Restaurants and bars constitute an exception – often excluded from the bans. High ETS exposure levels have been regularly recorded in restaurants and bars, constituting a health risk for workers,[8, 99] and costumers.[142]

Tobacco companies have claimed smoking bans in restaurants and bars will have a negative effect on revenues from the sector, and have used this argument to convince hospitality chambers and associations to oppose regulations.[134] However, meta-analysis of the effect of bans on revenues have shown either null or even a positve effect, except in those studies funded by tobacco companies.[143] Recently, developed countries have modified their legislation to ban smoking in restaurants and bars, thereby successfully reducing ETS exposure.[122, 125] A future challenge to develop similar regulations across the globe, and not only in developed countries, lies ahead. Moreover, continuous efforts will be required to expand and maintain smoking bans across the world, facing constant opposition from tobacco companies.

Most estimates of ETS exposure prevalence are quantifications of passive or involuntary smokers, that is, non-smokers who are exposed to ETS. However, this definition does not consider people exposed to ETS because of their own active smoking. Smokers are exposed to ETS, and aside from smoke directly inhaled on each puff, they carry an additional risk that depends on environmental concentrations of smoke.[144] This fact must be divulged among smokers: separating areas, that is reducing areas to create smoking sections without changing ETS generation rates, can only result in even higher health-risks for smokers.[145] Setting aside the observations of reduction in active smoking,[129] smoke-free policies will have a direct impact on smokers' health through the reduction of surrounding ETS levels.

As recognized by the WHO only an integral approach to tobacco control could lead to the elimination of ETS from all environments. Even while focalized interventions could help to reduce exposure, steps taken at higher levels are essential to eliminate ETS: active smoking reduction, increased taxation, elimination of advertisement, and smoking bans are some examples.[7] A fundamental change in the way we conceptualize smoking is required to channel social efforts to control tobacco smoke, i.e. there is more than individual free-will involved in smoking. Smoking is a profitable activity defended at all costs by tobacco companies, and what is disguised as a mainly individual decision is the product of years of research and manipulation of social roles, mass-media, information, and even science to present tobacco as an acceptable and desirable medium. Public discussion must be fostered to unveil health risks concealed by tobacco companies and create awareness on their manipulation of the public opinion. Hopefully, society at large will be able to weight smokers' freedom to smoke against non-smokers' right to attain the best level of health possible, pushing forward a consistent and rational policy to eliminate smoking and ETS.

In the US, racial disparities in exposure to pollution triggered the environmental justice movement, which consistently highlighted the unfairness of contaminants distribution, and more importantly, pushed society to find solutions.[146] Independently of which factor is associated with higher odds of exposure, the unfair distribution of contaminants experienced by individuals, groups, and even nations has a common denominator: power imbalance. Ethnic minorities, poor countries or non-smoking women share a similar profile when it comes to protecting themselves from unfair exposure to pollution: lack of resources, support, voters, money, education or knowledge, among others. Over the societal board vulnerable groups are constantly facing a more resourceful opposite, requiring a structural change, a modification in the balance of power, to alter the state of things. The environmental justice movement is a good example of the collective effort that will be required to equalize risk and exposure among different population groups exposed to ETS, not over the sole basis of a focalized intervention, but over a larger social movement aiming to eliminate exposures and reduce disparities.

References

[1] U.S. Department of Health and Human Services. The health consequences of involuntary exposure to tobacco smoke: A report of the Surgeon General. Atlanta, GA: U.S. Department of Health and Human Services; 2006.

[2] Environmental Protection Agency. *Respiratory Health Effects of Passive Smoking: Lung Cancer and Other Disorders.* US Department of Health and Human Services; 1993.

[3] Repace JL, Lowrey AH. An enforceable indoor air quality standard for environmental tobacco smoke in the workplace. *Risk Anal.* 1993;13:463-475.

[4] World Health Organization. International consultation on environmental tobacco smoke (ETS) and child health. Geneva: World Health Organization. 1999.

[5] Wipfli H, Avila-Tang E, Navas-Acien A, et al. Secondhand smoke exposure among women and children: Evidence from 31 countries. *Am. J. Public Health.* 2008;98:672-679.

[6] Takala J. Introductory report: Decent work-safe work. *16th World Congress on Safety and Health, Vienna, May.* 2002;27.

[7] World Health Organization. WHO framework convention on tobacco control (WHO FCTC). Geneva: World Health Organization; 2003.

[8] Wortley PM, Caraballo RS, Pederson LL, Pechacek TF. Exposure to secondhand smoke in the workplace: Serum cotinine by occupation. *J. Occup. Environ. Med.* 2002;44:503-509.

[9] Navas-Acien A, Peruga A, Breysse P, et al. Secondhand tobacco smoke in public places in Latin America, 2002-2003. *JAMA.* 2004;291:2741-2745.

[10] Corrao MA, Guindon GE, Cokkinides V, Sharma N. Building the evidence base for global tobacco control. *Bull. World Health Organ.* 2000;78:884-890.

[11] Samet JM, Yang G. Passive smoking, women and children. In: Samet JM, Yang G, eds. *Women and the Tobacco Epidemic: Challenges for the 21st Century.* Canada: The World Health Organization; 2001:17-45.

[12] Walsh D, Sorensen G, Leonard L. Gender, health, and cigarette smoking. In: Amick B, :Levine S, Tarlov A, Walsh D, eds. *Society and Health.* Oxford University Press; 1995:131-171.

[13] Gehrman CA, Hovell MF. Protecting children from environmental tobacco smoke (ETS) exposure: A critical review. *Nicotine Tob. Res.* 2003;5:289-301.

[14] Moore RS, Lee JP, Antin TM, Martin SE. Tobacco free workplace policies and low socioeconomic status female bartenders in San Francisco. *J. Epidemiol. Community Health.* 2006;60 Suppl 2:51-56.

[15] The GTSS Collaborative Group. A cross country comparison of exposure to secondhand smoke among youth. *Tob Control.* 2006;Jun;15 Suppl 2:4-19.

[16] MMWR. Exposure to secondhand smoke among students aged 13-15 years worldwide. *JAMA.* 2001;66:4921-4925.

[17] Barrientos-Gutierrez T, Reynales-Shigematsu LM, Avila-Tang E, Wipfli H, Lazcano-Ponce EC. Exposición a humo de tabaco ambiental en hogares de la ciudad de México: Análisis de nicotina ambiental y en cabello de niños y mujeres. *Salud Pública Mex.* 2007;49:S224-S232.

[18] Preston AM, Rodriguez C, Rivera CE, Sahai H. Determinants of environmental tobacco smoke in a population of Puerto Rican children. *Nicotine Tob Res.* 2001;3:61-70.

[19] Blackburn CM, Bonas S, Spencer NJ, Coe CJ, Dolan A, Moy R. Parental smoking and passive smoking in infants: Fathers matter too. *Health Educ. Res.* 2005;20:185-194.

[20] Vardavas CI, Athanasopoulos D, Balomenaki E, Niaounaki D, Linardakis MK, Kafatos AG. Smoking habits of Greek preschool children's parents. *BMC Public Health.* 2007;7:112.

[21] Jurado D, Munoz C, Luna Jde D, Fernandez-Crehuet M. Environmental tobacco smoke exposure in children: Parental perception of smokiness at home and other factors associated with urinary cotinine in preschool children. *J. Expo Anal. Environ. Epidemiol.* 2004;14:330-336.

[22] Bono R, Russo R, Arossa W, Scursatone E, Gilli G. Involuntary exposure to tobacco smoke in adolescents: Urinary cotinine and environmental factors. *Arch Environ. Health.* 1996;51:127-131.

[23] Jordaan ER, Ehrlich RI, Potter P. Environmental tobacco smoke exposure in children: Household and community determinants. *Arch Environ. Health.* 1999;54:319-327.

[24] Ownby DR, Johnson CC, Peterson EL. Passive cigarette smoke exposure of infants: Importance of nonparental sources. *Arch Pediatr Adolesc. Med.* 2000;154:1237-1241.

[25] Mannino DM, Caraballo R, Benowitz N, Repace J. Predictors of cotinine levels in US children: Data from the third national health and nutrition examination survey. *Chest.* 2001;120:718-724.

[26] Scherer G, Kramer U, Meger-Kossien I, et al. Determinants of children's exposure to environmental tobacco smoke (ETS): A study in southern Germany. *J. Expo. Anal. Environ. Epidemiol.* 2004;14:284-292.

[27] Schuster MA, Franke T, Pham CB. Smoking patterns of household members and visitors in homes with children in the United States. *Arch Pediatr. Adolesc. Med.* 2002;156:1094-1100.

[28] Soliman S, Pollack HA, Warner KE. Decrease in the prevalence of environmental tobacco smoke exposure in the home during the 1990s in families with children. *Am. J. Public Health.* 2004;94:314-320.

[29] Knight JM, Eliopoulos C, Klein J, Greenwald M, Koren G. Passive smoking in children. racial differences in systemic exposure to cotinine by hair and urine analysis. *Chest.* 1996;109:446-450.

[30] Wilson SE, Kahn RS, Khoury J, Lanphear BP. Racial differences in exposure to environmental tobacco smoke among children. *Environ Health Perspect.* 2005; 113: 362-367.

[31] Perez-Stable EJ, Herrera B, Jacob P, Benowitz NL. Nicotine metabolism and intake in black and white smokers. *JAMA.* 1998;280:152-156.

[32] Sexton K, Adgate JL, Church TR, et al. Children's exposure to environmental tobacco smoke: Using diverse exposure metrics to document Ethnic/Racial differences. *Environ Health Perspect.* 2004;112:392-397.

[33] Kaneita Y, Yokoyama E, Miyake T, et al. Epidemiological study on passive smoking among Japanese infants and smoking behavior of their respective parents: A nationwide cross-sectional survey. *Prev. Med.* 2006;42:210-217.

[34] Johansson A, Halling A, Hermansson G. Indoor and outdoor smoking: Impact on children's health. *Eur. J. Public Health.* 2003;13:61-66.

[35] Hofhuis W, de Jongste JC, Merkus,P J F M. Adverse health effects of prenatal and postnatal tobacco smoke exposure on children. *Arch Dis. Child* 2003;88:1086-1090.

[36] Windham GC, Eaton A, Hopkins B. Evidence for an association between environmental tobacco smoke exposure and birthweight: A meta-analysis and new data. *Paediatr Perinat. Epidemiol.* 1999;13:35-57.

[37] Hegaard HK, Kjaergaard H, Moller LF, Wachmann H, Ottesen B. The effect of environmental tobacco smoke during pregnancy on birth weight. *Acta Obstet Gynecol. Scand.* 2006;85:675-681.

[38] Ahluwalia IB, Grummer-Strawn L, Scanlon KS. Exposure to environmental tobacco smoke and birth outcome: Increased effects on pregnant women aged 30 years or older. *Am. J. Epidemiol.* 1997;146:42-47.

[39] Anderson HR, Cook DG. Passive smoking and sudden infant death syndrome: Review of the epidemiological evidence. *Thorax.* 1997;52:1003-1009.

[40] Brooke H, Gibson A, Tappin D, Brown H. Case-control study of sudden infant death syndrome in Scotland, 1992-5. *BMJ.* 1997;314:1516-1520.

[41] Adgent MA. Environmental tobacco smoke and sudden infant death syndrome: A review. *Birth Defects Research Part B: Developmental and Reproductive Toxicology.* 2006;77:69-85.

[42] Kum-Nji P, Meloy L, Herrod HG. Environmental tobacco smoke exposure: Prevalence and mechanisms of causation of infections in children. *Pediatrics.* 2006;117:1745-1754.

[43] Cook DG, Strachan DP. Health effects of passive smoking. 3. Parental smoking and prevalence of respiratory symptoms and asthma in school age children. *Thorax.* 1997;52:1081-1094.

[44] Strachan DP, Cook DG. Health effects of passive smoking. 1. Parental smoking and lower respiratory illness in infancy and early childhood. *Thorax.* 1997;52:905-914.

[45] Cook DG, Strachan DP. Health effects of passive smoking. 3. Parental smoking and prevalence of respiratory symptoms and asthma in school age children. *Thorax.* 1997;52:1081-1094.

[46] Stein RT, Holberg CJ, Sherrill D, et al. Influence of parental smoking on respiratory symptoms during the first decade of life: The Tucson children's respiratory study. *Am. J. Epidemiol.* 1999;149:1030-1037.

[47] Li JS, Peat JK, Xuan W, Berry G. Meta-analysis on the association between environmental tobacco smoke (ETS) exposure and the prevalence of lower respiratory tract infection in early childhood. *Pediatr Pulmonol.* 1999;27:5-13.

[48] Strachan DP, Cook DG. Health effects of passive smoking. 6. Parental smoking and childhood asthma: Longitudinal and case-control studies. *Thorax*. 1998;53:204-212.
[49] Cook DG, Strachan DP. Parental smoking, bronchial reactivity and peak flow variability in children. *Thorax*. 1998;53:295-301.
[50] Moshammer H, Hoek G, Luttmann-Gibson H, et al. Parental smoking and lung function in children: An international study. *American Journal of Respiratory and Critical Care Medicine*. 2006;173:1255.
[51] Dezateux C, Stocks J. Lung development and early origins of childhood respiratory illness. *Br. Med. Bull.* 1997;53:40-57.
[52] Willers S, Skarping G, Dalene M, Skerfving S. Urinary cotinine in children and adults during and after semiexperimental exposure to environmental tobacco smoke. *Arch Environ Health*. 1995;50:130-138.
[53] Stocks J, Dezateux C. The effect of parental smoking on lung function and development during infancy. *Respirology* 2003;8:266-285.
[54] Tang D, Warburton D, Tannenbaum SR, et al. Molecular and genetic damage from environmental tobacco smoke in young children. *Cancer Epidemiol. Biomarkers Prev.* 1999;8:427-431.
[55] Hecht SS, Ye M, Carmella SG, et al. Metabolites of a tobacco-specific lung carcinogen in the urine of elementary school-aged children. *Cancer Epidemiol. Biomarkers Prev.* 2001;10:1109-1116.
[56] Aycicek A, Erel O, Kocyigit A. Increased oxidative stress in infants exposed to passive smoking. *Eur. J. Pediatr.* 2005;164:775-778.
[57] Preston AM, Rodriguez C, Rivera CE, Sahai H. Influence of environmental tobacco smoke on vitamin C status in children. *Am. J. Clin. Nutr.* 2003; 77:167-172.
[58] Sasco AJ, Vainio H. From in utero and childhood exposure to parental smoking to childhood cancer: A possible link and the need for action. *Hum. Exp. Toxicol.* 1999; 18:192.
[59] Boffetta P, Tredaniel J, Greco A. Risk of childhood cancer and adult lung cancer after childhood exposure to passive smoke: A meta-analysis. *Environ. Health Perspect.* 2000;108:73-82.
[60] Chang JS, Selvin S, Metayer C, Crouse V, Golembesky A, Buffler PA. Parental smoking and the risk of childhood leukemia. *Am. J. Epidemiol.* 2006;163:1091-1100.
[61] Strachan DP, Cook DG. Health effects of passive smoking. 4. parental smoking, middle ear disease and adenotonsillectomy in children. *Thorax*. 1998;53:50-56.
[62] Mackay J, Eriksen MP. *The Tobacco Atlas*. Geneva: World Health Organization; 2002.
[63] Janson C, Kunzli N, de Marco R, et al. Changes in active and passive smoking in the european community respiratory health survey. *Eur. Respir. J.* 2006;27:517-524.
[64] Curtin F, Morabia A, Bernstein M. Lifetime exposure to environmental tobacco smoke among urban women: Differences by socioeconomic class. *Am. J. Epidemiol.* 1998; 148: 1040-1047.
[65] Kurtz ME, Kurtz JC, Contreras D, Booth C. Knowledge and attitudes of economically disadvantaged women regarding exposure to environmental tobacco smoke: A Michigan, USA study. *Eur. J. Public Health*. 2003;13:171-176.

[66] Chen CM, Lee PH, Chou YH, Kuo SF, Hsu YH. Avoidance of environmental tobacco smoke among pregnant taiwanese women: Knowledge, self-efficacy, and behavior. *J. Womens Health (Larchmt)*. 2007;16:869-878.

[67] Evans D, Fullilove MT, Green L, Levison M. Awareness of environmental risks and protective actions among minority women in northern Manhattan. *Environ. Health Perspect.* 2002;110:271-275.

[68] Scarinci IC, Watson JM, Slawson DL, Klesges RC, Murray DM, Eck-Clemens LH. Socioeconomic status, ethnicity, and environmental tobacco exposure among non-smoking females. *Nicotine Tob. Res.* 2000;2:355-361.

[69] Greaves L, Jategaonkar N. Tobacco policies and vulnerable girls and women: Toward a framework for gender sensitive policy development. *J. Epidemiol. Community Health.* 2006; 60 Suppl 2:57-65.

[70] Pope CA, Xu X. Passive cigarette smoke, coal heating, and respiratory symptoms of nonsmoking women in china. *Environ Health Perspect.* 1993;101:314-316.

[71] Lam TH, Liu J, Hedley AJ, Wong CM, Ong SG. Passive smoking and respiratory symptoms in never smoking women in Hong Kong. In: Slama K, ed. *Tobacco and Health.* New York: Plenum Press; 1995:547-549.

[72] Baker D, Henderson J. Differences between infants and adults in the social aetiology of wheeze. the ALSPAC study team. Avon longitudinal study of pregnancy and childhood. *J. Epidemiol. Community Health.* 1999;53:636-642.

[73] Jindal SK, Jha LK, Gupta D. Bronchial hyper-responsiveness of women with asthma exposed to environmental tobacco smoke. *Indian J. Chest Dis. Allied Sci.* 1999;41:75-82.

[74] Whittemore AS, Perlin SA, DiCiccio Y. Chronic obstructive pulmonary disease in lifelong nonsmokers: Results from NHANES. *Am. J. Public Health.* 1995;85:702-706.

[75] Hirayama T. Non-smoking wives of heavy smokes have a higher risk of lung cancer: A study from Japan. *Bull. World Health Organ.* 2000;78:940-942.

[76] Kalandidi A, Trichopoulos D, Hatzakis A, Tzannes S, Saracci R. Passive smoking and chronic obstructive lung disease. *Lancet.* 1987;2:1325-1326.

[77] Simoni M, Baldacci S, Puntoni R, et al. Respiratory symptoms/diseases and environmental tobacco smoke (ETS) in never smoker Italian women. *Respir. Med.* 2007;101:531-538.

[78] Kurahashi N, Inoue M, Liu Y, et al. Passive smoking and lung cancer in Japanese non-smoking women: A prospective study. *Int. J. Cancer* 2008;122:653.

[79] Lee CH, Ko YC, Goggins W, et al. Lifetime environmental exposure to tobacco smoke and primary lung cancer of non-smoking Taiwanese women. *Int. J. Epidemiol.* 2000;29:224-231.

[80] Yang M, Pyo MY. Molecular epidemiology of lung cancer in female passive smokers. *J Environ Sci Health C Environ. Carcinog Ecotoxicol Rev.* 2005;23:75-97.

[81] Barnoya J, Glantz SA. Cardiovascular effects of secondhand smoke: Nearly as large as smoking. *Circulation* 2005;111:2684-2698.

[82] Hanaoka T, Yamamoto S, Sobue T, Sasaki S, Tsugane S. Active and passive smoking and breast cancer risk in middle-aged japanese women. *Int. J. Cancer* 2005;114:317-322.

[83] Miller MD, Marty MA, Broadwin R, et al. The association between exposure to environmental tobacco smoke and breast cancer: A review by the California environmental protection agency. *Prev. Med.* 2007;44:93-106.

[84] Lee PN, Hamling J. Environmental tobacco smoke exposure and risk of breast cancer in nonsmoking women: A review with meta-analyses. *Inhal. Toxicol.* 2006;18:1053-1070.

[85] Roddam A, Pirie K, Pike M, et al. Active and passive smoking and the risk of breast cancer in women aged 36-45 years: A population based case-control study in the UK. *Br. J. Cancer* 2007;97:434-439.

[86] Sagiv SK, Gaudet MM, Eng SM, et al. Active and passive cigarette smoke and breast cancer survival. *Ann. Epidemiol.* 2007;17:385-393.

[87] Hamajima N, Hirose K, Tajima K, et al. Alcohol, tobacco and breast cancer—collaborative reanalysis of individual data from 53 epidemiological studies, including 58,515 women with breast cancer and 95,067 women without the disease. *Br. J. Cancer* 2002; 87:1234-1245.

[88] Fukuda K, Shibata A. Exposure-response relationships between woodworking, smoking or passive smoking, and squamous cell neoplasms of the maxillary sinus. *Cancer Causes Control* 1990;1:165-168.

[89] He J, Vupputuri S, Allen K, Prerost MR, Hughes J, Whelton PK. Passive smoking and the risk of coronary heart disease--a meta-analysis of epidemiologic studies. *N. Engl. J. Med.* 1999;340:920-926.

[90] Kaur S, Cohen A, Dolor R, Coffman CJ, Bastian LA. The impact of environmental tobacco smoke on women's risk of dying from heart disease: A meta-analysis. *J. Womens Health (Larchmt).* 2004;13:888-897.

[91] Sandler DP, Comstock GW, Helsing KJ, Shore DL. Deaths from all causes in non-smokers who lived with smokers. *Am. J. Public Health* 1989;79:163-167.

[92] Bonita R, Duncan J, Truelsen T, Jackson RT, Beaglehole R. Passive smoking as well as active smoking increases the risk of acute stroke. *Tob. Control.* 1999;8:156-160.

[93] Zhang X, Shu XO, Yang G, et al. Association of passive smoking by husbands with prevalence of stroke among Chinese women nonsmokers. *Am. J. Epidemiol.* 2005;161:213-218.

[94] Law M, Morris J, Wald N. Environmental tobacco smoke exposure and ischaemic heart disease: An evaluation of the evidence. *Br. Med. J.* 1997;315:973-980.

[95] Stillman F, Navas-Acien A, Ma J, et al. Second-hand tobacco smoke in public places in urban and rural china. *Tob. Control.* 2007;16:229-234.

[96] Hammond SK, Sorensen G, Youngstrom R, Ockene JK. Occupational exposure to environmental tobacco smoke. *JAMA* 1995;274:956-960.

[97] Shavers VL, Fagan P, Alexander LA, Clayton R, Doucet J, Baezconde-Garbanati L. Workplace and home smoking restrictions and racial/ethnic variation in the prevalence and intensity of current cigarette smoking among women by poverty status, TUS-CPS 1998-1999 and 2001-2002. *J. Epidemiol.Community Health* 2006;60 Suppl 2:34-43.

[98] Moussa K, Lindstrom M, Ostergren PO. Socioeconomic and demographic differences in exposure to environmental tobacco smoke at work: The Scandia public health survey 2000. *Scand. J. Public Health* 2004;32:194-202.

[99] Siegel M. Involuntary smoking in the restaurant workplace. A review of employee exposure and health effects. *JAMA* 1993;270:490-493.

[100] Bates M, Fawcett J, Dickson S, Berezowski R, Garrett N. Exposure of hospitality workers to environmental tobacco smoke. *Tob. Control* 2002;11:125-129.

[101] Knutsson A, Nilsson T. Tobacco use and exposure to environmental tobacco smoke in relation to certain work characteristics. *Scand. J. Soc. Med.* 1998;26:183-189.

[102] Akbar-Khanzadeh F. Exposure to environmental tobacco smoke in restaurants without separate ventilation systems for smoking and nonsmoking dining areas. *Arch Environ. Health*. 2003;58:97-103.

[103] Cenko C, Pisaniello D, Esterman A. A study of environmental tobacco smoke in south Australian pubs, clubs and cafes. *Int. J. Environ. Health Res*. 2004;14:3-11.

[104] Gee IL, Watson AF, Carrington J, et al. Second-hand smoke levels in UK pubs and bars: Do the English public health white paper proposals go far enough? *J. Public Health (Oxf)*. 2006;28:17-23.

[105] World Health Organization. Policy recommendations on protection from exposure to second-hand tobacco smoke. Geneva:2007.

[106] Edwards R, Hasselholdt CP, Hargreaves K, et al. Levels of second hand smoke in pubs and bars by deprivation and food-serving status: A cross-sectional study from north west england. *BMC Public Health* 2006;6:42.

[107] Goodman P, Agnew M, McCaffrey M, Paul G, Clancy L. Effects of the Irish smoking ban on respiratory health of bar workers and air quality in Dublin pubs. *Am. J. Respir. Crit. Care Med.* 2007.

[108] Skogstad M, Kjærheim K, Fladseth G, et al. Cross shift changes in lung function among bar and restaurant workers before and after implementation of a smoking ban. *Occup. Environ. Med.* 2006;63:482-487.

[109] Steenland K. Risk assessment for heart disease and workplace ETS exposure among nonsmokers. *Environ. Health Perspect.* 1999;107 Suppl 6:859-863.

[110] Stoney CM, Lentino LM, Emmons KM. Environmental tobacco smoke: Association with cardiovascular function at rest and during stress. *Int. J. Behav. Med.* 1998;5:230.

[111] Dietrich DF, Schwartz J, Schindler C, et al. Effects of passive smoking on heart rate variability, heart rate and blood pressure: An observational study. *Int. J. Epidemiol.* 2007; 36:834-840.

[112] Pope III C, Eatough DJ, Gold DR, et al. Acute exposure to environmental tobacco smoke and heart rate variability. *Environ. Health Perspect.* 2001;109:711-716.

[113] Mahmud A, Feely J. Effects of passive smoking on blood pressure and aortic pressure waveform in healthy young adults--influence of gender. *Br. J. Clin. Pharmacol.* 2004; 57: 37-43.

[114] Kato T, Inoue T, Morooka T, Yoshimoto N, Node K. Short-term passive smoking causes endothelial dysfunction via oxidative stress in nonsmokers. *Can. J. Physiol. Pharmacol.* 2006;84:523-529.

[115] Hovell MF, Zakarian JM, Wahlgren DR, Matt GE. Reducing children's exposure to environmental tobacco smoke: The empirical evidence and directions for future research. *Br. Med. J.* 2000;9:40.

[116] Klerman LV. Protecting children: Reducing their environmental tobacco smoke exposure. *Nicotine Tobacco Res*. 2004;6:239-253.

[117] Emmons KM, Wong M, Hammond SK, et al. Intervention and policy issues related to children's exposure to environmental tobacco smoke. *Prev Med*. 2001;32:321-331.

[118] World Health Organization. WHO report on the global tobacco epidemic, 2008: The MPOWER package. Geneva:2008.

[119] Ashley MJ. Smoking in the home: Changing attitudes and current practices. *Am. J. Public Health*. 1998;88:797-800.

[120] Al-Delaimy WK, Crane J, Woodward A. Passive smoking in children: Effect of avoidance strategies, at home as measured by hair nicotine levels. *Arch Environ. Health*. 2001; 56:117-122.

[121] Johansson A, Hermansson G, Ludvigsson J. How should parents protect their children from environmental tobacco-smoke exposure in the home? *Pediatrics* 2004;113:e291-5.

[122] Mulcahy M, Evans DS, Hammond SK, Repace JL, Byrne M. Secondhand smoke exposure and risk following the Irish smoking ban: An assessment of salivary cotinine concentrations in hotel workers and air nicotine levels in bars. *Tob. Control*. 2005; 14: 384-388.

[123] Abrams SM, Mahoney MC, Hyland A, Cummings KM, Davis W, Song L. Early evidence on the effectiveness of clean indoor air legislation in New York State. *Am. J. Public Health* 2006; 96:296-298.

[124] Skeer M, Land ML, Cheng DM, Siegel MB. Smoking in Boston bars before and after a 100% smoke-free regulation: An assessment of early compliance. *J. Public Health Manag. Pract*. 2004; 10:501-507.

[125] Johnsson T, Tuomi T, Riuttala H, Hyvarinen M, Rothberg M, Reijula K. Environmental tobacco smoke in Finnish restaurants and bars before and after smoking restrictions were introduced. *Ann. Occup. Hyg*. 2006; 50:331-341.

[126] Gorini G, Gasparrini A, Fondelli MC, et al. Environmental tobacco smoke (ETS) exposure in Florence hospitality venues before and after the smoking ban in italy. *J. Occup. Environ. Med*. 2005;47:1208-10; author reply 1210.

[127] Eisner MD, Smith AK, Blanc PD. Bartenders'respiratory health after establishment of smoke-free bars and taverns. *JAMA* 1998;280:1909-1914.

[128] Juster HR, Loomis BR, Hinman TM, et al. Declines in hospital admissions for acute myocardial infarction in New York state after implementation of a comprehensive smoking ban. *Am. J. Public Health* 2007;97:2035-2039.

[129] Heloma A, Jaakkola MS. Four-year follow-up of smoke exposure, attitudes and smoking behaviour following enactment of Finland's national smoke-free work-place law. *Addiction*. 2003;98:1111.

[130] Drope J, Bialous SA, Glantz SA. Tobacco industry efforts to present ventilation as an alternative to smoke-free environments in North America. *Tob. Control* 2004;13 Suppl 1:i41-7.

[131] Beaglehole R. Science, advocacy and health policy: Lessons from the New Zealand tobacco wars. *J. Public Health Policy*. 1991;12:175-183.

[132] Cunningham R. *Smoke and Mirrors: The Canadian Tobacco War* Idrc; 1996.

[133] Glantz SA, Balbach ED. *Tobacco War: Inside the California Battles.* University of California Press; 2000.
[134] Dearlove JV, Bialous SA, Glantz SA. Tobacco industry manipulation of the hospitality industry to maintain smoking in public places. *Tob. Control.* 2002;11:94-104.
[135] Muggli ME, Hurt RD, Douglas Blanke D. Science for hire: A tobacco industry strategy to influence public opinion on secondhand smoke. *Nicotine Tobacco Res*. 2003;5:303-314.
[136] Ong EK, Glantz SA. Constructing "sound science" and "good epidemiology": Tobacco, lawyers, and public relations firms. *Am. J. Public Health*. 2001;91:1749-1757.
[137] U.S. Environmental Protection Agency. Respiratory health effects of passive smoking: Lung cancer and other disorders. *Washington, DC: Office of Health and Environmental Assessment.* 1993;93-3606:230-249.
[138] Ernster V, Kaufman N, Nichter M, Samet J, Yoon SY. Women and tobacco: Moving from policy to action. *Bull. World Health Organ*. 2000;78:891-901.
[139] Mannino DM, Siegel M, Rose D, Nkuchia J, Etzel R. Environmental tobacco smoke exposure in the home and worksite and health effects in adults: Results from the 1991 national health interview survey. *Tob. Control* 1997;6:296-305.
[140] McGhee SM, Adab P, Hedley AJ, et al. Passive smoking at work: The short-term cost. *J. Epidemiol. Community Health*. 2000;54:673-676.
[141] Tsai SP, Wen CP, Hu SC, Cheng TY, Huang SJ. Workplace smoking related absenteeism and productivity costs in Taiwan. *Tob. Control* 2005;14 Suppl 1:i33-7.
[142] Lazcano-Ponce E, Benowitz N, Sanchez-Zamorano LM, et al. Secondhand smoke exposure in Mexican discotheques. *Nicotine Tob. Res*. 2007;9:1021-1026.
[143] Scollo M, Lal A, Hyland A, Glantz S. Review of the quality of studies on the economic effects of smoke-free policies on the hospitality industry. *Tob Control*. 2003;12:13-20.
[144] Robinson J. Daily exposure to environmental tobacco smoke: Smokers vs. nonsmokers in California. *Am. J. Public Health* 1996;86:1303-1305.
[145] Siegel M, Husten C, Merritt R, Giovino G, Eriksen M. Effects of separately ventilated smoking lounges on the health of smokers: Is this an appropriate public health policy. *Tob. Control* 1995;4:22-29.
[146] Sexton K, Adgate JL. Looking at environmental justice from an environmental health perspective. *J. Expo Anal. Environ. Epidemiol*. 1999;9:3-8.

Dr. Barrientos-Gutierrez is partially supported by the Fogarty International Center Training Grant (3 D43 TW00644). Dr. Gimeno is supported by a National Institute on Ageing Grant (AG13196). We are thankful to Thuy-Duong Do-Quang for her assisstance in editing this chapter.

In: Topics in Prevalent Diseases
Editors: N. C. Chavez-Tapia and M. Uribe
ISBN 978-1-60456-959-9

Chapter 11

Tuberculosis in Minorities

Ahmet Emin Erbaycu*
Izmir Training and Research Hospital
for Thoracic Medicine and Surgery, Izmir, Turkey

Ethnic Minority

Minority populations may be defined as distinct groups within the general population distinguished from the majority by their racial or ethnic heritage [1].

There is epidemiologic evidence suggesting that minority populations are more susceptible to certain systemic illnesses, especially to diseases that involve the respiratory system. Several studies comparing minority with non-minority populations have reported differences in the incidence and natural history of some diseases including tuberculosis (TB). On the other hand there is a complex interplay of social, economic, behavioral and biologic factors those may cause varying disease patterns in minorities. An effort is required to address the enormous and complex challenge of the increasing burden of respiratory diseases in minorities [1].

There is evidence that there is under-notification of TB. Under-notification leads to an underestimation of the disease burden. This hinders implementation of appropriate prevention and control strategies as a disproportionate number of people who become infected are the most vulnerable in society, and are also groups less likely to be notified, including the poor, the homeless, refugees and ethnic minorities [2, 3].

The incidence of TB is increasing in many industrially developed countries, particularly among the poor, ethnic minorities, prisoners and other institutionalized persons, and the socially isolated groups. The high incidence of TB among ethnic minorities stems principally from the fact that many of them are immigrants from high-incidence countries who arrive in their new countries of residence already infected. Factors such as poverty and overcrowding may be of secondary importance [4,5].

* www.ahmeterbaycu.com, drerbaycu@yahoo.com, 0 232 4333333 / 2363, 0 505 5815631.

The Incidence of Tuberculosis

In 2006, a total of 13,767 TB cases (4.6 per 100,000 population) were reported in the United States (US), representing a 3.2% decline from the 2005 rate. It was noted that foreign-born persons and racial/ethnic minority populations have continued to be affected disproportionately by TB in the US. In 2006, the TB rate among foreign-born persons in the US was 9.5 times that of US-born persons. The TB rates among blacks, Asians, and Hispanics were 8.4, 21.2, and 7.6 times higher than rates among whites, respectively. The decline in the overall national TB rate has slowed in US and the disparities in TB rates between whites and racial/ethnic minority populations thought to threaten progress toward the goal of eliminating TB in the US [6]. The pediatric TB caseload in North Carolina doubled in 2002 compared with the previous several years, Stout et al. reported in a retrospective cohort and cross-sectional study. Transmission among adults in poor communities, including US-born black citizens and a growing immigrant population, will likely contribute to new pediatric cases in the future [7]. Myers et al., in an ecological study of TB transmission in California, in 2006, confirmed that TB in California continues to be a disease of poverty and racial/ethnic minorities [8].

Among US-born persons, the number and rate of TB cases continued to decline in 2006. TB rate was 2.3 per 100,000 population (5,924 or 43.3% of all cases with known origin of birth), representing a 7.0% decline in rate since 2005 and a 68.6% decline since 1993. Among foreign-born persons, the number of TB cases increased in 2006, but the rate decreased. TB rate in 2006 was 21.9 per 100,000 population, representing a 0.5% decline in rate since 2005 and a 35.8% decline since 1993 (Figure-1).

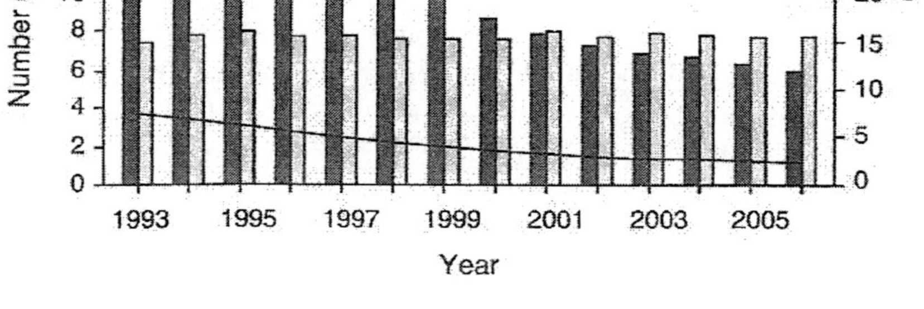

Figure 1. Number of rate of TB cases among US- and foreign-born persons, by year reported – US, 1993-2006 [6].

Table 1. Comparison of sociodemographic risk factors in US-born and foreign-born TB patients [8]

Risk factor	US-born (n=795) (no-%)	Foreign-born All (n=336) (no-%)	Foreign-born Asian (n=131) (no-%)	Foreign-born Hispanic (n=185) (no-%)
Ethnicity				
Black	446 (56.1)	11 (3.3)		
White	222 (27.9)	7 (2.1)		
Hispanic	115 (14.5)	185 (55)		
Asian	7 (0.9)	131 (39)		
Other	5 (0.6)	2 (0.6)		
Age, years				
<18	31 (3.9)	7 (2.1)	4 (3.1)	3 (1.6)
18-24	30 (3.8)	49 (14.6)	14 (10.7)	34 (18.4)
25-34	120 (15.1)	93 (27.7)	33 (25.2)	58 (31.4)
35-44	235 (29.6)	60 (17.9)	13 (9.9)	41 (22.2)
45-54	179 (22.5)	36 (10.7)	16 (12.2)	16 (8.7)
55-64	106 (13.3)	31 (9.2)	15 (11.5)	14 (7.6)
65-74	53 (6.7)	34 (10.1)	17 (13)	14 (7.6)
>75	41 (5.2)	26 (7.7)	19 (14.5)	5 (2.7)
Male	583 (73.3)	203 (60.4)	69 (52.7)	123 (66.5)
HIV seropositive	182 (22.9)	32 (9.5)	1 (0.8)	26 (14.1)
Alcohol use	499 (62.8)	122 (36.3)	33 (25.2)	87 (47)
Illicit drug use	421 (53)[a]	28 (8.3)	3 (2.3)[b]	22 (11.9)
Homelessness	214 (26.9)[c]	15 (4.5)	3 (2.3)	8 (4.3)
Incarceration	143 (18)[c]	3 (0.9)	2 (1.5)	1 (0.5)
High school diploma	413 (52)[c]	124 (36.9)	36 (27.5)[d]	73 (39.5)
Income < $10,000/year	482 (60.6)[a]	182 (54.2)	45 (34.4)[b]	126 (68.1)
Cigarette smoker	623 (78.4)[c]	134 (39.9)	46 (35.1)	77 (41.6)
Contact with known TB patient	309 (38.9)[c]	72 (21.4)	26 (19.8)	42 (22.7)
Travel outside the US in the previous 6 months	17 (2.1)[c]	49 (14.6)	13 (9.9)[d]	33 (17.8)

[a] $p<0.05$, in comparison of US-born and foreign-born patients.
[b] $p<0.01$, in comparison of foreign-born Asian and foreign-born Hispanic patients.
[c] $p<0.01$, in comparison of US-born and foreign-born patients.
[d] $p<0.05$, in comparison of foreign-born Asian and foreign-born Hispanic patients.

The foreign-born to US-born rate ratio increased 7.0%, from 8.9 in 2005 to 9.5 in 2006. 55.6% of TB cases in minorities were reported in persons from five countries: Mexico (1,912), the Philippines (856), Vietnam (630), India (540), and China (376). In summary of the 2006 report, in the US, the annual TB rate has decreased steadily while the rate of decrease has slowed. However, the proportion of TB cases among foreign-born persons has increased each year since 1993. It was concluded that, as the global TB pandemic remains unmitigated, eliminating TB in the US will be increasingly difficult because most foreign-born persons who progress from latent TB infection to TB disease initially became infected with TB abroad [6].

In an analysis of general characteristics of US-born and foreign-born patients with TB; the male to female ratio in black, Hispanic and white ethnic groups varied from 1.8:1 to 4:1. The two groups differed significantly in many TB risk factors. Foreign-born patients were significantly more than US-born patients to be Hispanic or Asian, HIV seronegative, have traveled outside of the US in the six months preceding the onset of TB, and have an annual income >$10,000. They were significantly less likely than US-born patients to use cigarette, alcohol and illicit drugs, to have a history of homelessness or incarceration, have contact with a known TB patient, to have graduated from high school (Table-1) [9].

The TB case rate among foreign-born persons was three to four times that of Spanish-born persons, between 2002 and 2004, in Madrid, Spain. Inigo et al. reported that foreign-born persons were much less likely to be clustered, suggesting a higher percentage of infection before arriving in Spain, that they were likely to be younger than Spanish-born TB patients, and that an extensive transmission between Spanish- and foreign-born populations, caused mainly by autochthonous strains, was taking place in Madrid. It was also marked that foreign-born TB patients less likely to be diagnosed in prison, to use injection drug, to be HIV positive, where there was no difference for homelessness, the incidence of extra-pulmonary TB, resistance to any drug, resistance to isoniazid and gender [10].

The report of active surveillance for TB in Wales, 1996-2003, revealed the mean annual incidence of TB as 2.3 per 100 000 children. Most of the patients were white children, but the proportion among non-white children increased. The greatest increase was seen in black African children, followed by Pakistani children. The authors concluded that cases of TB in black African children are rising even in low incidence areas, and may be associated with school outbreaks (Figure-2) [2].

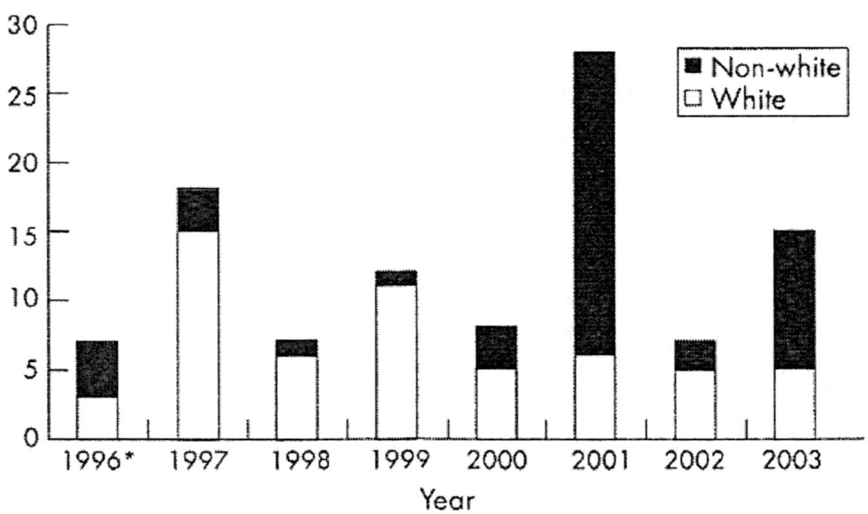

(* Part year).

Figure 2. Number of cases of tuberculosis in children by ethnic group, Wales, 1996-2003 [21].

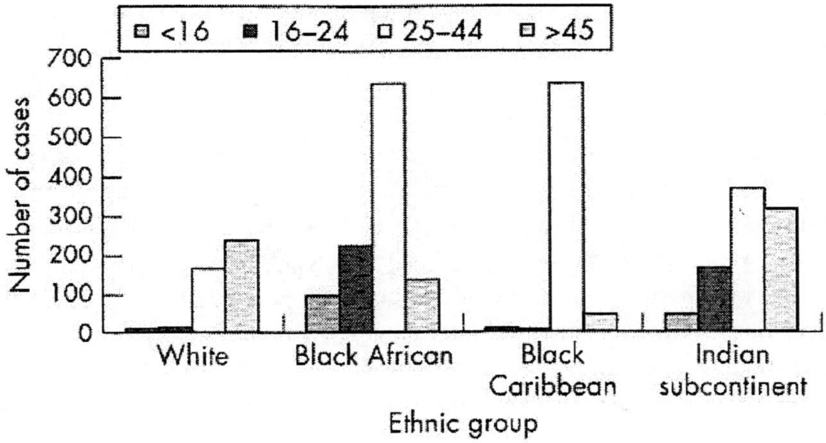

Figure 3. Number of patients with tuberculosis in London by age and ethnic group, 2003 [22].

Bakhshi et al. aimed to describe the epidemiology of TB in Birmingham, United Kingdom (UK), by ethnic group and to evaluate the implications of the findings for future trends in TB in the UK, in 1997. The authors concluded that the different epidemiology of TB in the Caucasian and Asian populations in the UK suggests that from about the second decade of the next century, TB in the UK will almost be entirely a problem of ethnic minorities and that even if new infection was eliminated now in Asian people, cases due to reactivation would continue to occur until the third quarter of the next century [11].

Siddiqi et al. notified, in 2001, that the rising incidence of TB in the UK in the last decade had been attributed mainly to the persistently high TB rates amongst ethnic minority groups. The authors concluded that there was a link between TB and deprivation in South Asian ethnic minority groups in West Yorkshire, the UK [12].

Anderson et al. reported that 75% of patients with TB in London were born abroad, nearly half have lived in the UK for < 5 years, but a third for > 10 years. And 86% were from an ethnic minority group and the incidence is highest in black Africans at 283/100 000 compared with 141, 141 and 8/100 000 for Pakistanis, Indians and whites, respectively. In other words, a third of patients with TB in London are from Africa and nearly a third from the Indian subcontinent. London reflects the worldwide rise in TB, with increasing incidence in ethnic minorities. Most patients were aged 25-44 years while the white population was aged > 45 years. There was a mix of middle and old aged patients in ethnic minorities (Figure-3) [3].

Despite the observation that TB case rates are higher among ethnic minorities, it is believed to be affected by the socioeconomic status (SES). Cantwell *et al.* studied the impact of SES using six indicators: crowding, income, poverty, public assistance, unemployment and education. They reported that SES impacted TB incidence via both a strong direct effect of crowding, manifested predominantly in overcrowded settings, and a TB-SES health gradient, manifested at all SES levels. It was concluded that SES accounted for much of the increased risk of TB previously associated with race/ethnicity [13]. Given the high rates of TB among various subpopulations commonly associated with low SES, the homeless, alcoholics, intravenous drug users, persons who have been incarcerated, and persons living in medically-underserved urban area, persons with TB have long been assumed to be of relatively lower SES than their demographic and geographic counterparts [13-15].

The increased TB incidence in the Netherlands during the last decade was mainly caused by immigration from countries of high TB prevalence [16,17]. In 2003, Hesselink *et al.* reported that 78.6% of all patients with culture-proven TB to be of foreign descent, where the national data of 1985 showed 30% of all TB cases to be of foreign descent [17,18].

The incidence of TB in France, has been stable at around 10/100.000 per year since 1997, Che et al. reported in 2006. Incidence rates of TB vary according to the geographic origin. The rate was highest among the ethnic group of sub-Saharan Africa (166.7/100.000 compared with 5.0/100.000 for those born in France) [19].

Minorities in the US and the foreign-born appear to be at increased risk for extra-pulmonary TB and its association with minority status or birth in a foreign country are even stronger than that for pulmonary TB. In 1986, 17.5% of all US TB cases were extra-pulmonary and 71.2% of these cases occurred among racial/ethnic minorities [20]. In an analysis of TB localization in ethnic groups, pulmonary TB (47%) was the most common presentation (Table-2) [2].

Human Immunodeficiency Virus Infection

Human immunodeficiency virus (HIV) infection is the strongest predictor of progression from latent to active TB with an annual risk of active disease of about 8% [21]. The greater prevalence of HIV infection leads to the greater incidence of TB in some minority groups. This is primarily responsible for the increased rates of TB reported nationally [22].

Table 2. Site of TB disease by ethnic group, Wales, 1996-2003 [21]

Site of TB Disease	White (No.-%)	Indian Subcontinent (No.-%)	Black African (No.-%)	Other (No.-%)	Total (No.-%)
All respiratory	36 (64)	14 (70)	12 (63)	6 (86)	68 (67)
Pulmonary	25 (45)	10 (50)	9 (47)	4 (57)	48 (47)
Intra-thoracic lymph nodes	10 (18)	3 (15)	3 (16)	2 (29)	18 (18)
Pleura	1 (2)	1 (5)	0 (0)	0 (0)	2 (2)
All non-respiratory	15 (27)	2 (10)	4 (21)	0 (0)	21 (21)
Extra-thoracic lymph nodes	4 (7)	1 (5)	2 (11)	0 (0)	7 (7)
Central nervous system	7 (13)	1 (5)	0 (0)	0 (0)	8 (8)
Miliary	2 (4)	0 (0)	1 (5)	0 (0)	3 (3)
Other	2 (4)	0 (0)	1 (5)	0 (0)	3 (3)
Not known	5 (9)	4 (20)	3 (16)	1 (14)	13 (13)
Total	56 (100)	20 (100)	19 (100)	7 (100)	102 (100)

Among socially and culturally marginalized groups, such as minority injection drug users (IDU), the toll on health status is even greater. Hepatitis B virus, HIV infection and acquired immunodeficiency syndrome (AIDS), hepatitis C virus and *Mycobacterium tuberculosis* are endemic in many populations of IDUs throughout the US. They often have co-occurring infections of at least two of these diseases and they are an important transmission link for HIV/AIDS, hepatitis B virus, hepatitis C virus and TB among their sexual partners, their future children and other IDUs. For only two of these diseases, hepatitis B virus and TB, are there efficacious interventions to prevent or cure the disease [23]. Minorities in general, and minority IDUs in particular, have higher death rates from AIDS and more complications from hepatitis B virus, hepatitis C virus and TB than non-Hispanic whites and the drug-free population [24]. In 2000, 2.5% of 16,377 TB cases in the US were among IDUs [25]. Historically, African Americans and other minority groups have had higher incidences of TB and higher mortality from TB than non-Hispanic whites [26,27]. In the mid-1990s, outbreaks of drug-resistant strains of TB were reported among IDUs in New York, San Francisco and San Juan, Puerto Rico [28-30]. Estrada marked the primary problem among IDUs and minorities as the lack of adherence to TB treatments, which increases the probability of multidrug-resistant TB (MDR-TB), increases costs of treatment, and increases morbidity and mortality, especially among people with HIV. He advised two harm reduction strategies that would help reduce high-risk behaviors among minority IDUs, syringe-exchange programs and community-based behavioral interventions [23].

Genetic Structure

Genetic factors may affect the susceptibility to TB, but no specific genes governing susceptibility have been identified [31]. Genetic polymorphisms conferring altered susceptibility or resistance to TB have been documented in various populations. After an epidemic of TB occurred in a community of Aboriginal Canadians between 1987-1989, significant linkage of TB to chromosome 2q35 loci, including NRAMP1 [32]. It was also reported that genetic variation in NRAMP1 affects susceptibility to TB in West Africans [31]. In a study, searching for variation in the vitamin D receptor gene, homozygotes for a polymorphism at codon 352 were significantly underrepresented among those with TB. This genetic variant, which predisposes to low bone mineral density in many populations, may confer resistance to certain infectious diseases [33].

Wilkinson et al. marked the role of dietary factors, notably vegetarianism that affects the serum levels of vitamin D, a vitamin known to be involved in protective immunity in TB. Vitamin D deficiency in a mainly vegetarian Gujarati population in London was associated with an increased risk of active TB and the relation between vitamin D and susceptibility to TB in this ethnic group was affected by genetic factors [34].

Strain Clustering and Drug Resistance

In a population-based, prospective, active surveillance and molecular epidemiology study, Bruyn et al. reported the molecular epidemiologic patterns of TB cases among ethnic minorities in Houston, Texas. 1139 culture-positive patients were enrolled for whom isolates of their culture specimen were available. Of these, 910 were part of an ethnic minority. The authors concluded that factors significantly associated with TB strain clustering were birth in the US, a history of homelessness, infection with the HIV, pulmonary disease, infection with a TB strain from principal genetic group 1 or 3, living in a residence with five or more persons present, and use of public transportation more than once weekly. Ethnicity was not a significant covariate for strain clustering after adjustments for factors related to socio-economic status [35].

In the analysis of 969 TB patients, in the city of Houston, for whom resistance information was available, there was a significantly higher rate of drug resistance among foreign-born (15.4%) than among US-born patients (8.4%). Isolates of foreign-born patients were significantly more likely to be resistant to at least isoniazid (8.6% versus 3%) and to be multidrug resistant (2.4% versus 0.7%) than were isolates cultured from US-born patients [9]. In a New Jersey study, comparing US-born and foreign-born patients, the resistance to isoniazid was 8.3% and 14% where the resistance to isoniazid plus rifampin was 2.7% and 3.6% [36].

The rising international prevalence of MDR-TB raises concerns for importation of such strains and transmission to the local population. In the study, analyzing TB in Houston ethnic minorities, although MDR-TB was most common in Asians, there was no evidence of transmission of MDR strains between foreign-born and US-born patients [35]. In 2005, a total of 124 cases of MDR-TB were reported in the US. It is obvious that MDR-TB continued to disproportionately affect foreign-born persons, who accounted for 101 (81.5%) of 124 MDR-TB cases [6].

In the US, the number of extensively drug-resistant TB (XDR-TB) cases among foreign-born persons did not change, while the percentage increased from 39% (12 cases) in 1993-1999 to 76% (13 cases) in 2000-2006 as the number of XDR-TB cases among US-born cases decreased [37].

Dahle *et al.* described the strain of first outbreak of MDR-TB in Norway originated from abroad, most likely from Somalia, but acquired MDR and spread further within the immigrant population in Norway. This was likely due to deficiencies in the Norwegian TB control system when applied to a population with a different social and ethnic background. The incidence of TB varies greatly between different groups within a society. It appears that contact tracing and TB prevention work may be more efficient if applied differently to these different groups [38].

In an analysis aiming to investigate risk factors associated with resistance to anti-TB drugs in British Columbia, Canada, 10% of the patients with TB were drug-resistant. Significant risk factors for resistance were younger age, foreign birth, ethnicity, reactivated TB and place of initial diagnosis. Foreign-born subjects were three times more likely to present with resistance than Canadian-born ones. Among ethnic groups, Chinese, South-East Asian and Other Asian subjects were 2-4 times more likely to present with resistance than

Caucasians. The authors concluded that the findings on risk factors for resistance have direct implications for TB control programs in industrialized countries where an increased proportion of subjects with TB are foreign-born. Clinicians should consider prescribing a regimen of four drugs as an initial treatment for these high-risk groups until drug susceptibility testing allows a more individual regimen [39].

Sreevatsan et al. described three principal genetic groups of *Mycobacterium tuberculosis* (MTB) on the basis of polymorphisms located at katG codon 463 and gyrA codon 95 [40]. Analysis of isolates from global sources has suggested that principal genetic group 1 organisms are common in many Asian countries, where it is rare in Central and South America. In the study, reported by El Sahly *et al.*, isolates infecting foreign-born patients were significantly more likely to belong to principal genetic group 1 than were isolates of US-born patients [9].

Treatment

Liu et al. evaluated physician prescribing practices in New Jersey for the initial treatment of TB and reported that, although the rate of drug resistance did not differ significantly between non-Hispanic white and non-Hispanic black patients, the former were about twice as likely to be treated with fewer than four drugs as were the latter after adjusting for other potential risk factors. Asians, those had had a high level of isoniazid resistance (17.3%), were also more likely to be treated with fewer than four drugs than were non-Hispanic black patients [36].

Nonadherence to drug therapy of tuberculosis appears to be the main risk factor for the development of drug resistance. Patients those fail to complete therapy are usually homeless or unstably housed. The deterioration of the public health infrastructure is a specific risk factor [41]. Recent immigrants (< 1 year since arrival) appear to have a lower TB treatment completion rate [42].

Wong et al. reported no difference for TB cure rate in Chinese (91.6%) and non-Chinese (87.2%) TB patients [43]. In the Denver study, Asian minorities seemed to have better adherence [44].

Future Strategies

Immigration has an impact on the epidemiological features of TB of the host countries. In many cases, it is difficult to measure this impact because most molecular epidemiology studies are not performed at the time when changes in the patterns of TB due to immigration are occurring [10]. An approach to the reduction of the incidence of TB in immigrants is to screen them on arrival in their new country of residence or in their country of origin before their departure. This strategy, unfortunately, met limited success. It is obvious that no single screening system is likely to be universally successful [4,45]. It is needed to work with international partners, including the Stop TB Partnership, to strengthen TB control in countries with high TB incidence [6]. The public health community needs better tools for targeting socioeconomically disadvantaged communities in a culturally appropriate and supportive way to screen for latent TB infection and TB and to gain acceptance of proven treatment and prevention options [7].

Much of the increased risk of TB among racial/ethnic minorities is due, not to intrinsic genetic differences but rather, to confounding by social and economic factors that increase risk of exposure to TB [13, 14, 46].

With the increased incidence and mortality of TB in minority populations, public awareness campaigns and education programs targeted toward high-risk groups and their health care providers are mandatory to curb this potentially lethal epidemic. Effective use of media, print, and television may disseminate information about TB using community, minority and ethnic sources. Baseline information of these individuals is vital to direct future educational interventions and preventive strategies [47-49]. In a survey analysis in Kansas City Metropolitan area, it was found that 92% of healthy minority population had heard of TB, 43% of them had a little information about TB, where 17% knew nothing and 10% knew a lot. The authors uncovered knowledge deficits about the etiology, transmission and treatment of TB within the inner city, including the lack of appreciation and knowledge that effective treatment of this infection is available [47].

The major concern to decrease TB rate must be to intensify the measures for TB control in these particular groups and the places where the TB transmission occurs [10].

A country needs for a strategy of screening for TB infection and case finding among the foreign-born population in their first contact with the health system. This strategy will allow decreasing incidence rates, but global TB control will be required to advance towards the elimination of the disease [10]. Tuberculosis control and prevention strategies should be mindful of the changing epidemiology and provide information, diagnosis and treatment tailored to the specific needs of the capital and its at-risk groups [3].

References

[1] The National Heart, Lung and Blood Institute Working Group. Respiratory diseases disproportionately affecting minorities. *Chest* 1995; 108: 1380-92.

[2] Fathoala B, Evans MR, Canmpbell IA, Sastry J, Alfaham M. Active surveillance for tuberculosis in Wales: 1996-2003. *Arch Dis. Child* 2006; 91: 900-4.

[3] Anderson SR, Maguire H, Carless J. Tuberculosis in London: a decade and a half of no decline. *Thorax* 2007; 62: 162-7.

[4] Grange J, Story A, Zumla A. Tuberculosis in disadvantaged groups. *Curr. Opin. Pulm Med.* 2001; 7: 160-4.

[5] Hawker JI, Bakhshi SS, Ali S, Farrington CP. Ecological analysis of ethnic differences in relation between tuberculosis and poverty. *Br. Med. J.* 1999; 319: 1031-4.

[6] Centers for Disease Control. Trends in tuberculosis incidence – United States, 2006. *MMWR* 2007; 56 (11): 245-50.

[7] Stout JE, Saharia KK, Nageswaran S, Ahmed A, Hamilton CD. Racial and ethnic disparities in pediatric tuberculosis in North Carolina. *Arch Pediatr Adolesc. Med.* 2006; 160: 631-7.

[8] Myers WP, Westenhouse JL, Flood J, Riley LW. An ecological study of tuberculosis transmission in California. *Am. J. Public health* 2006; 96: 685-90.

[9] El Sahly HM, Adams GJ, Soini H, Teeter L, Musser JM, Graviss EA. Epidemiologic differences between United States – and foreign-born tuberculosis patients in Houston, Texas. *J. Infect Dis.* 2001; 183: 461-8.

[10] Inigo J, de Viedma DG, Arce A, Palenque E, Rodriguez NA, Rodriguez E, Serrano MJR, Andres S, Bouza E, Chaves F. Analysis of changes in recent tuberculosis transmission patterns after a sharp increase in immigration. *J. Clin. Microbiol.* 2007; 45: 63-9.

[11] Bakhshi SS, Hawker J, Ali S. The epidemiology of tuberculosis by ethnic group in Birmingham and its implications for future trends in tuberculosis in the UK. *Ethn. Health* 1997; 2: 147-53.

[12] Siddiqi K, Barnes H, Williams R. Tuberculosis and poverty in the ethnic minority population of West Yorkshire: an ecological study. *Commun. Dis. Public health* 2001; 4: 242-6.

[13] Cantwell MF, McKenna MT, McCray E, Onorato IM. Tuberculosis and race/ethnicity in the United States: Impact of socioeconomic status. *Am. J. Respir. Crit. Care Med.* 1998; 157: 1016-20.

[14] Comstock GW, Cauthen GM. Epidemiology of tuberculosis. In: Reichman LB, Hershfield E, editors. Tuberculosis: A Comprehensive International Approach. Marcel Dekker, New York, 1992; 23-48.

[15] Centers for Disease Control and Prevention. Screening for tuberculosis infection in high-risk populations and the use of preventive therapy for tuberculosis infection in the United States. *MMWR* 1990; 39: 1-12.

[16] Broekmans JF, Herwaarden CLA van. De behandeling van tuberculose: korter en krachtiger. Ned Tijdschr Geneeskd 1996; 140: 2160-3.

[17] Index tuberculosis 1998. The Hague: The Royal Netherlands Tuberculosis Association, 1999.

[18] Hesselink DA, Yoo SM, Verhoeven GT, Brouwers JW, Smit FJ, van Saase JLCM. A high prevalence of culture-positive extrapulmonary tuberculosis in a large Dutch teaching hospital. *Netherlands J. Medicine* 2003; 61: 65-70.

[19] Che D, Bitar D, Desenclos JC. Epidemiology of tuberculosis in France. *Presse Med.* 2006; 35: 1725-32.

[20] Rieder HL, Snider DE Jr, Cauthen GM. Extrapulmonary TB in the US. *Am. Rev. Respir. Dis.* 1990; 141: 347-53.

[21] Selwyn PA, Hartel D, Lewis VA, Schoenbaum EE, Vermund SH, Klein RS, Walker AT, Friedland GH. A prospective study of the risk of tuberculosis among intravenous drug users with human immunodeficiency virus infection. *N Engl. J. Med.* 1989; 320: 545-50.

[22] Centers for Disease Control. Tuberculosis morbidity in the United States, 1990; final data. *MMWR* 1992; 40: 23-8.

[23] Estrada AL. Epidemiology of HIV/AIDS, hepatitis B, hepatitis C, and tuberculosis among minority injection drug users. *Public Health Rep.* 2002; 117: S126-134.

[24] Murrain M. Differential survival in blacks and Hispanics with AIDS. *Ethn. Health* 1996; 1: 373-82.

[25] Centers for Disease Control and Prevention. Reported tuberculosis in the United States, 2000. Atlanta (GA): National Center for HIV, STD and TB Prevention, Division of Tuberculosis Elimination; Reviewed January 28, 2002. Available from: URL: http:// www.cdc.gov/tb/surv/surv2000/default.htm.

[26] Sumaya CV. Major infectious diseases causing excess morbidity in the Hispanic population. *Arch Intern. Med.* 1991; 151: 1513-20.

[27] McBride D. Tuberculosis in African-American and minority populations: historic epidemiology of a nonclassic contagious process. *J. Assoc. Academ. Minor. Phys.* 1994; 5: 11-5.

[28] Friedman CR, Quinn GC, Kreiswirth BN, Perlman DC, Salomon N, Schluger N, et al. Widespread dissemination of a drug-susceptible strain of Mycobacterium tuberculosis. *J. Infect Dis.* 1997; 176: 478-84.

[29] Reyes JC, Robles RR, Colon HM, Marrero CA, Castillo X, Melendez M. *Mycobacterium tuberculosis* infection among crack and injection drug users in San Juan, Puerto Rico. *Puerto Rico Health Sci. J.* 1996; 15: 233-6.

[30] Frieden TR, Sterling T, Pablos-Mendez A, Kilburn JO, Cauthen GM, Dooley SW. The emergence of drug-resistant tuberculosis in New York City. *N Engl. J. Med.* 1993; 328: 521-6.

[31] Bellamy R, Ruwende C, Corrah T, McAdam KP, Whittle HC, Hill AV. Variations in the NRAMP1 gene and susceptibility to tuberculosis in West Africans. *N Engl. J. Med.* 1998; 338: 640-4.

[32] Greenwood CM, Fujiwara TM, Boothroyd LJ, Miller MA, Frappier D, Fanning EA, Schurr E, Morgan K. Linkage of tuberculosis to chromosome 2q35 loci, including NRAMP1, in a large aboriginal Canadian family. *Am. J. Hum. Genet.* 2000; 67: 405-16.

[33] Bellamy R, Ruwende C, Corrah T, McAdam KP, Thursz M, Whittle HC, Hill AV. Tuberculosis and chronic hepatitis B virus infection in Africans and variation in the vitamin D receptor gene. *J. Infect Dis.* 1999; 179: 721-4.

[34] Wilkinson RJ, Llewelyn M, Toossi Z, Patel P, Pasvol G, Lalvani A, Wright D, Latif M, Davidson RN. Influence of vitamin D deficiency and vitamin D receptor polymorphisms on tuberculosis among Gujarati Asians in west London: a case-control study. *Lancet* 2000; 355: 618-21.

[35] De Bruyn G, Adams GJ, Teeter LD, Soini H, Musser JM, Graviss EA. The contribution of ethnicity to *Mycobacterium tuberculosis* strain clustering. *Int. J. Tuberc. Lung Dis.* 2001; 5: 633-41.

[36] Liu Z, Shilkret KL, Finelli L. Initial drug regimens for the treatment of tuberculosis. Evaluation of physician prescribing practices in New Jersey, 1994 to 1995. *Chest* 1998; 113: 1446-51.

[37] Centers for Disease Control. Extensively drug-resistant tuberculosis – United States, 1993-2006. *MMWR* 2007; 56 (11): 250-3.

[38] Dahle UR, Sandven P, Heldal E, Mannsaaker T, Caugant DA. Deciphering an outbreak of drug-resistant Mycobacterium tuberculosis. *J. Clin. Microbiol.* 2003; 41: 67-72.

[39] Moniruzzaman A, Elwood RK, Schulzer M, Fitzgerald JM. A population-based study of risk factors for drug-resistant TB in British Columbia. *Int. J. Tuberc. Lung Dis.* 2006; 10: 631-8.
[40] Sreevatsan S, Pan X, Stockbauer KE, Connell ND, Kreiswirth BN, Whittam TS, Musser JM. Restricted structural gene polymorphism in the *Mycobacterium tuberculosis* complex indicates evolutionarily recent global dissemination. *Proc. Natl. Acad. Sci. USA* 1997; 94: 9869-74.
[41] Brudney K, Dobkin J. A tale of two cities: tuberculosis control in Nicaragua and New York City. *Semin. Respir. Infect* 1991; 6: 261-72.
[42] Abubakar I, Crofts JP, Gelb D, Story A, Andrews N, Watson JM. Investigating urban-rural disparities in tuberculosis treatment outcome in England and Wales. *Epidemiol. Infect* 2008; 136: 122-7.
[43] Wong MY, Leung CC, Tam CM, Lee SN. Directly observed treatment of tuberculosis in Hong Kong. *Int. J. Tuberc. Lung Dis.* 2005; 9: 443-9.
[44] Burman WJ, Cohn DL, Rietmeijer CA, Judson FN, Sbarbaro JA, Reves RR. Noncompliance with directly observed therapy for tuberculosis: epidemiology and effect on the outcome of treatment. *Chest* 1997; 111: 1168-73.
[45] Melzer M, Storring RA, Bagg LR. Tuberculosis in an area bordering east London: significant local variations when compared to national data. Infection 2000; 28: 103-5.
[46] Long ER. Constitution and related factors in resistance to tuberculosis. *Arch Pathol.* 1941; 32: 122-62.
[47] Marinac JS, Willsie SK, McBride D, Hamburger SC. Knowledge of tuberculosis in high-risk populations: survey of inner city minorities. *Int. J. Tuberc. Lung Dis.* 1998; 2: 804-10.
[48] Centers for Disease Control and Prevention. Prevention and control of tuberculosis in US communities with at-risk minority populations and prevention and control of tuberculosis among homeless persons. *MMWR* 1992; 41: 1-23.
[49] Klein SJ, Naizby BE. New linkages for tuberculosis prevention and control in New York City: Innovative use of non-traditional providers to enhance completion of therapy. *J. Community Health* 1995; 20: 5-13.

In: Topics in Prevalent Diseases
Editors: N. C. Chavez-Tapia and M. Uribe
ISBN 978-1-60456-959-9

Chapter 12

Parasitic Diseases of Infants

B.R. Mirdha and *Nishat Ahmad
Department of Microbiology,
*Department of Obstetrics and Gynaecology
All India Institute of Medical Sciences, New Delhi-110029, India

The burden of diseases and injury attributed to under nutrition, poor water supply, poor sanitation and inadequate personal and domestic hygiene accounts for almost 23% of the disability-adjusted life years (DALYs) from all causes world-wide and for 26% of DALYs in developing regions. [1] In addition, the upsurge of infectious disesases and the emergence of new ones also add to the burden. International initiatives are mostly targeted towards diseases that cause increased mortality such as HIV/AIDS, Malaria, tuberculosis and some vaccine preventable diseases. However, there is a strong need to focus attention on controlling other diseases that have public health importance. Among the infectious vector-borne diseases, malaria continues to be worsen in many areas and there are now an estimated 300 million to 500 million cases of malaria world wide each year with 2 million to 4 million deaths. In similar context, about 25% of world population is infected with round worm, 20% with hookworm, 17% with whipworm and 3% to 4% with schistosome [2]. Infection by soil transmitted helminthiasis has been increasingly recognized as an important public health problem, particularly in developing countries. Total of three soil transmitted infection (*Ascaris lumbricoides*, Hook worm and *Trichuris trichiura*) and schistosomiasis is 43.5 million life years lost, which is second only to tuberculosis (46.5 million) and well ahead of malaria (34.5 million) and measles (34.1 million) [3]. These parasitic infection are associated with malnutrition and impaired growth and development (due to decrease appetite, nutrient loss, malabsorption and decreased nutrient utilization), iron deficiency anaemia, decreased physical fitness and work capacity and impaired cognitive function.[4] However, what has happened over the past 25 years is the recognition that these helminthic infections that have serious health consequences. The formal recognition of the health consequences of worm infestation came in May 2001 when the 54th World Health Assembly passed a resolution affirming that the control of soil-transmitted helminthiasis should be considered as a public health priority.

More than two billion people world-wide suffer from parasitic infections. As far as can be determined, there are over 1,000 species of parasites that can infect humans. Humans play host to more than 130 different kinds of parasites, ranging from microscopic protozoal organisms to sizeable macroscopic tapeworms. Projections for the year 2025 suggest that more than half of the 8.3 billion people on earth at that time will be infected with at least one parasitic disease. Furthermore, some parasites can remain in the body for more than thirty years. This was proven when World War II Prisoner's of War (POW)'s were examined thirty years later. It was found that 15% were still infected with *Strongyloides* acquired during war period. More recently, when more than 500,000 American troops returned from Desert Storm, they were told not to donate blood because they had been exposed to *Leishmania.* Without question, thousands of Vietnam's war veterans are still suffering from undiagnosed parasitic infections. Parasites causing human infections are from four large phyla in the animal kingdom, namely, Protozoa (of the kingdom Protista), the Platyhelminthes (flatworms), the Nematodes (roundworms), and the Arthropoda (arachnids, crustaceans, insects, etc.). Parasites are organisms which live in or on another living organism called a "host" benefiting in some way at the host's expense, particularly in their plunder of nutrients. A host will suffer some degree of damage, ranging from slight discomfort to death. Parasites are much more complex than viruses and bacteria because their individual reproductive cycle makes it difficult to formulate an accurate diagnosis to many complaints.

Humans become hosts to parasites in several ways:

1. Via infected food or water
2. Via insect vectors: (mosquitoes---filariasis and malaria), (fleas---dog tapeworm), (houseflies--- Intestinal amoebiasis), and the (sandfly---leishmaniasis). Close contact with animals significantly increases the likelihood of parasite infections especially in children.
3. Via sexual contact: Trichomoniasis, Giardia, and amoebas.
4. Via penetration of skin and by inhalation: Hookworms; Ascaris Ova and oocysts of *Toxoplasma gondii* can be inhaled from contaminated dust.

Limiting the idea that disease-causing parasites are found only in tropics and sub-tropics is dangerously idealistic. Widespread travel, immigration, pollution, increased use of day cares and other institutional settings, increased popularity of household pets, the indiscriminate use of antibiotics and other immunosuppressive drugs, multiple sex partners with expanding anal/oral practices, and a general rise in population has seen to it that almost all people can now expect to be faced with the possibility of harboring at least one parasite at some point in their lives. Secondly, parasitic diseases, whether vector borne, food-borne, water borne or soil transmitted tend to affect certain vulnerable groups, such as children and the women of child bearing age [5]. Other vulnerable groups in the society are indigenous populations and minority ethnic groups, infants and pre-school children, the elderly, those with physical limitations and immunocompromised people who can be highly burdened with certain parasitic diseases. Among young children, infants are also vulnerable to many parasitic diseases. In the first year and a half of life, an infant needs at least 7 or more medical visits to accomplish all of the preventive services and assessments recommended. As an example, infants are vulnerable to malaria from the age of approximately three months, when immunity acquired from the mother is wearing off. Hospital series studies showed that in areas of intense malaria transmission, most cases of severe malaria anaemia and death occur in infants [6]. In addition, infants infected with HIV and malaria are at particular risk of anaemia during the first year of life [7]. Interestingly, studies have shown that exposure to infection like toxoplasmosis may be a risk factor for development of schrizophrenia, changes in personality and symptoms of psychosis including delusions and auditory hallucinations [8].

Infections at different times at one's life have different impact on the intensity of morbidity, mortality in strict medical terms. In addition, many infections have its impact on overall development, social and economic impact. In this context, infections affecting the infant are often clinically inapparent, subtle presentation and are difficult to diagnose and interpret. Because abnormalities may only become obvious as the child develops and fails to achieve desired developmental growth. It is of paramount importance to examine thoroughly and carefully to infants because parasitic diseases of infants are often neglected except for established/important diseases. Relative immaturity of the immune system is often the cause of increased risk of infection in infants. Infections in infants can be broadly classified into - congenital infection (infection *in -utero*) and infection acquired during infancy.

So vast is the field of human parasitology so many and far-reaching discoveries made, that it is not possible to do justice to the whole subject. Additionally, parasites, such as worms, are unusual in infants until they reach the toddler stage when they can and do put anything and everything into their mouths. Infants in most countries are breast-fed for most of their early months and thus, have little or no exposure to parasites. Thus, parasitic infections are relatively uncommon in the child less than 12 months old. However, institution-raised children have very different exposures. They are fed formula made with water, often live in very crowded circumstances with children of varying ages and are often weaned to solid foods at younger ages than breast-fed babies. All such children are at risk for intestinal parasites. The scope of this article encompasses diseases of parasitic origin in infants. The incidence of infectious diseases due to parasites among infants has been extrapolated from various studies.

Toxoplasmosis

Toxoplasmosis refers to the disease state that result from infection with the obligate protozoan parasite, *Toxoplasma gondi (T.gondii)*. *T.gondii* is a coccidian protozoa that is ubiquitous in nature, and the cat is the definitive host. The organism exists in three different forms i.e (i) an oocyst, in which sporozoites are formed within the intestinal tract of the cat and is shed in feces, (ii) a tachyzoite, that is the proliferative form and was formerly referred to as trophozoite. Tachyzoites are metabolically active and can proliferate rapidly in all mammalian cell types. They are the pathogenic stage of the parasite and are susceptible to both immune surveillance and killing by physical and pharmacological agents. Lastly, (iii) a tissue cyst that has an intra-cystic form termed as bradyzoite. Non-feline mammals or birds ingest infective oocysts from the contaminated soil. Tissue cysts then accumulate in the organs and skeletal muscle of these animals. The possible routes of transmission from animal to human are direct contact with cat feces, ingestion of undercooked meat containing infective oocysts, and ingestion of fruits or vegetables that have been in contaminated soil. Reactivation of toxoplasmosis is another important mechanism of infection in the immunocompromised host and also in the congenitally infected infant. Congenital infection results from placental infection and subsequent hematogenous spread to the fetus.

Toxoplasmosis is distributed worldwide. High prevalence of infection has been documented in Europe, Central America, and parts of Africa. However, sero-prevalence rates differ considerably from one country to another, from one region of a country to another, and even from one ethnic group to another in the same region. These widely disparate sero-prevalence rates among different populations throughout the world have been explained by differences in eating habits and sanitation practices that contribute to acquisition of infection. Among women of child-bearing age in the United States of America, the prevalence of antibody to *T. gondii* varies from approximately 3% to 30%, depending on the region of the country [9,10]. Toxoplasmosis of 3 to 10 per live births have been reported in Paris and Vienna, where maternal sero-prevalence rates of about 70% and 40% respectively have been observed.[11]

Congenital Toxoplasmosis

Infection of the fetus occurs as a consequence of maternal primary infection during pregnancy or, rarely, just before conception [12]. Reactivation of latent *Toxoplasma* infection during pregnancy does not lead to fetal infection except among immunocompromised women such as those infected with human immunodeficiency virus (HIV).[13,10] In addition, maternal re-infection may result in congenital toxoplasmosis. [14] Acute maternal infection which is usually acquired early in pregnancy may lead to fulminant fetal infection resulting in stillbirth, non-immune fetal hydrops, pre-term birth, and perinatal death. [15] On the other hand, chronic toxoplasma infection rarely has been associated with sporadic abortion. [16] Infection of the fetus occurs transplacentally during maternal parasitaemia. Placental infection is an important intermediary step, and up to 16 weeks may elapse between placental infection and subsequent infection of the fetus. This time lag has been termed as the prenatal incubation period. [10] Congenital toxoplasmosis has also occurred in twins and triplets. [17] In monozygotic twins, the clinical manifestations are usually similar, whereas in dizygotic twins, discrepancies in clinical findings are common.

Approximately 40% of infants born to mothers who acquired toxoplasmosis during pregnancy are infected with *T.gondii.* The rate of vertical transmission varies according to the trimester in which the mother is infected and fetal infection rates increases as pregnancy advances. Specifically, when maternal infection occurs in the first trimester, 15% of infants are infected, whereas maternal infection in the second and third trimesters results in transmission rates of 30% and 60%, respectively. The severity of clinical manifestation is greatest, however, when maternal infection is acquired early in pregnancy. Maternal infection in the first trimester results in severe disease in as many as 40% of infected fetuses, and in stillbirth or peri-natal death in an additional 35% of infants. Only about 15% of newborns have sub-clinical disease. However, maternal infection in the third trimester is rarely if ever associated with severe fetal disease or stillbirth, and about 90% of infants in such situations have sub-clinical infection. When a pregnant woman acquires *T.gondii*, tachyzoites are spread haematogenously to the placenta. The organism can then be spread transplacentally directly to the fetus during gestation or at birth. It is possible that differences in rates of transmission during gestation depend on placental size, virulence of the organism and genetic difference of the host in susceptibility.

The majority of newborns with congenital toxoplasmosis lack clinical signs of infection. This could probably because, infants frequently show specific immunologic tolerance in perinatal period.[10,18] However, thorough evaluation may demonstrate eye or neurologic abnormalities in about 20% of cases. Clinically apparent disease is present in only about 10% to 25% of infected infants.[11,19] The clinical manifestations of toxoplasmosis are often indistinguishable from those seen with other congenital infections, such as congenital cytomegalovirus infection and congenital syphilis. Approximately one third of infants present with generalized form of the disease that principally involves organs of the reticulo-endothelial system. The abnormalities include hepatosplenomegaly, jaundice, pneumonitis, generalized lymphadenopathy, rash, chorioretinitis, anaemia, thrombocytopenia, eosinophilia, and abnormal cerebrospinal fluid (CSF) indices.[12,20] The other two thirds of infected infants principally manifest neurologic disease.

Central nervous system(CNS) involvement is the hallmark of congenital *Toxoplasma* infection. Chorioretinitis, intracranial calcifications, and hydrocephalus are the most characteristic findings, occurring in approximately 86%, 37% and 20% of symptomatic infants, respectively.[2,10] This constellation of findings has been referred to as the "classic triad" of congenital toxoplasmosis. Chorioretinitis secondary to congenital toxoplasmosis can manifest at any stage. Regardless of age at diagnosis, most chorioretinitis due to toxoplasmosis is a consequence of congenital infection. It usually manifests as strabismus in infants, and in older children, defects in visual acuity are more common. Typically, the eye lesion consists of a focal necrotizing retinitis that is often bilateral with involvement of the macula and even the optic nerve. Complications include blindness, iridocyclitis, and cataracts. Intracranial calcifications may be single or multiple but typically are generalized and located in the caudate nucleus, choroid plexus, meninges, and sub-ependyma.[13, 21] They are visualized best by computed tomography (CT) but are often detected on ultrasonography as well. Intracranial calcifications may resolve with appropriate antimicrobial therapy. Hydrocephalus may be the only manifestation of disease. Microcephaly, when present, indicates severe brain injury. *T.gondii* has been detected in the inner ear and mastoid, with the associated inflammation resulting in deafness. Ascending flaccid paralysis with myelitis has also been reported. [14, 22]

Other, less common manifestations of congenital toxoplasmosis are nonimmune hydrops fetalis, myocarditis, nephritic syndrome, and immunoglobulin abnormalities with both hypergrammaglobulinemia and hypogammaglobulinemia have been described. A variety of endocrine abnormalities may occur, including hypothyroidism, diabetes insipidus [15, 23], precocious puberty and growth hormonendeficiency. The prognosis of congenital toxoplasmosis is much better than before because infants with infection but without disease manifestation can be diagnosed by ante-natal diagnosis and thereafter administration of specific treatment may avoid the fatal outcome.

Congenital toxoplasmosis should be suspected in any infant with symptoms or signs that have been mentioned in clinical presentation. If congenital toxoplasmosis is suspected, a fundoscopic examination and CT scan should be performed, because chorioretinitis and cerebral calcifications are frequently present in symptomatic illness.

Isolation of *T. gondii* from body fluids and tissues provides definitive evidence of infection. The organism can be isolated from placenta, amniotic fluid, fetal blood obtained by cordocentesis, umbilical cord blood, infant's peripheral blood, and from CSF by means of intraperitoneal and subcutaneous inoculation into laboratory mice.[16,24] Mouse inoculation may require as long as 4 to 6 weeks for demonstration of the parasite. Although it is not a practical method, isolation of the organism should be attempted whenever possible. It is usually performed at Reference Laboratory. In addition, tissue culture has been used to isolate *T. gondii* from amniotic fluid. Histopathologic examination of the placenta as well as tissues obtained at postmortem examination or by biopsy from stillborns or infants should also be performed because the specimens may demonstrate the presence of tachyzoites. Serologic assays for measurment of antibodies to *T. gondii* in serum and body fluids are the most widely used methods of diagnosing congenital toxoplasmosis.[25, 26] Serologic methods are most commonly used for confirming the diagnosis of *Toxoplasma* infection . The presence of Ig M antibodies to *Toxoplasma* in the infant's blood or CSF is diagnostic of congenital infection. IgM antibodies may be detected by the indirect immunofluorescence antibody (IFA) test or Enzyme Linked Immunosorbent Assay (ELISA). The IgM antibodies appear in the first week of infection and peak at approximately 1 month. These antibodies persist for several months to over 1 year. Diagnosis of congenital toxoplasmosis by IgG antibody requires serial measurements of the antibody titre over the first several months of life: therefore, this method of diagnosis does not allow for prompt institution of appropriate therapy. Transplacentally acquired IgG antibodies persists upto 12 months or longer, however, in the absence of infection, the antibody titer usually decreases by the second or third month of life. The IFA and ELISA tests are widely available, and when performed in an appropriate reference laboratory. Tests that detect *T. gondii* - specific IgM are (1) the double sandwich IgM ELISA, which has a sensitivity of 75% to 80% and a specificity of 100% [16], (2) the IgM immunosorbent agglutination assay (ISAGA), which is the most sensitive test but should not be performed on umbilical cord blood, because even small quantities of maternal IgM antibodies contaminating the specimen will yield a false-positive result [27] and (3) the IgM immunofluorescent antibody test. The last test is not recommended because it has both a much lower sensitivity than either the IgM ELISA or IgM immunosorbent agglutination assay and poor specificity secondary to rheumatoid factors and anti-nuclear antibodies, contributing to false-positive results. An additional assay that may assist in ruling out maternal infection acquired in the first 3 months of pregnancy is the IgG avidity test performed by the ELISA technique. This test is based on the principle that although the antibody-binding avidity or affinity for an antigen is initially low after primary antigenic stimulation, IgG antibodies that are present from previous antigenic stimulation are usually of high avidity. Therefore, a high avidity result in the first trimester would exclude an infection acquired in the previous 12 weeks. Because the majority of adults with acquired *Toxoplasma* infection are asymptomatic, evaluation of the pregnant woman and newborn is usually prompted by either seroconversion or an elevated maternal *Toxoplasma* IgG titer. [28, 29] The latter may reflect chronic or past infection, so the accuracy of the maternal infection is determined serologically. If recent maternal infection is documented by seroconversion or rising IgG antibody titers, the fetus should be evaluated by ultrasonography, and amniotic fluid should be tested for specific toxoplasma DNA with polymerase chain reaction (PCR). Postnatally, serologic testing of paired maternal and infant sera should be performed at a reliable laboratory that will include assays for *Toxoplasma* IgG and IgM antibodies. Neonatal serum for *Toxoplasma* IgA determination by ELISA also should be considered because it may yield the only positive result in some infants.

PCR analysis has been used successfully to detect *Toxoplasma* DNA in amniotic fluid, placenta, CSF, brain tissue, urine, and fetal and infant blood. PCR performed on amniotic fluid obtained by amniocentesis has become one of the preferred methods of confirming *in-utero* infection.False-negative results have been reported, however, and inter-laboratory variability in performance of PCR assays has been documented.PCR performed on neonatal CSF is recommended for the evaluation of possible central nervous system involvement.[30, 31]

The presence of neonatal IgM antibody in serum or CSF, or a positive PCR result for blood or CSF indicates congenital infection. In addition, at risk infants should undergo serologic follow-up to detect rising serum IgG titers during the first year of life or persistence of IgG antibody beyond 12 to 15 months of age, when maternal IgG antibody has disappeared.[32] Uninfected infants show a continuous decline in *Toxoplasma* IgG titer with no detectable IgM or IgA antibodies.

Low IgG titers that indicate remote maternal infection do not require further evaluation of the mother or infant unless the mother is infected with HIV. Because fetal infection do occur during chronic *Toxoplasma* infection in HIV-infected pregnant women, their infants should be evaluated serologically at birth for evidence of congenital infection. It has been suggested that HIV-infected pregnant women who have low CD4+ T lymphocyte counts and who are seropositive for *Toxoplasma* antibody should receive prophylaxis to prevent fetal infection.[33, 34] Nevertheless, if such women previously have had toxoplasma encephalitis, prophylaxis with pyrimethamine, sulfadiazine, and leucovorin (folinic acid) should be considered.[35]

It is currently recommended that fetuses and infants who are infected with *T. gondii* receive specific therapy effective against this pathogen, even if they have no clinical signs of disease. On the basis of comparison with untreated historic controls, outcome is improved substantially by maternal, fetal, and neonatal treatment. Spiramycin has been used in pregnant women with acute toxoplasmosis to reduce transplacental transmission of *T. gondii.* If fetal infection is confirmed after the 17th week of pregnancy, however, treatment with pyrimethamine, sulfadiazine, and folinic acid is recommended. Prenatal treatment of congenital toxoplasmosis reduces the clinical severity of infection in the newborn while shifting the disease to a more sub-clinical form. This effect in turn may ameliorate the long-term neurologic complications that are commonly seen among infants who have clinical manifestations in the neonatal period. Neonatal treatment has also resulted in reductions in sensorineural hearing loss and neurodevelopmental and visual handicaps. In infants with congenital toxoplasmosis, the treatment consists of pyrimethamine, sulfadiazine, and folinic acids. [36] The actual duration of therapy is not known, although prolonged courses, at least 1 year, are preferred. Most experts recommend combined treatment until the patient is one year old. [10] Complete blood cell counts and platelet determination must be monitored closely while the patient is receiving therapy. Current therapies are not effective against encysted bradyzoites and therefore may not prevent reactivation.

Among infants born with congenital toxoplasmosis, the mortality rate has been reported to be as high as 12%. In addition, infants with congenital toxoplasmosis are at high risk for ophthalmologic, neurodevelopmental, and audiologic impairments, including mental retardation (87%), seizures (82%), spasticity and palsies (71%), and deafness (15%). [36, 37] Neonatal screening for IgM antibody has also been advocated so that asymptomatic infants can be detected and treated before neurologic symptoms develop.

Malaria

An estimated 3 billion people, almost half of the world's population live in areas where malaria transmission occurs and malaria is endemic in 107 countries and territories in tropical and subtropical regions. The human toll of malaria is staggering between 350 million and 500 million epoisodes of clinical malaria each year leading to an estimated 1 million death, most in sub-Saharan Africa. [38] Malaria is one of the leading killers of children under age five, accounting for almost 1 death in 10 (8%) world-wide and nearly 1 death in 5 (18%) in sub-Saharan Africa. [39] Some 50 million pregnant women a year are exposed to malaria-at least 60% of them in Africa. [40]

Of the four species of human malaria, *Plasmodium vivax* (*P. vivax*) has the widest distribution, but *P. falciparum* tends to predominate in tropical areas. Infections with *P. malariae* and *P. ovale* have restricted distribution. Malaria spread to humans by the bite of female anopheline mosquitoes. After the bite of the mosquito, sporozoites are injected into the bloodstream but are cleared within half an hour. The parasites mature in the parenchymal cells of the liver and form mature schizonts, which contains 7500 to 40,000 merozoites depending on the species. The release of the merozoites results in the appearance of the ring stage in erythrocytes in the peripheral blood. Within hours, the parasite assumes an amoeboid asexual form and is referred to as a trophozoite. The sexual form is called gametocyte. In infections with *P. vivax, P. malariae* and *P. ovale*, all forms are seen in the peripheral blood from early ring forms through mature schizonts and gametocytes. In infections with *P. falciparum,* usually only rings and gametocytes are found in the peripheral blood. In addition to trasmission by the bite of mosquitoes, malaria can be transmitted by transfusion of blood products.

In infants, this has occurred after simple transfusion as well as after exchange transfusion [41, 42]. Malaria parasites survive in blood for weeks. Relapse due to malaria can occur from *P. vivax* for up to 2 years and rarely for up to 4 years. Relapses from *P. malariae* have occasionally occurred. Malaria may also be transmitted by syringes and needles and can spread by this route among heroin addicts. Infection in heroin addicts who become pregnant can result in congenital infections [43].

In highly endemic areas of stable malaria transmission, where infection is common, the population can develop some immunity. However, in these areas children and pregnant women are at greater risk of developing severe symptoms and dying from malaria. Whereas in areas of low, epidemic or unstable malaria transmission, few people can have some natural immunity and thus adults are also at risk of becoming seriously ill with malaria. In cases of stable malaria, most adult women develop natural immunity that makes infection due to malaria asymptomatic. In such situation the main impact of malaria infection is malaria-related anaemia in the mother and the presence of parasites in the placenta, contributing to low-birth weight, a leading cause of impaired development and infant mortality. [44] Children under age five are most likely to suffer from severe effects of malaria because they have insufficient naturally acquired immunity to the parasite. A severe infection can kill a child within hours.[45]

Placental Malaria

The pathophysiology of the malaria infected placenta is caused by accumulation of parasitized erythrocytes within the intervillous spaces. [46] Placental infected erythrocytes are a distinct parasite form that binds to chondroitin sulfate A (CSA) on syncitiotrophoblast and inner villous spaces. Placental infected erythrocytes do not adhere to CD36, a ubiquitous receptor on the microvasculature endothelium that commonly supports adhesion of infected erythrocytes from non-pregnant individuals. Adhesion to CSA allows parasites to sequester in the placenta, where dense accumulation can often occur with little or no parasitaemia detectable in the peripheral blood. Because CSA binding parasites do not commonly infect non-pregnant women as they lack immunity to this parasites form prior to the first pregnancy. [47] Finding by Stevenson *et al.* suggest that placental malaria decreases susceptibility in the offspring of primigravida and increases susceptibility in the offspring of multigravida. Among primigravida, the pronounced inflammatory response to placental malaria could confer protection for example by reducing parasitaemia and thereby preventing congenital transmission. [47] Alternately, sensitization of the fetal or neonatal immune system may be modulating immunity in a way that modifies susceptibility to parasitaemia such as inducing regulating T (Treg cells) which have been related to malaria susceptibility in rodents. Inflammatory signals inhibit the development of T regulatory cells and the inflammatory responses are common in primigravida but not in multi-gravida Women with placental malaria could lead to different effects of sensitization in their offspring. [48,49] Direct destruction of placental syncytium can alter placental integrity allowing parasitized erythrocytes to enter the feto-maternal unit and perhaps establish route for congenital transfer. [50]

Bruce-Chwatt [50] found that when the placenta was infected, infant weight at birth was an average of 145 g less than the weight of infants born to women with uninfected placentas. Similarly, Archibald [51] found infant weight at birth to be 170 g less. In 1925, Blacklock and Gordon [52] noted that 35% of infants born to mothers with infected placentas died within the first 7 days of life, whereas only 5% of those born to mothers with uninfected placentas died during this period. In 1958, Cannon [53] found that the mortality among infants was 6.9% for those whose mothers' placentas were infected compared with 3.4% for those whose mothers' placentas were uninfected, suggesting that malaria has an important influence on birth weight as well as on infant survival. Malaria therefore contributes to fetal loss, still birth, prematurity and neonatal death.

Effect of Malaria during Pregnancy

Malaria during pregnancy is estimated to cause tens of thousands or hundred of thousands of infant death each year. These estimates are extrapolated from the incidence of malaria-related outcome such as low birth weight, maternal anaemia that increases infant mortality risk. [54] Malaria during pregnancy reduces birth weight, and low birth weight is a major determinant of infant mortality. Luxemburger et al.[55] estimated the impact of malaria during pregnancy on infant mortality in Karen population living in Thailand. Between 1993 and 1996, a cohort of 1,495 mothers and their infants were followed weekly from admission of the mother to antenatal clinics until one year. Both falciparum malaria and vivax malaria during pregnancy were associated with low birth weight. The other major adverse effect of malaria in pregnancy on the mother was anaemia. Malaria causes anaemia through haemolysis and increased splenic clearance of infected and uninfected erythrocytes and cytokine induced dyserythropoeisis. In malarious areas, malaria and anemia are likely to act together to reduce birth weight. Their independent effects are difficult to distinguish. In a study conducted in a highly malarious area of Papua New Guinea, severe maternal anaemia was associated with low birth weight in primigravidae, whereas there was no obvious consistent association between parasite positivity and low birth weight. [56]

Premature birth results commonly from symptomatic malaria and is usual in severe malaria. In sub-Saharan Africa where malarial transmission is generally much higher and maternal malaria is rarely associated with symptoms, two studies have demonstrated that there were different consequences on the newborn infant, depending on the timing of infection. Parasitaemia in the antenatal period was associated with intrauterine growth retardation, whereas cord blood parasitaemia, probably reflecting a recent active infection, was associated with premature birth.[57, 58] It is further estimated that in sub-Saharan Africa up to 35% of preventable low birth weight is the result of placental malaria. [59] Both the density and the prevalence of parsitaemia are increased in pregnant women compared with women who are not pregnant but who reside in the same geographic area. For *P. falciparum*, Campbell et al. found a parasite density of 6896 per mm^3 in pregnant women and 3808 per mm^3 in non-pregnant women; for *P. vivax,* the parasite density was 3564 per mm^3 for pregnant women. The prevalence as well as the density of the parasitaemia decreased with increasing parity. [60]

Infants who have parasites demonstrable in their cord blood appear to be more severely affected than those who do not have parasitaemia at the time of delivery. Recent studies from Kenya using PCR have indicated that cord blood samples showed PCR prevalence of 32%, 23% and 21% for *P.falciparum, P.malariae* and *P. ovale* respectively. The reported cord blood parasitaemia in Kenya was 10.4%. These findings indicate that cord blood infections are common in sub-Saharan Africa.However, the presence of discordant malaria parasite strain between maternal and cord samples in 57% indicate that cord malaria parasites were acquired antenatally by transplacental transmission of infected erythrocytes.[61,62]

Influence of Maternal Antibody on Risk of Infection

Antimalarial antibodies are transferred from the mother to the infant. The prevalence of precipitating antibody to *P. falciparum* within 24 hours of birth in Gambia was 87% in newborns and 87.5% in their mothers. The prevalence of antibody in these newborns reflected the extent to which malaria had been controlled in the area in which their mothers lived. In infants born in the provinces with more malaria, 97% had antibodies to malaria. Antibodies decrease in the period from birth to 25 weeks of age, subsequently, as a result of postnatal acquisition of infection, endogenous antibody synthesis begins and antibody levels rise. [63] Infants less than 3 months of age have a lower than expected incidence of clinical disease, death from malaria and parasitaemia. This has been attributed to a variety of factors. However, the two most important causes are probably the fact that the level of serologic immunity is high at this age and that fetal hemoglobin is present in the circulating red blood cells. [65] Sehgal et al. [64] studied the role humoral immunity in acquired malaria infection among newborns in Papua New Guinea. Among 104 newborns in their study, there was a 3.8 per cent incidence of congenital malaria, and a cumulative incidence of acquired malaria of 3 per cent at 12 weeks and 38% by 48 weeks of age. Ninety per cent of infants lost maternal antibody between 4 and 7 months, and the majority of asymptomatic malaria occurred among infants with detectable malaria antibody. The rise in prevalence of parasitaemia corresponded with a fall in the amount of fetal hemoglobin in the red blood cells. [66] The fact that cells containing fetal hemoglobin are poor hosts for the malarial parasite and had been previously suggested as one of the reasons for the selective advantage of sickle cell anaemia and sickle cell trait in areas in which malaria is endemic.

Congenital Malaria

There has been no consistently accepted definition of congenital malaria. Some have taken the position that parasites must be demonstrable in the peripheral blood of the infant during the first day of life; while others have accepted cases that were confirmed within the first 7 days of life. [67] In areas in which malaria is endemic, infants are exposed to mosquitoes and may become infected by this route at a very young age. Thus, it may be difficult to distinguish congenital cases from acquired cases. However, a sufficient number of cases of congenital possibility of postnatal transmission, to establish the fact that the clinical onset of disease in a congenitally infected infant can be delayed for weeks or rarely even for months. [42]

Clinical congenital malaria was described before Laveran discovered the malaria parasite itself. [69] Women and their foetus remain at particularly high risk of malaria-attributable morbidity. Each year, an estimated 75,000-200,000 infants die as a direct result of pregnanacy associated malaria. In a recent study in Thailand at least 210 cases of malaria in infants have been reported. [70] Singh et al. [71] carried out a study in women and infants aged 15 days to 8 months in Central India and were successfully followed–up. Malarial infection was recorded in 218 infants. Infection with *P.vivax* was common amongst infants. No clinical symptoms were reported in infants aged less than or equal to 3 months. Some of the Infants with *P.falciparum* infection had fatal outcome. Malaria during first few months of life may be due to transplacental transfer of parasitized maternal erythrocytes. Although IgG and IgM antimalarial antibodies can be detected in maternal blood, only IgG antibodies are present in the infant's blood. These antibodies can delay and modify the onset of clinical manifestations. Congenital malaria can be acquired by transmission of parasites from mother to child during pregnancy or perinataly during labour. [59] Studies, however, suggest that incidence of congenital malaria has increased and values between 0.3 to 33% have been observed from both endemic and non-endemic areas. Although placental infections with *P. falciparum* have been described [72], the role of other species especially *P. vivax*, which exists in good proportion in some countries, is not known. In a study conducted in Central India, although 2.2% women were placenta positive for *P. vivax* or mixed infection, but none of the infants developed parasitaemia up to 6 months of age. [72] Congenital malaria in *P. vivax* has been described from Sri Lanka, Italy, Singapore and Thailand. [73-77]

Despite massive involvement of the placenta, it is generally agreed that clinically apparent congenital infections are rare in areas where malaria is endemic and levels of maternal immunity are high. Covell reviewed cases of congenital malaria that had been reported up to 1950 and estimated the incidence at 16 (0.3%) infections per 5324 live births. For women having an over attack of malaria during pregnancy, the rate of congenital infection was higher and was estimated to be 1 to 4%. [64] Congenital malaria is more common in infants of women who have immigrated to areas in which malaria is endemic than in women who have been raised to maturity in such areas because their levels of immunity are lower than those of the native population. Conversely, congenital malaria is also more common among women who immigrate from areas in which malaria is endemic to areas that are free of malaria. Loss of immunity results from lack of frequent exposure. Although rare, congenital malaria may also occur as a result of maternal infection by chloroquine-resistant *P. falciparum*. A number of reported cases of chloroquine-resistant congenital malaria in Africa and Indonesia responded to treatment with intravenous quinine. [78, 79]

Clinical Presentation

It has been reported that clinical symptoms are rarer in younger infants and absence of febrile episodes has been described. This has been attributed to transplacentally acquired antibodies (IgG), which confer transient protection to infant and thus manifestations are mild. Although IgG and IgM antimalarial antibodies can be detected in maternal blood, only IgG is normally found in the infant's blood. Asymptomatic presentation has also been described. [71] Children with congenital malaria can present with fever, irritability, feeding problems, hepato-splenomegaly, anaemia and jaundice. A case of congenital malaria is reported in a six weeks old male infant who presented with irritability, decreased feeding and jaundice for four days. [78] The most common clinical findings in cases of congenital malaria are fever, anaemia and splenomegaly, which are present in more than 80% of cases. The anaemia, which may be accompanied by pallor, is associated with a reticulocytosis in about half of the cases. Jaundice and hyperbilirubinemia are found in about a third of the cases. Either the direct or the indirect bilirubin may be elevated, depending on whether liver dysfunction or hemolysis is the most important process in an individual case. Hepatomegaly also may be present but is less common than splenomegaly. Nonspecific findings include failure to thrive, poor feeding, regurgitation and loose stools. In developing countries, when malaria occurs during the first few months of life, it is frequently complicated by other illnesses such as pneumonia, septicemia and diarrhoea.

As the findings in infants are non-specific, the clinical distinction from other congenital infection rests primarily on the absence of a skin rash and a maternal history of exposure to malaria. The detection of malaria parasites in the infant's blood is essential for diagnosis, although blood smears can be negative if there are low parasite count (<50/µl blood). It has also been considered that three repeated smears over 48 hours should be reported negative before excluding the diagnosis. [68]

Chagas' Disease

Chagas' disease, also known as American sleeping sickness, is caused by infection with protozoan *Trypanosoma cruzi*. The illness is endemic in Mexico, Central America and South America. It is estimated that 15 to 16 million people are infected with *T. cruzi* in Latin America and 75 to 90 million people are exposed to infection. When *T. cruzi* is transmitted to man through the feces of triatomes, at bite sites or in mucosa, through blood transfusion or orally through contaminated food, it invades the bloodstream and lymphatic system and becomes established in the muscle and cardiac tissue, the digestive system and phagocytic cells. The other mechanisms for transmitting Chagas' infection can be primarily due to handling infected animals, organ transplantation and laboratory accidents. [80, 81]. This causes inflammatory lesions and immune responses, particularly mediated by CD4+, CD8+, interleukin-2 (IL-2) and IL-4, with cell and neuron destruction and fibrosis, and leads to blockage of the cardiac conduction system, arrhythmia, cardiac insufficiency, aperistalsis, and dilatation of hollow viscera, particularly the esophagus and colon. Fever, general lymphadenopathy, edema, hepatosplenomegaly, myocarditis, and meningoencephalitis are observed in severe cases. This is followed by chronic phase. Most of the cases present as indeterminate form (asymptomatic, with normal results from electrocardiogram and x-ray of the heart, esophagus, and colon), which may involve either cardiac or digestive form (megaesophagus and megacolon), or cardiac and digestive forms together. There is great regional variation in the morbidity due to Chagas' disease, and severe cardiac or digestive forms may occur in 10 to 50% of the cases, or the indeterminate form in the other asymptomatic cases, but with positive serology. Several acute cases have been reported from the Amazon region, most of them by *T. cruzi*. The infection may become reactivated such that it spreads as a severe disease causing diffuse myocarditis and lesions of the central nervous system. Approximately five percent of patients, usually young children and immunocompromised – develop a fatal infection. The so-called congenital form mentioned earlier may also occur, by means of transmission across the placenta or through the birth canal during deliverey, and this may give rise to abortion, prematurity or organic lesions in the fetus. [83, 84] The prognosis for Chagas' disease may also be very poor in the congenital form, which may lead not only to abortion and prematurity but also to organic lesions in the liver, spleen, heart and central nervous system with neurological sequelae and mental deficiency. Many cases may be asymptomatic and remain in the indeterminate form. The congenital form of Chagas' disease seems to occur solely in pregnant women who have a lesion in the placenta that favors penetration by *T. cruzi* as far as the chorionic villi, where amastigote forms multiply (probably in Hofbauer cells) and subsequently invade the fetal circulation.

The congenital transmission of Chagas' disease was evaluated in 57 pregnant women with Chagas' disease and their 58 offspring in three hospitals in São Paulo City. The transmission of Chagas' disease at fetal level was confirmed in three (5.17%) of the 58 cases studied and one probable case of congenital Chagas' disease. Two infected infants were born to chagasic women with HIV infection and were diagnosed by parasitological assays in both the cases placenta revealed *T. cruzi* and HIV p24 antigen were detected by immunohistochemistry. The Western blot method using trypomastigote excreted/secreted antigens of *T. cruzi* was positive for IgG antibodies in 54/55 newborns and for IgM in 1/55 newborns. One of the two newborns with circulating parasites had however, no detectable IgG or IgM antibodies. The analysis showed a linear correlation between maternal and newborn IgG antibody titers at birth. [85]

Prevalence of antibodies against *T. cruzi* in puerperal women were assessed to study possible congenital transmission of Chagas' disease in Peru. The overall prevalence of Chagas' disease in the 3000 puerperal women studied was only 0.73%. No cases of intrauterine congenital transmission were found. However, it has been recommended that studies on prenatal detection should be carried out to evaluate possible congenital transmission of Chaga's infection. However, the estimates in Argentina of congenital cases are at least 10 times more frequent than the acute cases by vector transmission. [85, 86] Several experimental studies have been done in an attempt to determine the possible mechanisms involved in congenital transmission, taking into account that only 2 to 10% of infected mothers transmitted the infection to their babies. [87, 88] Determining causes of congenital diseases such as parasitic factors, such as the strain of *T. cruzi* or the parasitic load, and about host factors, such as immunological or nutritional status of pregnant women, obstetrical history and maternal stage of disease but none of these factors have yet been conclusively demonstrated. The incidence of congenital transmission has always been determined in women during the indeterminate or chronic period of infection [89]. During these phases of the disease, the parasitaemia is low and recurrent, undetectable by direct parasitological methods and only detectable in some cases by xenodiagnosis or hemoculture. There are few previous reports on acute infection of pregnant woman. In fact, Rassi et al. [90] in Brazil in 1958, reported a case, subsequently reviewed by Brabin. [91] Three cases of congenital transmission were studied by Moya et al.[89]. It is interesting to note that in both non-infected cases the maternal infection took place during the third trimester of pregnancy, while in the case in which the newborn was infected, the infection occurred in the earlier period of pregnancy. The finding suggests that the time of infection could be a risk factor for *T. cruzi* transmission during the acute infection of the mother. Diagnosis of infection is made by clinical, epidemiological and parasitological parameters. The parasitological methods used were the microhematocrit centrifuge technique, Strout and hemocultures, essentially performed as previously described. The classical serological methods (ELISA, indirect immunofluorescence and indirect hemagglutination) were performed for immunodiagnosis. For histological examination, the placental tissue is stained with hematoxylin-eosin and examined. The following microscopic alterations are observed in the placenta i.e. granulomatous changes, inflammatory infiltrates and focal necrosis in the chorionic villi. The fibrinoid layer was thicker in some modified villi in which syncytial modifications such as edema and calcification foci were present. Vascular thromboses were also seen.[92]

Leishmaniasis

Leishmaniasis, a protozoal disease is transmitted by the bite of some species of sandflies (*Phlebotomus* and *Lutzomyia* species) and affects various age groups depending on the infecting Leishmania species, geographic location, disease reservoir, and host immunocompetence. Leishmaniasis is seen in almost all parts of the world with the only exception of Australia and Antarctica. The prevalence is the highest in central and South America, Southern Europe, Central Africa and parts of southern and central Asia. [93] In the human host, *Leishmania* are intra-cellular parasites that infect the mononuclear phagocytes. The extent and presentation of the disease depend on several factors, including the humoral and cell-mediated immune response of the host, the virulence of the infecting species, and the parasite burden. Pathogenesis appears related to T-cell cytotoxicity, and control of disease depends on the magnitude of T helper 1 and multiple cytokine responses early in the course of infection. During progressive *Leishmania* infection in mice, Th2-type CD4 T cells expand and secrete interleukin-4, resulting in polyclonal B-cell activation. [94] Current data indicate that susceptibility to leishmaniasis is genetically determined. [95] In cutaneous leishmaniasis (CL), the amastigotes replicate in the dermis and do not spread beyond the site of the vector's bite. The lesion often heals spontaneously. In visceral leishmaniasis (VL), the amastigotes replicate in macrophages of the mononuclear phagocyte system and then spread to the entire reticuloendothelial system, resulting in "kala-azar" or they replicate and spread in the naso-oropharyngeal mucosa, resulting in mucocutaneous leishmaniasis (ML). Children are at greater risk than adults in endemic areas. Malnutrition contributes to the development of disease, and incomplete therapy of initial disease is a risk factor for recurrence of leishmaniasis. Children usually present with intermittent fever, anaemia, weight loss, and abdominal distension. Splenomegaly, hepatomegaly, lymph node enlargement. Thrombocytopenia, anaemia, leucopenia and hypergammaglobulinemia are the most common findings. [96] In developing countries, malnourished children are extremely susceptible to develop progressive infection. In these areas, the disease has an insidious onset with pyrexia, which is continuous or remittent and becomes intermittent at a later stage. Occasionally, the disease may present with an acute onset. Children presenting later in the course of the disease may demonstrate oedema caused by hypoalbuminemia, haemorrhage due to thrombocytopenia or growth failure related to the presence of chronic infection. [97] VL is endemic in tropical and sub-tropical areas including the Mediterranean basin. The vast majority of cases are recorded in the Indian subcontinent, East Africa and northeastern Brazil, where *L. donovani* and *L. infantum* are the main aetiological agents. Occasional non-vector transmissions have been reported through blood transfusions, sexual intercourse, organ transplants, excrements of dogs, and sporadic cases outside the endemic areas.

Recently, visceral leishmaniasis has received increasing attention, as a result of the parasite emerging as an opportunistic pathogen among HIV-infected patients[96.] VL is a chronic parasitic infection that infects approximately 400,000 individuals annually, with a predilection towards early childhood. Three epidemiological forms affecting children have been recognised. In India and Brazil where an animal reservoir has not been identified, VL is found in all age groups. This epidemiological form was first described in India, and is known as the Indian type of visceral leishmaniasis. In this form of the disease, children between 5 and 15 years of age are affected. *L. donovani* is the predominant parasite of this form of Leishmaniasis in India while, in the New World, the disease is predominantly caused by *L. chagasi*. In areas with animal reservoirs, such as the Mediterranean Basin, VL mainly affects children of 1 to 4 years of age; it is caused mainly by *L. infantum*, transmitted by phlebotomine sandflies, and dogs are the most important reservoir. The African type of VL is again caused by *L. infantum* affecting older children and young adults and rodents are the reservoir hosts. Prospective studies in northeastern Brazil have shown that approximately 12% of infected children develop typical VL. It has been reported that the median age at diagnosis of Mediterranean VL is less than 3 years and infants are frequently affected. Typical VL usually occurs after an incubation period, which can vary widely from 2 weeks to 8 months (usually 2-6 months), depending on the patient's age and immune status, and the species of *Leishmania*. [95]

Intermittent fever, pallor, refusal to feed or anorexia, weight loss, abdominal distension, cough, vomiting and diarrhoea are the commonest presenting complaints. Massive splenomegaly was almost universally encountered in this study population. Hepatomegaly, lymph node enlargement and ecchymoses or gingival bleeding are the other common manifestations noted on physical examination. Certain unusual manifestations in the form of tachycardia, cardiac murmur, petechiae or ecchymoses, and jaundice are also seen in children in different studies. [98,99] Skin lesions and mucosal lesions in the mouth and nose although rare have been described. Rare manifestations of VL include haemophagocytic syndrome, acute hepatitis, cholecystitis, and Guillain-Barré syndrome. Also, post–kala azar CL has been reported from India. [96] It is said to occur in approximately 10% of cases after the treatment of VL. Lesions can develop as late as 1-2 years after treatment for the original disease and manifest on the face, trunk or extremities, and may persist for as long as 20 years. In Africa, it has been reported that dermal lesions occur in only 2% of cases.

Skin lesions are the hallmark of CL and these skin lesions heal spontaneously within 2-10 months. In ML, known as *espundia* in South America, mucosal ulcerations usually develop by metastasis rather than by local spread, and causes disfiguring lesions over the face. It destroys the mucous membranes of the nose, mouth, and throat. Secondary infection plays a prominent role in the size and persistence of these ulcers. Children are rarely affected and the progression of the disease is slow and steady but it carries a significant mortality rate [95].

Congenital Leishmaniasis

Vertical transmission of leishmaniasis is possible and the institution of treatment is imperative in cases of pregnant women with kala-azar. During pregnancy the disease is life-threatening for the mother and may have consequences for the fetus. Symptomatic or asymptomatic mother with Leishmania infection may get reactivated by pregnancy, and then congenitally transmitted to the child. Cases of infantile VL have been reported since 1950. [100] Subsequently, various indigenous cases of infantile kala-azar have also been reported from India, [99] Britain, [100] Brazil.[101,104] Report of infantile VL kala-azar contracted during visits to leishmania endemic geographical area have been reported from many developed countries like Sweden [102] and Germany. [103] Cases of American VL also have affected most under-five urban children with overall mortality of 9.2% to 21.2%. Mortality was related to low age, signs of severe disease and concomitant infection. [106] Between 1989 and 1998, fifty patients from rural areas of Palestine with VL were studied. Forty-nine (98%) were younger than 6 years old, the youngest being 9 months. The findings indicate that an active focus of potentially fatal VL exits in the Jenin district of the West Bank follows the pattern of a predominantly infantile disease. [105] In Tunisia, CL was studied in 166 children with age ranging from 5 months to 15 years. Leishmaniasis affected grown-up children in 74.5 percent of the total cases. Involvement of face was in 76.5 percent of cases and mucosal leishmaniasis was present in 9 children (6.8%). [106] Similar report from specific geographic area in Italy was considered to be probably responsible for infantile leishmaniasis has been described. [107]

In children, however, definite diagnosis of VL relies on the demonstration of Leishmania in tissue specimens (bone marrow, or splenic aspirates or peripheral blood) or tissue culture. Microscopy of bone marrow aspirates is the safest diagnostic approach for paediatric patients, with amastigotes seen in more than 90% of cases by an experienced observer. Repeated sampling, however, may be required. In adult patients, bone marrow microscopy is less sensitive (~70%). The higher diagnostic efficacy of the bone marrow examination in children is probably related to the heavier parasitisation encountered in children. Microscopic examination of splenic aspirates offers the highest sensitivity (up to 98%), but is associated with the risk of life-threatening haemorrhage in cases with profound thrombocytopenia. In immunocompetent individuals, serological assays (direct agglutination, enzyme-linked immunosorbent assay, and indirect immunofluorescence) are considered to be sensitive for the diagnosis of visceral leishmaniasis. A strip test employing the recombinant K39 antigen of *L. chagasi* has been developed. This strip test has a sensitivity of 100% and a specificity of 98% among patients tested in India. However, in a study from Sudan, which compared the use of the recombinant K39 strip test with that of the recombinant K39 enzyme-linked immunosorbent assay and the direct agglutination test, the former gave limited sensitivity [67% versus 100%, and 91% (at > 1:1600 cut-off) respectively]. The interpretation of serological results is complicated by high titres observed for months or years after successful treatment and in cases of asymptomatic infection. Moreover, serological tests are positive in only half of HIV infected patients with Leishmaniasis. [108] Over the past 5 years, the value of polymerase chain reaction (PCR) for the diagnosis of VL has been assessed using different clinical specimens (peripheral blood, bone marrow, and spleen). The detection of persistent parasite DNA in infected tissues by means of PCR may also be used as a marker for the risk of relapse after initial cure. Currently, PCR should be regarded as a promising tool, with the potential advantage of using blood specimens rather than the conventional invasive procedures such as splenic aspirate, bone marrow aspiration and liver biopsy. The available treatment includes pentavalent antimony: meglumine antimoniate (Glucantime) or sodium stibogluconate (Pentostam), however these drugs are poorly tolerated and resistance similar to that has been observed in the treatment of Indian VL . Liposomal amphotericin B is being used instead of antimony for treatment of VL in children in France and is well tolerated. Liposomal amphotericin B is almost 100% effective. It can be administered in six intravenous injections of 3-4 mg/kg/dose (days 1 to 5 then on day 10). A two-day protocol (10 mg/kg/d) that would reduce overall cost by shortening the duration of hospitalization is now being studied. Another oral drug, i.e., miltefosine, has been successfully used for treatment of visceral leishmaniasis in India.[108]

Intesinal Protozoa

Entamoeba histolytica

Asymptomatic colonization of neonates with various species of ameba is common in areas of high endemicity. Infection probably results from ingestion of fecal material at birth, from unsterile oral fluids given as a supplement to breast-feeding or from close contact with infected mothers. [109] Rates of acquisition and shedding of amebic infections, appear to be independent of age. [110] On rare occasions, fatal intestinal amoebiasis with colitis has been reported in infants. [111] Extraintestinal complications mostly amoebic liver abscess and other have also been reported in infants. [112] The lesion may be single or multiple. The size, location and number of abscesses determine appropriate treatment. Immunochromatographic tests for direct antigen detection and PCR assays may be used also with liver abscess fluid.

Diagnosis can be established by stool examination and possibly by serologic studies. Differentiation between *E. histolytica* and *E. dispar* can also be achieved by stool antigen detection. Several antigen detection tests using ELISA are now commercially available, most of these cross-react with *E. dispar,* while other specifically recognize only *E. histolytica.* Recently, many PCR-based assays have been developed for direct detection of *E. histolytica* and *E. dispar* in biological samples using DNA or ribosomal RNA amplification, but most of these cannot be performed in field studies. Metronidazole is the drug of choice for both intestinal and extra-intestinal amoebiasis.[113, 114]

Giardiasis

Giardia lamblia, also known as *Giardia intestinalis* or *Giardia duodenalis*, is a flagellated protozoan that infects the gastrointestinal tract. It is spread by the fecal-oral route after ingestion of cysts. In industrialized countries, Giardiasis has a prevalence of 2% to 5%in developed nations whereas in developing countries prevalence is 20% to 30%. Rates of infection are highest in areas of poor sanitation. Food-borne transmission and water-borne transmission also occur. Infection is often asymptomatic. However, the younger the patient when infected, it is more likely that symptomatic infection will occur. [115] High-risk groups include children, previously uninfected adults and travelers, and immunocompromised persons. Giardiasis is being increasingly recognized as a cause of chronic diarrhoea or malabsorption, especially among children. Day-care center outbreaks reflecting person-to-person spread have demonstrated the high infectivity. [116,117] The growing number of reports of giardiasis in infants, [118, 119] especially those who are not breast-fed, suggests that infants are at risk as soon as they eat or drink from a contaminated environment. In a study of lactating mothers and their infants, it was observed that 82% of mothers and 42% of infants excreted *Giardia* at least once during the study period, some infants were as early as 3 months of age. Of these infected infants, 86% had diarrhoea, suggesting that the first exposure to the parasite results in disease. [118] In a prospective study of diarrhea conducted in Mexico, infants were frequently infected with *Giardia* from birth to 2 months, with a crude incidence rate of first *Giardia* infection of 1.4 infections per child-year in the infants form birth to 2 months of age. Breast-feeding is believed to protect against symptomatic giardiasis. This protection may be mediated by both cellular and humoral immunity and nonspecifically by the anti-giardial effects of unsaturated fatty acids. However, giardiasis should be considered among the treatable causes of chronic diarrhoea, especially when associated with symptoms of malabsorption or malnutrition in infants. [119, 120] Some cases have been recognized by stool or duodenal fluid examination in the first 4 weeks of life. The diagnosis of giardiasis can be made on the basis of demonstration of cysts or trophozoites in feces; or of trophozoites in duodenal fluid or, less frequently, on duodenal biopsy. Detection of antigen is also useful for giardiasis. The drug of choice is oral metronidazole. It usually is given three times daily for 5 to 7 days with a cure rate of 80% to 95%.

Cryptosporidiosis

Cryptosporidium is a coccidian protozoon that is known to be an important cause of chronic diarrhea in patients with acquired immunodeficiency syndrome (AIDS) and of acute diarrhea in immunocompetent patients, particularly young children. [121] The species infecting humans and most other mammals is *Cryptosporidium parvum*. *Cryptosporidium* infects a wide variety of animal species; there is often a history of animal contact among infected individuals. Person-to-person spread, particularly in household contacts and day-care centers, [122] is well-documented and suggests that the organism is highly infectious. Water-borne outbreaks also occur. The life cycle involves ingestion of thick-walled oocysts, release of sporozoites, which penetrate intestinal epithelium, and development of merozoites. There is both asexual and sexual reproduction, with the latter resulting in formation of new oocysts that can be passed in stools. High-risk populations include children in tropical developing areas and immunocompromised individuals. Outbreaks secondary to food-borne transmission occur in more affluent countries. Infection is self-limiting in immunocompetent hosts; diarrhoea may lasts approximately 10 to 14 days without therapy. Whereas in immunocompromised hosts often have a prolonged course with chronic diarrhea and wasting and involvement of the biliary and pancreatic ducts. The clinical manifestations of illness in immunocompetent persons resemble those of *Giardia* infection but are somewhat shorter in duration. Symptoms and signs include watery diarrhoea, abdominal pain, myalgia, fever and weight loss. Although infection in the first month of life has been described, no reports have yet focused specifically on the neonate with cryptosporidiosis. The fact that symptoms resolve before excretion of oocysts suggests that a newborn whose mother has been ill with cryptosporidiosis in the month before delivery ought to be at risk even if the mother is asymptomatic at the time of the child's birth. Furthermore, with the increasing frequency of AIDS, it is likely that women with symptomatic cyptosporidiosis will occasionally be delivered of infants who will become infected. Infants infected early in life may develop chronic diarrhoea and malnutrition. [123]

The diagnosis of cryptosporidiosis is most typically made by examination of fecal smears using Giemsa's stain, Ziehl-Neelsen stain, auramine-rodhamine stain. Sheather's sugar flotation, an indirect immunofluorescence procedure, a modified concentration – sugar flotation method, or an ELISA and in recent times by PCR. Because illness is usually self-limited in the normal host, attention to fluid, electrolyte and nutritional status usually suffices. Enteric isolation of hospitalized infants with this illness is appropriate because of the high infectivity. Several studies suggest that the risk of infection early in life may be decreased by breast-feeing. Hyper immune bovine colostrum raised against *Cryptosporidium* oocysts and sporozoites and monoclonal antibodies have reduced cryptosporidial infection in animals. [123,124] Because cryptosporidiosis is self-limiting in most cases, treatment consists of maintaining adequate hydration and supportive care. In severe cases and in immunocompromised patients, however, several treatment options could be considered. Nitazoxanide is the drug of choice. Paromomycin, a nonabsorbed aminoglycoside, has been shown to decrease stool excretion of oocysts. Paromomycin also has been used in combination with azithromycin for 4 weeks, followed by paromomycin alone for another 8 weeks with some improvement in clinical symptoms and decrease in oocysts passage.

Isospora and Cyclospora

Isospora belli is endemic in much of the tropics, whereas it is rare in temperate climates. Infection of the immunocompetent is uncommon; this disease is commoner, however, in immunosuppressed individuals who visit endemic areas. The disease is transmitted faecal-orally, the organisms invade duodenal cells and replicate predominantly sexually. After a round of sexual replication, persistent spores are produced. Although the spores are detectable in the stools, flotation methods to concentrate the stool sample improve detection rates. Co-trimoxazole is an effective treatment but relapses are common. [125, 126]

Cyclospora cayetanensis has a worldwide distribution and is endemic in Nepal, Peru, and Haiti. The organisms identified in the stools are larger than *cryptosporidium. Cyclospora* causes intermittent watery diarrhoea in the immunosuppressed. Organisms of the genus *Cyclospora* that are similar to cryptosporidia have been shown to cause diarrhea, but their importance in neonates is unknown. [127] In immunocompetent hosts, *C.cayetanensis* and *I.belli* produce self-limiting infections, but in immunocompromised hosts chronic diarrhoea and anorexia can cause serious sequelae. The treatment for both infections is Trimethoprim-sulfamethoxazole (TMP-SMX) twice daily for 7 to 10 days. In patients with AIDS, treatment should be the continuation of TMP-SMX three times per week as prophylaxis. [128]

Microsporidium

Human microsporidial infection was a rarity. It was first described to cause diarrhoea in a French patient in the early 1980s and subsequently it was demonstrated that up to one third of patients with pathogen-negative diarrhoea harboured microsporidium as the likely cause of symptoms. [129] Most infections were with *Enterocytozoon bieneusi*, which was originally thought to be only capable of growing in human intestinal mucosa. A smaller number of patients are also infected by a different species of *Enterocytozoon.* In the milieu of the duodenal fluid, microsporidial spores, which are highly resistant, project a long tube-like structure that penetrates the mucosal cell. The contents of the spore are extruded into the cell and there the microsporidial organisms use the cellular mitochondria as an energy source to undergo their replicative cycle. Severe villous atrophy results from infection. Microsporidiosis appears to be a late manifestation of HIV infection [130] usually in individuals with a CD4+ cell count below 100 cells/mm^3. The original diagnosis of microsporidia could only be made with electron microscopy, which is still used for accurate speciation. However, a variety of special stains have been developed as well as ultra-thin sections, providing a reliable diagnosis by light microscopy. Special techniques that stain spores in the faeces are able to distinguish these spores from bacteria, which are very similar in size, and this provides an accurate diagnosis. The most commonly used stain is chromatrope and calcofluor. Recent molecular techniques have been used to detect DNA of the organism directly from the clinical specimens. Albendazole has been shown to reduce stool volumes in microsporidial diarrhoea but eradication of *E. bieneusi* does not occur. [131]

Free-living Amoebae

Naegleria fowleri, *Acanthamoeba* spp. and *Balamuthia mandrillaris* are free-living amoebae that may occasionally induce pathology in humans and other mammals. [132] Central nervous system disease due to *N. fowleri*, called primary amoebic meningoencephalitis occurs in previously healthy children or young adults after exposure to polluted water at home or in swimming pools, rivers, ponds or lakes. The vegetative forms reach the CNS directly through the nostrils and via the olfactory neuroepithelium.Incubation period is short (3-6 days) and the clinical course is acute or fulminant,characterized by necrotizing haemorrhagic meningoencephalitis,involving mainly the base of the brain,brain stem and cerebellum. Large clusters of trophozoites are recovered microscopically in histological specimens of the CNS parenchymal lesions; often around the vessels. [133] *N. fowleri* has three biological stages in its life cycle: the trophozoite, the flagellate form and the cyst. The trophozoite (15-25 μm) shows a single vesicular nucleus with a large, central karyosome. A pulsative vacuole is often seen in the cytoplasm. If a change in the ionic concentration of the environment occurs, the vegetative form transforms into a pear-shaped biflagellate stage which usually reverts back into the trophozoite stage very rapidly. The smooth-walled spherical cyst (7-15 μm) is the environmentally resistant stage, with a bilaminar wall interrupted by round pores covered by a mucous plug through which the trophozoite may excyst. *B. mandrillaris* and *Acanthamoeba* spp. are pathogenic "opportunistic" free-living species that cause a form of granulomatous amoebic encephalitis (GAE). GAE is usually diagnosed in debilitated or malnourished subjects, in pathologically or iatrogenically immunocompromised individuals, and in AIDS patients. The primary foci of these amoebae are often located in the lungs and skin and they reach the CNS and other organs via a haematogenous route in cases of disseminated infections. *Acanthamoeba* species. more frequently also cause severe, subacute non-or bilateral keratitis mainly in contact lens wearer. [134] *Acanthamoeba* spp and *B. mandrillaris* show only two morphological stages: the trophozoite and the cyst. The main morphological features of *Acanthamoeba* trophozoites (15-45 μm) are the presence of fine, spine-like ectoplasmic projections (acanthopodia) on the surface of the cell, an endoplasmic pulsative vacuole, and a single nucleus with a large, centrally located karyosome. The cystic form (15-20 μm) shows a bilaminar wall, with an outer wrinkled ectocyst and an inner polygonal, stellate or oval endocyst. Pores are located at the points of contact beween the two layers and usually are covered by an operculum, also known as an "ostiole". *B. mandrillaris* vegetative forms have a mean length of 40 μm. The main morphological feature is the branched shape, with some pseudopodia ejected in various directions. The granular endoplasm contains a conspicuous, single nucleus with a large karyosome. The cystic forms are spherical or oval with a mean diameter of 15 μm (range 10-30 μm), mono- or binucleated with a trilaminar wall: an inner thin endocyst, an outer wrinkled ectocyst and a thick amorphous, fibrillar middle layer (mesocyst). [132, 135]

To date, several hundred cases of free-living amoebic infections have been reported in the literature with a prevalence of *N. fowleri* meningoencephalitis and acanthamoebic keatitits. [136-138] In HIV-positive subjects, almost all CNS or disseminated infections are due to *Acanthamoeba* spp. or *B. mandrillaris.* [139]

The definitive diagnosis of primary amoebic meningoencephalitis, GAE, and subacute keratitis relies on the direct microscopic identification of amoebic trophozoites and/or cysts in the cerebrospinal fluid (CSF), brain tissue or corneal stroma. In cases of infection caused by *N. fowleri*, the CSF is purulent and on light microscopic examination, motile amoebic trophozoites with ectoplasmic pseudopodia (lobopodia) can be identified. Organisms are better seen in phase-contrast microscopy. Smears prepared from CSF can also be stained with various techniques. However, in cases of *Acanthamoeba* or *Balamuthia* cerebral infections, the CSF is clear and amoebic trophozoites or cysts are not microscopically seen. The definitive diagnosis may be made with recovery of trophozoites and/or cystic forms in autoptic histological specimens or with stereotactic cerebral biopsy. To isolate *N. fowleri* and *Acanthamoeba* spp., the biological specimens (CSF, brain, lungs, skin, corneal scrapings etc.) can be cultured on 1.5% - 3% non-nutrient agar plates that have been coated on the surface with gram-negative bacteria (e.g. *Escherichia coli*, *Enterobacter aerogenes*), incubated at 37°C and microscopically inspected every day. The biological specimen can be obtained aseptically and processed as soon as possible. After 2-3 days of incubation, amoebae begin to multiply towards the periphery of the agar plate, while the centrally located forms tend to encyst. Various synthetic liquid media are also available for *in- vitro* axenic growth for both *Naegleria* and *Acanthamoeba* spp. These media are also useful for experimental pharmacological tests. *B. mandrillaris* cannot grow on agar plates, but only on some cellular lines or in an elective axenic chemical medium. The diagnosis can be made also with transmission electon microscopy and scanning electron microscopy. Immunohistological techniques such as IIF assay with rabbit antisera specific for the various free-living amoebic species and isoenzyme characterization are important diagnostic tools for species identification, along with light and ultra-structural morphological features. [132]

Nematode Infections in Infants

Nematodes are the most common helminthes of humans and infections with nematodes are most prevalent in the tropics. Nematodes are bilaterally symmetrical worms that are attenuated at both ends. They have a characteristic cuticle that encompasses the worm in a relatively impervious but elastic and semi permeable shield. These cuticles are shed through a series of moltings by larvae. This has implications for both antigenic properties as well as associated immune response to the nematode parasite, because each larval stage may have quite distinct expression of specific antigens. In addition, larvae and adult worms shed secretory-excretory molecules thrugh cuticular pores, which often provoke host immunologic responses. In contrast to most free living nematodes, parasitic nematodes have varying requirements for support and shelter from the external environment. Filarial nematodes are highly adapted to human hosts that no life cycle stage is free-living. Other parasitic nematodes, such as hookworms and *Ascaris spp.* retain a free-living portion of their life cycle as either eggs or larvae. Humans may be either the definitive host, intermediate host or accidental host for parasitic nematodes. [140] The life cycle of nematodes is often complex, requiring intermediate hosts for particular larval stages. However, the typical life cycle includes oviposition by gravid females, maturation of eggs with subsequent release of larvae, and development of larvae through a typical series of various stages, resulting in creation of fecund adult male and female worms. These worms mate to create fertile embryos (except *Strongyloides stercoralis,* where the female are parthnogenic (i.e., do not require a male worm to produce fertile eggs). Infection occurs either through ingestion of mature eggs or larvae or through penetration of skin by nematode larvae or by insect bites. The symbiotic relationship between nematode and humans usually results in varying degrees of harm to the human host. Usually the infective stage for mammals is the third larval stage. There is often an arrest in the development of larvae after their entry into human hosts [141]. Intestinal infections due to nematodes are often subclinical, and disease is usually apparent only in heavily infected individuals. Clinical spectrum for intestinal parasites ranges from nonspecific abdominal symptoms to malabsorption, iron deficiency anaemia (hookworm), and acute conditions of the abdomen (ascariasis and trichuriasis). Mortality is usually attributable to complications of high parasitic burden. Some of the primary intestinal nematodes may also manifest extra-intestinal manifestation such as granulomas (visceral larva migrans and angiostrongyliasis) and dermatologic manifestations (cutaneous larva migrans, larva currens). Rarely more serious disease occurs because of nematode larval invasion of neurologic (angiostrongyliasis and gnathostomiasis), subcutaneous (onchocerciasis) and lymphatic tissues (filariasis). In many cases, the host immune response is contributory to tissue damage from parasite passage or entrapment.

Nematode infections have been shown to adversely affect physical growth, development, and nutritional status of children. Infection with one intestinal worm can also predispose to infections with other helminth species, such as other nematodes or possibly even trematodes. Helminth infections may even predispose to superinfection and transmission of bacterial disease. It is apparent that there is yet more to be learned about the ecology and impact of nematode infections, especially their impact on an immunologically and nutritionally vulnerable population of preschool-age children [142]. The nematodes can be categorized broadly into: soil-transmitted nematode infections, vector-borne nematode infections, and foodborne nematode infections.

Soil-transmitted Nematode

The soil-transmitted nematodes are distributed in both temperate and tropical regions. Humidity, type of soil, temperature and rainfall are the determining factors. Additionally, the soil-transmitted nematodes thrive among impoverished populations living under crowded and unsanitary conditions. [142] Most soil-transmitted nematodes cause intestinal infections. Humans acquire these infection by ingestion of embryonated eggs of *Ascaris lumbricoides, Trichuris trichiura* and *Enterobius vermicularis* from fecally contaminated material or by penetration of skin by free-living infective filariform larvae (*S. stercoralis and hookworm). Ascaris lumbricoides,* hookworm and *S. stercoralis* adult worms reside within the small intestine. Other nematodes live the in ceacum (*E. vermicularis)* and the large intestine (*T. trichiura).*

Immunology

The immune responses to nematodes depend in large part on the location and stage of the parasite. Generally the most immunogenic phase is during larval invasion of tissues. More commonly, individuals manifest premunition, the ability of the body to protect against concomitant or massive infection once an adult worm has established residence. A form of acquired immunity exists in populations with endemic transmission of nematodes; the intensity of infection decreases sharply after the second decade of life, returning slightly at older ages. The mechanisms of protection against nematodes have been subject of intense investigation. Features seen in characteristic responses of mammalian hosts to intestinal and tissue nematodes include local and systemic eosinophilia and local and systemic IgE production. These aspects suggested an allergic or immediate type of hypersensitivity pattern in controlling nematode infections. Work done with mouse models of nematode infection showed that these responses required the presence of T cells (gut-associated lymphoid tissue [GALT]), and there appears to be selective proliferation of particular CD4+ T cells (Th_2 subset) in many intestinal nematode infections. Subsequent study showed that particular T cell – derived lymphokines (interleukin-4 [IL-4], interlukin-5 [IL-5], and interleukin-3 [IL-3]) were the dominant mediators of local and systemic responses [143]. Similar responses have been detected in human nematode infections. Depletion of these Th_2 cytokines did not result in decreased immunity; thus, whether these responses are truly host protective is still a matter of debate. In contrast, in certain mouse models, engendering a counter-Th_1 response results in protection. Other areas regarding immunity to nematodes are under investigation. What causes these responses seems to be worm-derived products; the appearance of these antigens may be key in generating a protective *vs.* a diverted host response. Effector mechanisms to kill nematode parasites include oxygen and nitric oxide radicals and complement. The parasites have in most cases evolved means to evade these destructive responses. The puzzle of immunity to nematodes may be part of the "discontinuous variations in resistance"; some individuals are able to develop effective responses against (intestinal) nematodes, whereas others seem incapable of doing so [144, 145, 146].

Ascariasis

Ascaris lumbricoides is one of the largest and most common parasites of humans. Humans contract ascariasis by ingestion of embryonated eggs through faecal contamination. Because the eggs are invariably sticky, they may be found adhering to utensils, furniture, money, fruit, vegetables, door handles and fingers in endemic areas. As infective eggs can occur in the air and household dust, there is risk of exposure by inhalation. When eggs hatch in the duodenum, the larvae migrate through the liver, lungs and upper alimentary tract. When they reach the small intestine they mature into adult worms. Many of the larvae are destroyed on their journey through the host as they are lost in appropriate tissues. The cycle from ingestion of eggs to the production of fertilized eggs by mature *A. lumbricoides* takes 2-3 months. Adult worms can survive for 1-2 years and female worms can generate eggs for a period of one year although some may continue as long as 20 months [147].

Ascariasis is most common in children of pre-school or early school age. The most common clinical manifestations are non-specific abdominal colic and sometimes abdominal distention. High intensities of infection may result in obstruction of the small bowel by tangled masses of adult worms; this complication occurs in approximately 1 in 1,000 infected individuals and may reprsent 30% to 50% of children who have acute obstruction in endemic areas. Clinical manifestations during larval migration in the lungs are generally minimal in endemic areas; however, Loeffler's pneumonitis, with eosinophilia, wheezing and pulmonary infiltrates may occur in areas with seasonal transmission of Ascariasis. Prevalence and intensity of *Ascaris lumbricoides* infection have been analyzed by many cross-sectional studies in children.In one study population of 387 children under two years of age and one hundred mothers of children under one year of age were analysed. Prevalence was 3.3% (95% CI:1.0-7.8) for children under one year,30.7% (95%CI:25.4-36.4)for one-year-olds,and 42.3% (95% CI: 33.0-51.9) for mothers of children under one were observed. These results indicated that ascariasis was an important problem in the first year of life and demonstrated the need for research in the area of maternal and infantile ascariasis [148]. Report on two infants who presented with massive hematemesis have been reported by Sangkhathat et al [148]. In the first patient, a gastroduodenoscopy was performed and roundworms were found adhering to an oozing duodenal ulcer. The second case was hematemesis together with peritonitis. Finding suggests that the intestinal ascariasis can be a cause of massive gastrointestinal bleeding. Most Ascaris infections are of a chronic form and are widely considered to significantly impair childhood nutrition, especially in areas where poor growth and ascariasis are common; the infection is most likely to affect bodily growth, fat absorption, vitamin A absorption, iodine absorption, lactose digestion, and protein absorption [149]. However, some studies have implicated Ascaris infections in impairments of mental processing and impaired cognitive function. [150, 151]

The diagnosis is made by quantitative examination of the stools for distinctive golden-coated ovoid embryonated or unembryonated eggs; concentration techniques are rarely needed for examination. Adult worms may sometimes be passed per rectum or coughed up through the nose or mouth. Eosinophilia may be evident during pulmonary migration of third stage; in uncomplicated intestinal infections, eosinophils do not exceed 10% of total white blood cell count. Treatment is with mebendazole for uncomplicated intestinal ascariasis. Pyrantel pamoate may be used for heavy infestations [150].

Trichuriasis (Whipworm)

Trichuris trichiura is also transmitted by ingestion of eggs contaminating the soil or foods. The eggs are extremely resistant to the external environment and mature after 3 weeks. After ingestion, larvae mature to adult forms during their passage through the gut. On arrival at the large intestine, adult worms are whip shaped with a narrow anterior end buried in intestinal mucosa and a coiled thicker posterior segment exposed to the lumen. Adult size ranges from 30 to 50 mm. Trichuris worms cause minute blood losses (0.005 mL/worm/daily) from trauma and proteolysis at their sites of attachment to mucosa. Inflammation secondary to these worms may be significant and even systemic. Adult females shed approximately 13,000 eggs/worm/daily.The entire life-cycle in humans is contained within the intestinal environment. It is reasoned that Trichuris must be a very efficient parasite because worm fecundity is relatively low. Humans are the principal host, although pigs, lemurs and monkeys have also been reported to be infected.[152] *Trichuris trichiura*, the whipworm,is most common in the warm,moist, tropical and subtropical countries,where prevalences in children can be over 90%,although it is also found in temperate climates.An estimated 1049million persons harbour Trichuris including 114million preschool-age children, and 233million school-age children 5-14 years.Trichuriasis has been estimated to cause 6.4million disability-adjusted life-years(DALYs) to be lost.[153]Trichuriasis (whipworm) affects especially children 5 to10 years old. In hyperendemic areas severe infections may develop into dysentery-like syndrome with tenesmus ,right-sided abdominal pain, bloody diarrhea. Severe inflammation of the colon and rectum with heavy infections can result in significant losses of water and electrolytes. A large worm burden may build up in the rectal vault; persistent straining, coupled with deceased muscle tone, may result in rectal prolapse [154]. Stunted growth and severe anaemia are well recognized in severe cases of trichuriasis, often complicated by multiple parasitic infections. Subtle deficits in school performance have been associated with moderate infections. Very high prevalences have been reported in the following population groups: 98% in school children living in urban slums in Ujung Pandang, South Sulawesi, Indonesia, and 97% in rural primary school children on the Kenya Coast; 94% in persons of all ages in Ha Nam province, Vietnam, in which night soil is used routinely as fertilizer [154,155]. Studies from Malaysia report a higher incidence of heavy *T. trichiura* infections amongst Indian children than in Malays. The reason for this is, as yet, unknown but it indicates that ethnic factors, most likely ethnic differences in behaviour help to determine the intensity of infection. Heavy infections of *T. trichiura* have long been known to be associated with anaemia, protein-energy malnutrition and chronic diarrhoea and dysentery. Thus, trichuriasis can cause enough blood loss in heavy infections to produce anaemia, although it does not always do so, and heavily infected children often are severely anaemic when seen in hospitals. However, in relatively well-nourished children with lighter infections, anaemia is unlikely to develop solely from the infection. Whether or not Trichuris is related to iron status in a particular study will vary with intensity and duration of infection [156,157].

The diagnosis of trichuriasis is established by finding characterisitic barrel-shaped, twin plugged eggs in stool. Direct examination of stool may be unreliable in light infections, and concentration techniques may be required. Diagnosis can be confirmed by visualization of adult worms at proctoscopy. Moderate peripheral eosinophilia (5% - 15% of total white blood cell differential) may be seen after infection. Mebendazole and pyrantel pamoate are the drugs of choice for treatment of trichuriasis.[155,154]

Enterobiasis (Pinworm)

Enterobiasis (threadworm, a pinworm disease) is caused by the small nematode *Enterobius vermicularis.* While usually considered a nuisance, rather than a cause of serious disease, morbidity (especially in children) is significant. Infection usually occurs by ingestion of eggs by contaminated hands, food and less commonly water. Subsequently four methods of transmission exist: (a) direct infection from the anal and perianal regions by fingernail contamination (auto-infection), and soiled night clothes; (b) exposure to viable eggs on soiled bed linen and other contaminated environmental objects; (c) by contaminated dust containing embryonated eggs (from bed clothes, toys, furniture, and cat and dog fur) and (d) retroinfection; after hatching on the anal mucosa, larvae migrate into the sigmoid colon, and caecum. Humans are the only host. In temperate climates, transmission is facilitated by decreased washing, increased clothing and contact, and prolonged survival of eggs. The short-lived female worm resides in the cecum but wanders out into the perineal area to deposit eggs. Rarely adult worms may migrate to other sites such as the vulva, peritoneum, and appendix. Pinworm eggs mature very quickly, so there is further potential for wide transmission of the parasite. In addition, retroinfection may result from larvae that hatch from eggs and return to the caecum [158]. Infection is most common in young school children (5-10 years) living in overcrowded conditions (it is unusual at <2 years); rates of infection of 80-90% have been reported at summer camps and various institutions. Sex incidence is equal. No social class is exempt. In Iraq, 9% infections were recorded, most being in those <5 years old. In a south India fishing community, infection rate was 74.3%; after mass antihelmintic chemotherapy, some subjects re-acquired a significantly higher level of infection. [159] Adult worms migrate from the female genital tract to the peritoneum; they can also enter the peritoneal cavity through a perforated bowel wall, for example, appendicitis, diverticulitis, or intestinal malignancy. Direct migration has been recorded after abdominal operation. Migration to an ectopic site(s) can give rise to diagnostic difficulty. Sites of ectopic infection include: the liver, spleen, kidney and lung. Chronic pelvic peritonitis has been described. The occasional presence of *E. vermicularis* in the appendix has been recognized since 1724; it has been implicated in the pathogenesis of acute appendicitis since 1907. At Allahabad, India, 2921 appendicectomies (all specimens were subjected to histological examination) were carried out during a 25 year period [160]; in 153 (5%) a significant pathological abnormality was reported – in 75 (2.5%) a parasite: *E vermicularis (41), Entamoeba histolytica (17), Ascaris lumbricoides (13), A lumbricoides and Trichuris trichiura (2), and Taenia spp. (2)* was identified. Further spread to the environment from finger contamination and autoinfection follows local scratching. Routine examination of a faecal sample gives a positive diagnosis in 5-15% of infected subjects. Adult worms are occasionally visualized during colonoscopy. Diagnosis is dependent on accurate identification of adult worms or eggs, or both – which can be visualized in the perianal region (or less often vagina), usually at night. Cellophane tape applied to the perineum on awakening in the morning is used to detect eggs deposited on skin. Eggs are not usually seen on stool examination because of the low level of excretion; occasionally adult worms can be seen but are quite small (10 by 0.5 mm). Blood eosinophilia (6% - 12% white blood cell differential) may be associated with infection.

Toxocariasis (Visceral Larval Migrans)

Toxocara canis (dog roundworm) and *Toxocara cati* (cat round-worm) larvae are the causative agents of visceral larval migrans [161]. Infections are found worldwide in both temperate and tropical climates. Dogs and cats are carriers of adult worms, often after being infected with larvae *in-utero*; the roundworms complete its life cycles in the intestines of their hosts with the passage of ova. Infections in humans are acquired by ingestion of eggs shed by household pets or found outside the home (e.g., sandboxes). Release and limited development of larvae within the intestine after ingestion of eggs and larva penetration of the bowel wall, enter into the portal blood and then to the liver and lungs. They form granulomas within these viscera and induce prominent peripheral eosinophilia and IgE responses. Due to their small size, larvae may escape into the peripheral circulation to lodge in small vessels of other tissues (e.g., retina and brain). Clinical manifestions include tender hepatomegaly, hepatitis, or wheezing caused by larval migration. The extent of symptoms reflects the amount of ingested embryonated eggs and the intensity of host immune response to the larvae. Manifestation may also be occult, with constitutional symptoms of fever, night sweats, and anorexia. Symptoms may persist for months to years without resolution because the inciting larvae often remain alive but encapsulated within host granulomas [162]. Retinitis may develop as a result of subretinal trapped larvae. Diagnosis is usally made by serologic determination of toxocara titers by ELISA because cross-reactive antigens within the Ascaris group of nematodes makes indirect methods such as immunofluorescent antibody tests and indirect hemagglutination assay unreliable. Demonstration of the parasites in tissue is definitive. Ocular toxocariasis is typically a mono-ocular disease of young children. Clinical findings include posterior and peripheral retinochoroiditis, optic papiilitis and enophthamitis. The percentage of seroprevalence of anti-*toxocara* antibody, the method of diagnosis, has been shown to be higher in children. The higher value of anti-*toxocara* antibody in children could obviously be explained because of their frequent pica behaviour and contact with resident animals. [163]

Hookworm Infections

Hookworm are the vampires of the gut, feeding by sucking blood from the capillaries of the intestinal mucosa. Hookworm infection results from infection by *Ancylostoma duodenale* and *Necator americanus. Ancylostoma duodenale* (Old World hookworm) is found throughout the Mediterranean to India and some parts of Far East Asia. *Necator americanus (*New World hookworm), is widely distributed throughout North and South America, Africa, and Asia. Human hookworm infections have been associated with humans in the Old World for over 5,000 years. [164] Larvae hatch from eggs deposited on ground by infected humans. After maturation, larvae penetrate exposed skin or are ingested through drinking water. After entry into the venous circulation, infective larvae are carried to the lungs, penetrate alveoli, and enter the tracheal air space to be coughed and swallowed. Other modes of transmission, such as oral or transmammary passage of larvae, may account for some *Ancylostoma* infections. [165] The larvae then mature into adults, which attach to the jejunal mucosa. Buccal structures pierce the mucosa and anchor the worm, which sucks minute quantities of blood from intestinal capillaries. Endemicity of hookworm in an area is sustained by infections acquired by children and adolescents. [166] The major clinical manifestations of infection in children are iron deficiency anaemia and hypoalbuminemia resulting from chronic worm burden and poor host diet. Growth retardation is seen in children with heavy infections in the second decade of life. Minor clinical manifestations include pruritus, erythema, and vesicular rash (ground itch) resulting from larval invasion of skin and occasional gastrointestinal and respiratory complains. Symptoms may be more directly related to intensity of parasitic infection rather than host immune responses. The people or groups of people most at risk from hookworm infection will be those with impaired iron status or iron-deficiency anaemia. Adolescent girls, women of child-bearing age and those who are pregnant are vulnerable and any individuals with heavy worm burdens will also be at risk of hookworm-induced disease. What constitutes a heavy worm burden is difficult to define. On the basis of cross-sectional surveys of communities, the prevalence of infection is observed to rise steadily from infancy, to slow down or level off in later childhood and then remain stable during adulthood. Hookworm in infants goes back to 1946, when investigations of the species of hookworm found in 11 of 21 individuals necropsied at Military Govt Hospital were carried out.[165] Twenty cases of hookworm disease in early childhood on Guam were investigated. One of the remarkable features presented by seven fatal cases was the cardiac enlargement. [167] There has been much interest to know whether intestinal nematode infections have detrimental effects on cognition and educational achievement in children. The diagnosis is made from finding characteristic ovoid eggs in fecal examination. Rhabditiform larvae may hatch form embryonated eggs and should be differentiated from *Strongyloides* larvae (large buccal cavity, small genital primordium). Treatment is with mebendazole and supplemental iron salts.

Cutaneous Larva Migrans (Creeping Eruption)

Animal hookworm larvae, especially *Ancylostoma braziliense,* are responsible for dermatologic disease, which is being increasingly recognized. Infective larvae penetrate skin but are unable to pass through to the circulation and the lungs. Infection commonly manifests as dermatitis, typically on the extremities; the larvae move within the skin, resulting in migrating erythemas with pruritus. Treatment with topical thiabendazole is successful in controlling the rash and pruritus. Accidental ingestion of larvae may induce eosinophilic enteritis in humans. [165, 167]

Strongyloidiasis

Strongyloides stercoralis has a variety of disease manifestations from asymptomatic infection to disseminated fatal hyperinfections. Larvae in stool develop intro free-living adults or infective filariform larvae in the soil. The infective larvae penetrate skin to enter circulation, then pass to the lungs and finally to the upper small intestine, where they develop into adults. Adult worms produce eggs from which first-stage or rhabditiform larvae may hatch during transit through the bowel. In addition, *Stronglyoides* infections can result in autoinfection when rhabditiform larvae develop to infective larvae while still within the bowel. Because the infective larvae proceed through the lungs to reinfect the small intestine, the parasite is able to maintain infections for prolonged periods (over decades) [168]. This continuing cycle has the potential to increase dramatically when host immune status fails to control worm burden or invasion, resulting in hyperinfection (expansion of worms in lungs and intestine) and dissemination (penetration of viscera, e.g., liver and brain), respectively. Cases are also found among immigrants and other exposed populations, but severe infections are increasingly recognized among malnourished or immunosuppressed individuals. In patients with severe malnutrition or immunosuppression, disseminated strongyloidosis can manifest as acute abdominal distress, paralytic ileus, asthma, or sprue-like disease. Cases supporting a linkage between strongyloidiasis and human immunodeficiency virus (HIV) infections are being reported [169]. In endemic areas, children often have asymptomatic strongyloidiasis. Gastrointestinal symptoms (epigastric pain, vomiting and diarrhea) may be prominent in some individuals. A chronic malabsorption-like syndrome with weight loss and protein-losing enteropathy may develop in severe infections. Repeated exposure of skin to infective larvae results in typical skin lesions (*larva currens*). The diagnosis of stronglyloidiasis must be considered in any patient from an endemic region who is to be treated with immunosuppressive agents (e.g., chemotherapy and transplant drugs). Definitive diagnosis requires demonstration of characteristic rhabditiform larvae (short buccal cavity and large genital primordium), because eggs hatch within the intestine. Diagnosis of uncomplicated infection can be difficult because repeated stool examinations often fail to demonstrate larvae, even after concentration. Yield may be further improved using duodenal fluid recovered by the string test. In strongyloides hyperinfection, larvae may be readily recovered from sputum and other body fluids, as well as tool. Treatment of strongyloidiasis with thiabendazole is successful but has frequent side effects. Albendazole or ivermectin have been used for treatment of disseminated strongyloidiasis [170]. *Strongyloides fulleborni* is a parasite of primates that has been reported to cause human infections in Papua New Guinea and Africa. In these areas, there is a high incidence of infections among nursing infants resulting in hyperinfection, malabsorption, and often fatal disease. The parasite has been demonstrated in breast milk, supporting the possibility of transmammary transmission [170,171].

Vector-transmitted Nematode Infections

Filarial Infections

Filarial worms cause lymphatic (bancroftian and brugian filariasis) and subcutaneous disease (onchocerciasis, loiasis). Lymphatic disease caused by *Wuchereria bancrofti*, *Brugia malayi* and *Brugia timori* account for more than 90 million human cases throughout the tropics, far more than other filarid parasites combined. Filarial worms are long, thread-like parasites that reside in tissues or body cavities. Fertilized females extrude mature microfilariae; these highly motile forms circulate in the peripheral blood or move within the cutaneous tissues. Some filarial species maintain distinct periodic shifts in the density of microfilariae detected in the peripheral blood, where maximal densities occur at times synchronous with peak feeding cycles of primary arthropod vectors. Filariasis are non-fatal but often chronic infections that may lead to disfiguring and debilitating sequelae. Pediatric reports of clinical filarial diseases are uncommon. In most cases, treatment is effective but frequently requires follow-up and retreatment [172].

Bancroftian Filariasis

Wuchereria bancrofti is the most common filarial parasite in humans with a worldwide distribution but occurs predominately in urban coastal areas in tropical and subtropical regions. *Wuchereria bancrofti* is exclusively a human parasite with no known animal reservoir. In endemic areas, exposure begins early in childhood and continues throughout life; rates of mcirofilaraemia in children can be significant in areas of high transmission. Some innate immunity to filarial infection may exist, but most immunity is partial and increases with age and exposure; acquired immunity probably regulates chronic worm burdens and protects from super infection. Development of partial immunity coincides with the presence of adult worm antigens, elevated antifilarial IgE and IgG antibody levels, and skin test positivity to filarial antigens.Asymptomatic exposed individuals in endemic areas are protected against infective larvae by antibody-mediated immunity. In endemic areas, many infections occur without evident disease; individuals commonly remain asymptomatic despite detectable microfilaraemia. Pathologic conditions result from continual lymphatic irritation and are strongly associated with variable host immunologic responsiveness between early and chronic infections.[173] Generally lymphatic diseases can be divided into inflammatory manifestations (characterized by adenolymphangitis, lymphoedema, lymphatic ulceration orchitis, chyluria, and hydrocele) and obstructive manifestations associated with tissue fibrosis and skin thickening. Tropical pulmonary eosinophilia is asthma like disorder found in endemic populations, generally among young men [174]. It is also an occult filariasis associated with marked immunologic hyperresponsiveness to microfilarial antigens. Massive accumulation of activated eosinophils in the lung (Loeffler's syndrome) result in a chronic obstructive or restrictive pulmonary syndrome.

Malayan and Timorian Filariasis

Brugia malayi and *Brugia.timori* are related parasites with similar disease manifestations. Infections are limited to rural areas of Asia, with *B. malayi* being most common in Southeast Asia and *B. timori* restricted to southeastern Indonesia. Their life cycles resemble that of *W. bancrofti*, but varying microfilarial periodicities are found with *B. malayi* infection. Malayan and timorian filariasis manifest with inflammation of the lymphatics and recurrent acute symptoms. Acute episodes may occur with greater frequency and severity than in bancroftian filariasis. Elephantiasis usually affects areas below the knees and elbows. Inguinal lymphatic abscesses and scarring are common, whereas hydrocele and chyluria are very uncommon manifestations of disease [175].

In pediatric age groups, the drug of choice for lymphatic filariasis is diethylcarbamazine citrate (DEC), which kills blood-stage mcirofilariae. It has a short half-life and very low toxicity in humans. However, antihistamines or corticosteroids may be required to abrogate allergic reactions to antigens released by dying microfilariae. Ivermectin, a macrocyclic lactone antibiotic, can also reduce microfilaraemia, but like DEC, it may require re-treatment at 6 month intervals.

Onchocerciasis (River Blindness)

Onchocereca volvulus occurs in West and Central Africa, Yemen, and Central and South America. The worm is transmitted from person to person by the bites of female black flies (*Simulium* spp.) that breed in fast-flowing streams. Infection begins at an early age in endemic areas; children as young as 6 months have had detectable infections. [176] Infective larvae may require 12 months to develop into adult worms; fertile female parasites normally live up to 15 years and discharge millions of microfilariae. Microfilariae can persist in the skin, eyes and other tissues for up to 24 months. No known animal reservoirs exist. Adult worms in subcutaneous tissues are surrounded by characteristic fibrous nodules. Skin nodules can be easily detected, particularly over bony prominences, yet nodules will occur in deeper tissues with no observable signs in some cases. Nodules occur at lower frequency in children compared with adults. An immunologically mediated onchocercal dermatitis may accompany severe infections, causing intense rash and itching, changes in skin pigmentation and swelling, thickening and atrophy of the skin. In chronic infections, large numbers of microfilariae in the eyes eventually die and calcify; causing ocular lesions and impaired sight or blindness. Pathologic conditions are related to microfilarial density and the balance of host inflammatory and suppressor responses. Demonstration of microfilariae in skin snips or the isolation of adult worms from excised nodules is definitive. The Mazzotti reaction, based on an immediate hypersensitivity response to dying microfilariae after giving DEC tretment, gives further evidence of active disease. All palpable nodules should be surgically removed. Although DEC effectively kills microfilariae, Ivermectin is a safe and effective microfilaricidal drug, providing longer lasting control with fewer side effects [177].

Loaisis

Loa loa, the African eye worm, is confined to West and Central Africa. The worm is transmitted by several species of day-biting deer flies (*Chrysops* spp.). The prepatent period is about 6 months but may be considerably longer. Adult worms may live 17 years or more. Adult worms migrating in subcutaneous tissues can provoke a temporary inflammation ("Calabar swellings") in any part of the body. Commonly microfilaraemia is less often found in children than in adults, although adult worms are present. *Loa loa* may rarely invade the central nervous system (CNS), causing encephalitis or spinal cord damage. Loaisis is often diagnosed clinically because of the conspicuous transient swellings associated with fever and prominent eosinophilia. During acute phases of infection, microfilaria are frequently not detectable in peripheral blood. Thus, immunodiagnosis using an immunofluorescence antibody test is the preferred choice for detection of disease [178].

Zoonotic Filariases

Several species of *Dirofilaria* animal parasites have been reported to cause human pulmonary and cutaneous disease. Humans constitute dead-end hosts because microfilariae are not produced in these zoonotic infections. *Dirofilaria immitis,* dog heartworm, has been responsible for cases of human pulmonary disease. Transmission is mosquito borne. This infection has not been reported in children. [179]

Other Nematodes

Angiostrongyliasis

There are approximately 20 species of *Angiostrongylus;* but only *Angiostrongylus cantonensis* and *Angiostrongylus costaricensis* are foodborne and accidental parasites of humans. *Angiostronglylus cantonensis* lives in the pulmonary arteries of rats; female adult worms lay eggs, and first-stage larvae hatch and enter the alveoli. The larvae then migrate up the pulmonary tree, are swallowed, and are passed in the feces. Second-stage larvae then enter terrestrial or aquatic snails and develop into third-stage, or infective, larvae. When the mollusks are eaten by rats, these larvae are released, enter the intestinal tissues, and are carried by the circulation to the brain. They develop into young adult worms in the CNS and after 3 weeks migrate to the pulmonary arteries to complete their life cycle. When humans eat infected mollusks, infective larvae can enter the CNS and cause eosinophilic meningitis or eosinophilic meningoencephalitis. [180] *Angiostrongylus cantonensis* is reported from many parts of Asia, Pacific Islands, Australia, India, Parts of Africa, and a few of the Caribbean Islands. Most angiostrongyliasis patients in Taiwan are children, whereas most in Thailand are adults. [181, 182] Penetration of intestinal mucosa by the released larvae may cause nausea, vomiting, abdominal pain, and diarrhoea. A skin rash with itching has also been reported from some areas in Thailand. Mild fever, malaise, cough, sneezing, and rhinorrhoea may also occur. CNS manifestations (headache, fever, stiff neck, and paresthesisas of the trunk and extremities) may occur soon afterward, and cranial nerve palsies have also been observed. Coma is common in Taiwanese children but is not often seen in Thai patients. In cases of meningitis there is an eosinophilic pleocytosis, and worms may be recovered from spinal fluid, especially in children. The disease may persist for several weeks, and then symptoms eventually resolve. Deaths have been reported but are rare. A confirmed diagnosis requires the recovery of worms from cerebrospinal fluid or the eye. A presumptive diagnosis may be based on symptoms and history of ingestion of or association with snails form endemic areas. Serologic tests only support a presumptive diagnosis; antibody or antigen detection tests of sera and cerebrospinal fluid using monoclonal antibodies are of value. Radiographic scans (computed tomography and magnetic resonance imaging) are useful. Mebendazole and albendazole are reported to be effective in treating children in Taiwan. Supportive treatment and sometimes surgery are necessary when worms are present in the eyes. Infections are easily prevented by simply cooking the intermediate and paratenic hosts thoroughly before eating them [183].

Cestodes Infections

Cestodes have complex life cycles. Human serve as the definitive host for *Taenia saginata*, *Hymenolepis diminuta*, *Diphyllobothrium latum* and *Dipylidium caninum*. Whereas for *T. solium* and *Hymenolepsis nana* humans serve as both intermediate and definitive host. Adult tapeworm infection is not life-threatening but larval tapeworms can be serious. *Dypylidium caninum* infestation is infrequent. Additionally, often the infected patients are symptom less. A case of *D.caninum* infection in infant has been reported [184].

Cystic Echinococosis

In developing countries, cystic hydatidosis, caused by *Echinococcus granulosus* is both a medical and economic problem related to environmental hygiene and healthy veterinary practice. Hydatidosis is endemic in sheep and cattle raising areas world-wide. Cystic echinococcosis in children has been described from many countries. [185, 186] Hydatidosis in children in general is more common in male then female. It is also higher in rural populations than urban. Lung is the commonest organ involved in children. Fertile cysts from lungs having protoscoleces have been reported in infant from Uruguay. [187] A series of 29 histologically confirmed cases of intracranial and spinal hydatidosis from South India included 12 cases in pediatric age group. [188]

Neurocysticercosis (NCC)

Epilepsy is probably one of the common disorders in children. Age specific prevalence rates are highest in the 1st decade of life especially below the age of 2 years. There are several prevalence studies suggests that the prevalence rate is 5.59 per 1000 population with no gender or geographical differences. NCC is caused by the larval stage of *Taenia solium* and is a major public health problem in non-Islamic developing countries including India [189]. The natural history of the live cysticercus is variable. In children 60-76% are single parenchymal NCC granulomas. Calcifying lesions are much less common in children (15%) as compared to adults (55%). School-age children are most affected with a slight male preponderance. The youngest child described was 9 months of age. [190, 191] In a series of 558 children, 51% of symptomatic partial epilepsies were due to either active or inactive NCC.

Serology, CSF studies, stool examinations, and fundoscopy examination not useful in childhood epilepsy as the parasite load is not high. EEG is rather more useful for investigation. Anti-epileptic drugs are given till lesions resolve or become inactive [192].

Trematodes (Flukes) Infections

Flukes are uncommon in developed countries. However due to increase travels and adventure trips their importance is growing. One divides the flukes according to the place where they reside within the body sites of the host: Blood flukes, Liver flukes and Lung flukes.

Blood Flukes

There are three important blood flukes: *Schistosoma haematobium, Schistosoma mansoni* and *Schistosoma japonicum.*

Schistosomiasis: Schistosomiasis results from infection by flatworms. The disease has a low mortality rate, but has high morbidity and causes incapacitating sequelae in millions of people each year. Formerly known as bilharzias after Thedor Bilharz, who identified the parasite in Egypt in 1851, Shistosomiasis is acquired by humans through infection with *S. haematobium*, *S. intercalatum*, *S.japonicum*, *S.mansoni* and *S.mekongi*. World Health Organisation statistics estimate the mortality at 11,000 deaths and the burden of diseases representing 1.7 million DALY's annually. Eighty five percent of all cases occur in sub-Saharan Africa although parasites has also been isolated in South Africa, Egypt's Nile river valley, Brazil, Surinam, Venezuela, Iran, Iraq, Saudi Arabia, Southern China and many other places.[193] Human acquires schistosomiasis in fresh water bodies contaminated with infected human excretion. Feces and urine carry schistosoma eggs that hatch once in water and seek a host in the form of specific snail species. The parasite multiplies asexually by thousands and develop into a larval form that leaves the snail and is capable of infecting humans, who are exposed through ingestion, bathing, washing and numerous other activities involving fresh water. The worm penetrates the skin and grows inside the blood vessels, eventually producing eggs that migrate to the liver, intestines or bladder and are passed in excretion. In rare instances eggs disseminate to brains and spinal cord. Schistosomiasis symptoms represent an immune response to parasite eggs rather than to actual worm. A case of acute schistosomiasis is defined as the onset of fever or hypersensitivity symptoms after an exposure of 3 weeks and chronic schistosomiasis is mainly with involvement of genital, gastrointestinal and urinary system involvement. Chronic schistosomiasis occurs after contract of organisms for a period from 4 months to 3 years [194]. Diagnosis in acute schistosomiasis relies on serology [193], whereas detection of ova along with serology is the mainstay for disease diagnosis. Typical manifestation includes a rash or itchy skin several days after infection, followed by non-specific symptoms such as fever, muscle aches. People repeatedly infected over the course of many years develop liver, lung and urinary bladder damage. Schistosomiasis can also attribute to anaemia and stunted growth.

Food-borne Flukes

Currently, 601, 293.8, 91.1, and 79.8 million people are at risk for infection with *Clonorchis sinensis*, *Paragonimus* spp., *Fasciola* spp., and *Opisthorchis* spp., respectively. Residents living near freshwater bodies have a 2.15-fold higher risk (95% confidence interval 1.38-3.36) for infections than persons living farther from the water. Food-borne trematodiasis, which is caused by liver flukes (*Clonorchis sinensis, Fasciola spp.,*

Opisthorchis spp.), and intestinal flukes *(Echinostoma spp.*, *Fasciolopsis buski*, heterophyids), is an emerging public health problem. In China, clonorchiasis infections have more than tripled over the past decade; approximately 15 million people were infected with *C. sinensis* in 2004. [195] *C. sinensis* is also prevalent in Vietnam. Most of the trematode infection ensues in following manner; parasite eggs from infected humans or animals reach freshwater bodies through contaminated fecal matter e.g., through non-hygienic defecating habits of humans or the use of human feces for fertilizer (night soil). Once eggs have reached a suitable body of fresh water, they develop and release a miracidium. It enters an aquatic snail, which acts as first intermediate host. Inside the snail, within several weeks, the miracidium transforms into cercariae. They are released into the freshwater environment and attach, penetrate, and encyst as metacercariae in susceptible second intermediate hosts. Infection with foodborne trematodes is accomplished through ingestion of metacercariae.

Opisthorchis viverrini is endemic in Cambodia, the Lao People's Democratic Republic, Thailand, and Vietnam, and *O. felineus* is endemic in the former Soviet Union, Kazkastan, and Ukraine. An estimated 67.3 million people are at risk for infection with *O. viverrini* and 12.5 million are at risk for infection with *O. felineus* [196].

At least 292.8 million people are at risk for infection with *Paragonimus spp.*, with 195 million residing in China. Paragonimiasis also occurs in the Republic of Korea and the Philippines, parts of Africa (eastern Nigeria and Southwestern Cameroon), and South America (Ecuador and Peru) .No estimates are currently available regarding populations at risk for intestinal flukes. *F. buski* is common in Bangladesh, China, India, Indonesia, Malaysia, Taiwan and Thailand. Echinostomes have been reported in China, Indonesia, Malaysia, the Philippines, the Republic of Korea, Taiwan and Thailand. Among the heterophyids, *Heterophyes heterophyes and Metagonimus yokogawai* are the 2 species of greatest medial importance. They are prevalent in the Balkans, China, Egypt, India, Indonesia, the Islamic Republic of Iran, Israel, Japan, the Republic of Korea, the Philippines, Spain, Sudan, Taiwan, Thailand, Tunisia, and Turkey. [197]

Conclusions

The problems of parasitoses in the past, which mainly consisted of classic parasitoses, were generally regarded as a public health issue rather than an individual disease issue because of the large number of infected persons and the relatively mild pathogenicity of classic parasitoses. Nowadays, parasitoses are reemerging. We need to face them as diversified individual disease/s that often have serious outcomes. The process of parasitism involves a relationship in which both the host and the parasite can survive over time in the presence of a strong immune response of the host. We must therefore, renew our awareness of the fact that parasitic infections still exist all over the world and are now presenting many new problems that must be studied carefully and resolved appropriately.

References

[1] Murray CJL and Lopez AD. The Global burden of Diseases. Harvard University Press. Cambridge, MA, 1996.

[2] Montressor A, Crompton DWT, Gyorkos TW, Savioli L. Helminthis Control in School Age Children .World Health Organisation, Geneva, 2002.

[3] Taylor- Mascie CGN, Karim E. The burden of chronic diseases. *Science.* 2003; 302 (5652): 1921-22.

[4] Stephenson LS, Latham MC, Ottesen EA. Global Malnutrition. *Parasitology.* 2000; 121:S5- S22.

[5] Ramaiah KD, Radhamani MP. John KR, Evans DB, Guyatt H, Joseph A, Datta M, Vanamail P. The impact of lymphatic filariasis on labour inputs in Southern India: results of a multi-site study. *Ann. Trop. Med. Parasitol.* 2000; 94:353-64.

[6] Lawoyin TO. Infant & maternal deaths in rural southwest Nigeria: a prospective study. *Afr.J.Med. Med. Sci* 2007;36(3):235-41

[7] Karp CL, Auwaeter PG .Co-infection with HIV & tropical infectious diseases I protozoal pathogens.*Clin. Inf. Dis.* 2007; 145(9):1208-13.

[8] Desmonts G and Couvreur J. Congenital toxoplasmosis : A prospective study of the offspring of 542 women who acquired toxoplasma during pregnancy. In: Thalhammer O et al (eds): Perinatal medicine (Stuttgart, Germany,1979 p.51) .

[9] Villena I, Chemla C, Quereux C, Dupouy D, Leroux B, Foudrinier F, Pinon JM. Prenatal diagnosis of congenital toxoplasmosis transmitted by an immunocompetent woman infected before conception. Reims Toxoplasmosis Group. *Prenat. Diagn.* 1998;18(10):1079-81.

[10] Dunn D, Wallon M, Peyron F et al. Mother to child transmission of toxoplasmosis : Risk estimation and clinical counselling. *Lancet.* 1999;353:1829-33.

[11] Aspock H,Pollak A.Prevention of prenatal toxoplasmosis by serological screening of pregnant women in Austria.*Scand J.Inf. Dis.Suppl.* 1992;84:32-37

[12] Wong SY, Remington JS. Toxoplasmosis in pregnancy. *Clin. Infect. Dis.* 1994 ; 18 (6): 853-61.

[13] Remington JS, Newell JW, Cavanaugh E. Spontaneous abortion and chronic Toxoplasmosis. Report of a case, with isolation of the parasite. *Obstet. Gynecol.* 1964; 24: 25-31.

[14] Couvreur J, Thulliez T, Daffos F, Aufrant C, Bompard Y, Goumy P, Tournier G. 6 cases of toxoplasmosis in twins. *Ann. Pediatr* (Paris). 1991; 38(2): 63-8.

[15] Mc Leod R, Mack DG. Boyer KM et al. Phenotypes and functioning of lymphocytes in congenital toxoplasmosis. *J. Lab. Clin. Med.* 1990;116:623-25.

[16] Guerina NG, Ware J, Burbridge J et al. Neurodevelopmental outcomes for infants with congenital Toxoplasma infection from a new born serologic screening and treatment programme. *Pediatr Research* 1995, 37: 292A.

[17] Peyron F, Ateba AB, Wallon M et al. Congenital toxoplasmosis in twins: a report of fourteen congenital cases and comparison with published data. *Pediatr. Inf. Dis. J.* 2003; 22:695-701 .

[18] Arun V, Noble AG. Toxoplasmosis Study Group. Cataracts in congenital toxoplasmosis. *J. AAPOS.* 2007 ; 11(6):551-4.
[19] Tamma P. Toxoplasmosis. *Pediatr. Rev.* 2007 Dec;28(12):470-1.
[20] Oygur N,Yilmaz G,Ozkaynak C,Guven AG.Central diabetes insipidus in a patient with congenital toxoplasmosis. *Am. J. Perinatol.* 1998 ;15(3) :191-2
[21] Magann EF, Chauhan SP, Doherty DA, Lutgendorf MA, Magann MI, Morrison JC. A review of idiopathic hydramnios and pregnancy outcomes. *Obstet. Gynecol. Surv.* 2007; 62(12):795-802.
[22] Brooks RG, Sharma SD, Remington JS. Detection of Toxoplasma gondii antigens by a dot-immunobinding technique. *J. Clin. Microbiol.* 1985 ; 21(1):113-6.
[23] Jones JL, Kruszon-Moran D, Wilson M, McQuillan G, Navin T, McAuley JB.Toxoplasma gondii infection in the United States: seroprevalence and risk factors. *Am. J. Epidemiol.* 2001; 154(4): 357-65.
[24] Hofflin JM, Remington JS. Tissue culture isolation of Toxoplasma from blood of a patient with AIDS. *Arch. Intern. Med.* 1985 ;145(5):925-6.
[25] Daffos F, Forestier F, Capella-Pavlovsky M et al. Prenatal management of 746 pregnancies at risk for congenital toxoplasmosis. *N. Engl. J. Med.* 1988; 318:271-75.
[26] Foulon W. Congenital toxoplasmosis: is screening desirable? *Scand. J. Inf. Dis.* 1992; 84 (Suppl): 11-17
[27] Romand S, Chonsson M, Francek J et al. Usefulness of quantitative polymerase chain reaction fluid as early prognostic marker of fetal infection with T.gondii. *Am. J. Obst.Gynaecol.* 2001: 97(2):296-300.
[28] Robert-Gangneux F, Gavinet MF, Ancelle T, Raymond J, Tourte-Schaefer C, Dupouy-Camet J. Value of prenatal diagnosis and early postnatal diagnosis of congenital toxoplasmosis: retrospective study of 110 cases. *J. Clin. Microbiol.* 1999; 37 (9): 2893-8
[29] Beaman MH, Luft BJ, Remington JS. Prophylaxis for toxoplasmosis in AIDS. *Ann. Intern. Med.* 1992 ; 117(2):163-4.
[30] Remington JS, Thulliez P, Montoya JG. Recent developments for diagnosis of toxoplasmosis. *J. Clinical Microbiol.* 2004; 42(3):941-5
[31] Ciardelli L, Meroni V, Avanzini MA, Bollani L, Tinelli C, Garofoli F, Gasparoni A, Stronati M. Early and Accurate Diagnosis of Congenital Toxoplasmosis. *Pediatr. Infect .Dis. J.* 2008 ;27(2):125-9
[32] Eichenwald HF and Kotsevalvo. Immunologic response of premature and full term infants to infection with certain viruses. *Pediatrics* 1960;25:829-39
[33] McAuley JB, Boyer KM, Patel D, et al. Early and longitudinal evaluations of treated infants and children and untreated historical patients with congenital toxoplasmosis: The Chicago Collaborative Treatment Trial. *Clin. Infect Dis.* 1994; 18:38-72.
[34] Hohlfeld P, Daffos F, Costa JM, Thulliez P, Forestier F, Vidaud M. Prenatal diagnosis of congenital toxoplasmosis with a polymerase-chain-reaction test on amniotic fluid. *N. Engl. J. Med.* 1994; 331:695-99.
[35] Stray-Pedersen B. Toxoplasmosis in pregnancy. *Baillieres. Clin. Obstet. Gynaecol.* 1993; 7:107-37.

[36] Wilson CB, Remington JS, Stagno S, Reynolds DW. Development of adverse sequelae in children born with subclinical congenital toxoplasma infection. *Pediatrics.* 1980; 66: 767-74.

[37] de Roever-Bonnet H, Koppe JG, Loewer-Seger DH. Follow-up of children with congenital toxoplasma infection and children who became serologically negative after 1 year of age, all born in 1964-1965. In: Thalhammer O, Baumgarten K, Pollak A, eds. Perinatal medicine: Sixth European Congress, Vienna. Littleton, Massachusetts: PSG Publishing Company, 1979:61-75

[38] Lengeler C. Insecticide-treated nets for malaria control: real gains. *Bulletin. World. Health .Organ.* 2004; 82(2):84

[39] Smith T, Killeen G, Lengeler C, Tanner M. Relationships between the outcome of Plasmodium falciparum infection and the intensity of transmission in Africa. *Am. J. Trop. Med. Hyg.* 2004 ; 71(2 Suppl): 80-6

[40] Marchant T, Schellenberg JA, Nathan R, Abdulla S, Mukasa O, Mshinda H, Lengeler C. Anaemia in pregnancy and infant mortality in Tanzania. *Trop. Med. Int. Health* 2004; 9(2): 262-6.

[41] Piccoli DA, Perlman S, Ephros M. Transfusion-acquired Plasmodium malariae infection in two premature infants. *Pediatrics* 1983 ; 72:560-2

[42] Ghosh S, Patwari A, Mohan M et al. Clinical and hematologic peculiarities of malaria in infancy. *Clin. Pediatr.* (Phila) 1978; 17:369-71.

[43] Keitel HG, Goodman HC, Havel RJ et al. Nephrotic syndrome in congenital quartan malaria. *JAMA* 1956; 161:522-3.

[44] Uneke CJ. Impact of placental Plasmodium falciparum malaria on pregnancy and perinatal outcome in sub-Saharan Africa: I: introduction to placental malaria. *Yale. J. Biol. Med.* 2007 ; 80(2):39-50.

[45] Beeson JG, Reeder JC, Rogersonsen SJ, Bown GV. Parasitic adhesion and immune evasion in placental malaria. *Trends Parasitol.* 2001:17:331-37.

[46] Fried M, Duffy PE. Adherence of Plasmodium falciparum to chondroitin sulfate A in the human placenta. *Science.* 1996; 272(5267):1502-04.

[47] Stevenson MM, Riley EM. Innate immunity to malaria. *Nat. Rev. Immunol.* 2004; 4:169-80.

[48] Piccirillo CA, Shevach EM. Naturally occurring CD4+CD5+ immunoregulatory cells: Central players in the arena of peripheral tolerance. *Semin. Immunol.* 2004; 16:81-88.

[49] Croker IP, Tansinda DM, Baker PN. Syncytiotrophoblast degradation and the pathophysiology of malaria infected placenta. *Placenta* 2004; 25:273-82.

[50] Bruce-Chwatt LJ. Malaria in African infants and children in southern Nigeria. *Ann. Trop. Med. Parasitol.* 1952; 46:173- 78.

[51] Archibald HM. The influence of malarial infection of the placenta on the incidence of prematurity. *Bull. WHO* 1956; 15:842-87.

[52] Blacklock DB, Gordon RM. Malaria parasites in the placental blood. *Ann. Trop. Med. Parasitol.* 1925; 19:37

[53] Cannon DSH. Malaria and prematurity in western region of Nigeria. *Br. Med. J.* 1958; 2:877-83.

[54] Guyatt HI, Snow RW. Impact of malaria during pregnancy on low birth weight in Sub-Saharan Africa. *Clin. Microbiol. Rev*. 2004, 17:760-69.

[55] Luxemburger C, McGready R , Kham A, Morison L, Cho T, Tan C, White NJ . Nosten G. Effects of Malaria during Pregnancy on Infant Mortality in an area of Low Malaria Transmission. *Am. J. Epidemiol*. 2001; 154(5) :459-65.

[56] Brabin BJ, Ginny M, Sapau J et al. Consequences of maternal anaemia on outcome of pregnancy in a malaria endemic area in Papua New Guinea. *Ann. Trop. Med. Parasitol.* 1990; 84: 11-24.

[57] Steketee RW, Wirima JJ, Hightower AW et al. The effect of malaria and malaria prevention in pregnancy on offspring birth weight, prematurity and intrauterine growth retardation in rural Malawi. *Am. J. Trop. Med. Hyg*. 1996; 55 (Suppl 1):33-41.

[58] Menendez C, Ordi J, Ismail MR et al. The impact of placental malaria on gestational age and birth weight. *J. Infect. Dis*. 2000; 181:1740-5.

[59] Desai M, Ter Kuile FO, Nosten F et al. Epidemiology of malaria in pregnancy. *Lancet. Infect. Disease* 2007; 7:93-104.

[60] Campbell CC, Martinez JM, Collins WE. Seroepidemiological studies of malaria in pregnant women and newborns from coastal E1 Salvador. *Am. J. Trop. Med. Hyg*. 1980; 29:151-7

[61] Tobian AA, Mehrotra RK, Malhotra I et al. Frequent umbilical cord blood and maternal blood infections with Plasmodium falciparum, Plasmodium malariae and P. ovale in Kenya. *J. Inf. Dis*. 2000; 182:558-63.

[62] Malhotra I, Mungai P, Muchiri E et al. Umbilical cord-blood infections with Plasmodium falciparum malaria acquired antenatally in Kenya. *J. Inf. Dis*. 2006; 194: 176-83.

[63] Covell G. Congenital malaria. *Trop. Dis. Bull*. 1950; 47:1147.

[64] Sehgal VM, Siddiqui WA, Alpers MP. A seroepidemiological study to evaluate the role of passive maternal immunity to malaria in infants. *Trans. R. Soc. Trop. Med. Hyg*. 1989; 83(Suppl.):105-6

[65] Molineaux L, Cornille-Brogger R, Mathews HM et al. Longitudinal serological study of malaria in infants in the West African savanna. *Bull. WHO*. 1978; 56:573-8

[66] Menon R. Pregnancy and malaria. *Med. J. Malays*. 1972; 27:115-119

[67] Laveran A. Paludism. London, The New Sydenham Society 1893:104.

[68] Pengsaa K. Congenital malaria in Thailand. *Ann. Trop. Pediatr*. 2007; 27:133-39.

[69] Singh N, Mehra RK, Srivastava N. Malaria during pregnancy and infancy, in an area of intense malaria transmission in Central India. *Ann. Trop. Med. and Parasitol*. 2001; 95 (1):19-29.

[70] Hindi RD, Azimi PH. Congenital malaria due to *Plasmodium falciparum*. *Pediatrics*. 1980; 66: 977–9.

[71] Singh N, Saxena A, Shrivastava R. Placental Plasmodium vivax infection and congenital malaria in central India. *Ann. Trop. Med. Parsitol*. 2003; 97:875-8.

[72] De Silva DH, Mendis KN, Premarathne UN, Jayatilleke SM, Soyza PE. Congenital malaria due to Plasmodium vivax: a case report from Sri Lanka. *Tans. R. Soc. Trop. Med. Hyg*.1982; 76:33-35.

[73] Comellini L, Tozzola a, Baldi F, Brusa S, Serra L, Agostoni C, Scaglia m. Plasmodium vivax congenital malaria in a newborn of a Zairian immigrant. *Ann. Trop. Paediatr.* 1998; 18(1):41-3

[74] Lee WW, Singh M, Tan CL. A recent case of congenital malaria in Singapore. *Singapore. Med. J.* 1996; 37:541-43.

[75] Wivanitkit V. Congenital malaria in Thailand, an appraisal of previous cases. *Pediatrics Int.* 2006; 48:562-65.

[76] Valecha N, Bhatia S, Mehta S, Biswas S, Dash AP. Congenital malaria with atypical presentation: a case report from low transmission area in India. *Malar. J.* 2007; 6:43.

[77] Fischer PR. Malaria and Newborn. *J. Trop. Pediatr.* 2003; 49:132-34.

[78] Rampengan D, Rampengan TH. Congenital falciparum malaria with chloroquine resistance type II. *Paediatr. Indones.* 1989; 29(1-2):13-9

[79] Airede AI. Congenital malaria with chloroquine resistance. *Ann. Trop. Paediatr.* 1991; 11:267-9

[80] Coura JR, Junqueira ACV, Carvalho-Moreira CJ, Borges-Pereira J, Albajar PV 2007. Uma visão sistêmica da endemia chagásica. In AC Silveira, *La Enfermedad de Chagas a la Puerta de los 100 Años del Conocimiento de Una Endemia Americana Ancestral*, Organización Panamericana de la Salud y Fundación Mundo Sano, Buenos Aires, p. 25-35.

[81] Bittencourt AL. Possible risk factors for vertical transmission of Chagas' disease. Revista do Instituto de Medicina Tropical de São Paulo 1992 ; 34:403-8

[82] Carlier V, Torrico F (organizers) 2005. Colóquio Internacional Infección Congênita por *Trypanosoma cruzi*: desde los mecanismos de transmissión hasta una estratégia de diagnóstico y control. *Rev. Soc. Bras. Med. Trop.* 2005; 38 (Supl. II): 1-128.

[83] Nisida IV, Amato Neto V, Braz LM, Duarte MI, Umezawa ES. A survey of congenital Chagas disease carried out at three health Institutions in Sao Paulo City, Brazil. *Rev. Inst. Med. Trop. Sao Paulo* 1999; 41(5):305-11.

[84] Mendeoza Ticona CA, Cordova Benzaquen E, Ancca Juarez J et al. The prevalence of Chagas' disease in puerperal women and congenital transmission in an endemic area of Peru. *Rev. Panam. Salud Publica* 2005; 17(3):147-53.

[85] Gürtler RE, Segura EL, Cohen JE. Congenital transmission of *Trypanosoma cruzi* infection in Argentina. *Emerg. Inf. Dis.* 2003; 9:29-35.

[86] Kirchhoff L. American trypanosomiasis (Chagas' disease). A tropical disease now in the United States. *N. Eng. J. Med.* 1993; 329:639-44.

[87] Fretes RE, Fabro SP. *In vivo* and *in vitro* analysis of lysosomes and acid phosphatase activity in human chagasic placentas. *Exp. Mol. Pathol.* 1995; 63: 153-60.

[88] Sartori MJ, Lin S, Frank FM, Malchiodi E, Fabro SP. The role of placental alkaline phosphatase in the interaction between human placental Trophoblast and *Trypanosoma cruzi*. *Exp. Mol. Pathol.* 2000;72: 84-90.

[89] Moya P, Moretti E. Doenca de Chagas congenita. *In:* Fundação do Instituto Oswaldo Cruz. "Clinica e Terapeutica da doenca de Chagas: Uma abordagem pratica para o clinico geral". 1st edition, Rio de Janeiro1997;383-410.

[90] Rassi A, Borges C, Koeberle F, De Paula OH. Sobre a transmissão congênita da doença de Chagas. *Revista Goiania de Medicina* 1958; 4:319-32.

[91] Brabin Rabin L. The epidemiological significance of Chagas disease in women. *Memórias do Instituto Oswaldo Cruz* 87:73, 1992.
[92] Spellberg B, Edwards JE, Jr. Type 1/ type 2 immunity in infectious diseases. *Clin. Infect. Dis*. 2001; 32:76-102.
[93] Handman E. Leishmaniasis: current status of vaccine development. *Clin. Microbiol. Rev*. 2001; 14: 229-43.
[94] Peter CM. Leishmaniasis. In: Behrman RE, Kliegman RM, Jenson HB, editors. Nelson Textbook of Pediatrics. 16th edn. Philadelphia: WB Saunders; 2000.
[95] Bryceson A. Visceral leishmaniasis in India. *Lancet.* 2000;356:1933
[96] Pintado V, Martin-Rabadan P, Rivera ML, Moreno S, Bouza E. Visceral leishmaniasis in human immunodeficiency virus (HIV)-infected and non-HIV-infected patients. A comparative study. *Medicine* (Baltimore) 2001; 80:54-73.
[97] Figueiró-Filho EA, Duarte G, El-Beitune P, Quintana SM, Maia TL. Visceral leishmaniasis (kala-azar) and pregnancy. *Klin. Padiatr.*1995 ; 207(6):347-9.
[98] Zambrano E. Cases of infantile visceral leishmaniasis observed in the ten-year period 1939-49 in the Province of Brindisi. *Lattante.* 1950; 21(5):283-9.
[99] Mittal V, Sehgal S, Yadav TP et al. Congenital transmission of kala-azar. *J. Com. Dis.* 1987; 19: 84–5.
[100] Hill FG, Letsky EA. Infantile kala-azar in Britain. *Br. Med. J.* 1975; 3(5979):354-5.
[101] De Castro AS, Gondin A. Case of infantile kala-azar, first case observed in Rio de Janeiro. *J. Pediatr.* (Rio J) 1955; 20(9):517-29.
[102] Granert C, Elinder G, Ost A, Henter JI. Kala-azar in a one-year-old Swedish child. Diagnostic difficulties because of active hemophagocytosis. *Acta. Paediatr.* 1993; 82(9):794-6.
[103] Meinecke CK, Schottelius J, Oskam L, Fleischer B. Congenital transmission of visceral leishmaniasis (Kala Azar) from an asymptomatic mother to her child. *Pediatrics* 1999; 104(5):e65 .
[104] Rey LC, Martins CV, Ribeiro HB, Lima AA. American visceral leishmaniasis (kala-azar) in hospitalized children from an endemic area. *J. Pediatr. (Rio J).* 2005; 81(1):73-8.
[105] Abdeen ZA, Sawalha SS, Eisenberger CL. Khanfar HM, Greenblatt CL, Yousef O, Schnur LF, Azmi K, Warburg A, Bader KA, Jaffe CL. Baneth G. Epidemiology of visceral leishmaniasis in the Jenin District, West Bank: 1989-1998. *Am. J. Trop. Med. Hyg.* 2002 ;66(4):329-33.
[106] Kharfi M, Benmously R, El Fekih N, Daoud M, Fitouri Z, Mokhtar I, Ben Becher S, Kamoun MR.Childhood leishmaniasis: report of 106 cases. *Dermatol. Online. J.* 2004; Oct 15;10(2):6.
[107] Di Martino L, Gramiccia M, Occorsio P, Di Muccio T, Scalone A, Gradoni L. Infantile visceral leishmaniasis in the Campania region, Italy: experience from a Paediatric Referral Centre . *Parassitologia.* 2004; 46(1-2):221-3.
[108] Minodier P, Noël G, Blanc P, Uters M, Retornaz K, Garnier JM. Treatment of visceral leishmaniasis in children. *Med. Trop.* (Mars). 2007; 67(1): 73-8.
[109] Kotcher E, Mata LJ. Esquivel R et al. Acquisition of intestinal parasites in newborn human infants. *Fed. Proc.* 1965; 24:442-6.

[110] Knight R. Surveys for amoebiasis. Interpretations of data and their implications. *Ann. Trop. Med. Parasitol.* 1975; 69:35-48

[111] Hsiung CC. Amebiasis of the newborn: report of three cases. *Chin. J. Pathol.* 1958 ; 4:14- 17

[112] Dykes AC, Ruebush TK, Gorelkin L et al. Extraintestinal amebiasis in infancy: report of three patients and epidemiologic investigations of their families. *Pediatrics.* 1980 ; 65:799-803

[113] Tannich E, Burchard GD. Differentiation of pathogenic from nonpathogenic Entamoeba histolytica by restriction fragment analysis of a single gene amplified in vitro. 1991 *J. Clin. Microbiol.* 1991; 29:250-55

[114] Bruckner DA. Amebiasis. *Clin. Microbiol. Rev.* 1992 ; 5:356-69

[115] Black RE, Dykes AC, Sinclair SP et al. Giardiasis in day care centers. Evidence of person-to-person transmission. *Pediatrics.* 1977; 60:486-91

[116] Pickering LK, Woodward WE, DuPont HL et al. Occurrence of G. lamblia in children in day care centers. *J. Pediatr.* 1984; 104:522-26

[117] Monaghan H, Garvey RG, Egan-Mitchell B et al. Giardiasis in infancy diarrhoea. *Arch Dis. Child.* 1980; 55:715-16

[118] Islam A, Stoll BJ, Ljungstrom I, et al. *Giardia lamblia* infection in a cohort of Bangladeshi mothers and infants followed for one year. *J. Pediatr.* 1983; 103:996-1000

[119] Morrow AL, Reves RR, West MS et al. Protection against infection with *Giardia lamblia* by breast-feeding in a cohort of Mexican infants. *J. Pediatr.* 1992; 121:363-70

[120] Walterspiel JN, Morrow AL, Guerrero ML, Ruiz-Palacios GM, Pickering LK. Protective effect of secretory anti-*Giardia lamblia* antibodies in human milk against diarrhea. *Pediatrics.* 1994; 93:28-31

[121] Current WL, Garcia LS. Cryptosporidiosis. *Clin. Microbiol. Rev.* 1991; 4:325-58

[122] Alpert G, Bell LM, Kirkpatrick CE et al. Outbreak of cryptosporidiosis in a day care center. *Pediatrics.* 1986; 77:152-7

[123] Cruz JR. Cryptosporidiosis in infants. *J. Clin. Microbiol.* 1988 ;26 :88-91

[124] Ungar BL. Enzyme-linked immunoassay for detection of *Cryptosporidium* antigens in fecal specimens. *J. Clin. Microbiol.* 1990; 28:2491-95

[125] Mirdha BR, Kabra SK, Samantray JC. Isosporiasis in children. *Indian. Pediatr.* 2002; 39(10):941-4.

[126] Pape JW, Verdier RI, Jhonson WD Jr. Treatment and prophylaxis of Isospora belli infection in patients with Acquired immunodeficiency Syndrome. *N. Eng. J. Med.* 1989; 320: 1044-47.

[127] Madico G, McDonald J, Gilman RH. Carbera L, Sterling CR. Epidemiology and treatment of Cyclospora cayetanensis in Peruvian children. *Clin. Inf. Dis.* 1997;24:977-81

[128] Iyer RN. Cyclosporiasis in an infant. *Ind. J. Med. Res.* 2006;24(2):144-45

[129] Didier ES. Microsporidiosis. *Clin. Inf. Dis.* 1998; 27:1-7

[130] Kotler DP, Orenstein JM. Clinical syndromes associated with microsporidiosis. *Adv. Parasitol.* 1998; 40:321-349.

[131] Schuster H, Chiodini PL. Parasitic infections of the intestine. *Curr. Opin. Infect. Dis.* 2001; 14: 587-91.

[132] Visvesvara GS, Neafie RC, Martinez AJ. Pathogenic and opportunistic free-living amebae. In: Horsburgh CR, Nelson AM (eds) Pathology of emerging infections. ASM Press, Washington, 1997; p.257-267.

[133] Visvesvara GS. Laboratory diagnosis. In: Rondanelli EG (ed) Amphizoic amoebae. Human pathology. Piccin, Padova, 1987; p.193-215.

[134] Moura H, Wallace S, Visvesvara GS. Acanthamoeba healyi, N. sp. and the isoenzyme and immunoblot profiles of Acanthamoeba spp., group 1 and 3. *J. Parasitol.* 1992; 39:573-583.

[135] Stothard DR, Schroeder-Dietrich JM, Awwad MH, Gast RJ, Ledee DR, Rodriguez-Zaragoza S, Dean CL, Fuerst PA, Byers TJ. The evolutionary history of the genus Acanthamoeba and the identification of eight new 18S rRNA gene sequence types. *J. Eukaryot. Microbiol.* 1998; 45:45-54.

[136] Sison JP, Kemper CA, Loveless M, McSchane D, Visvesvara GS, Derensinki SC. Disseminated Acanthamoeba infection in patients with AIDS: Case report and review of literature. *Clin. Inf. Dis.* 1995;201:1207-16

[137] Martinez AJ, Visvesvara GS. Balamuthia mandrillaris infection. *J. Med. Microbiol.* 2001; 50:205-207.

[138] De Jonckheere JF, Brown S. Primary amebic meningoencephalitis in a patient with AIDS: unusual protozoological findings. *Clin. Infect. Dis.* 1997 ; 25(4):943-4.

[139] Vookin MH, Howe DK, Visvesvara GS, Mc Langhlin GC. Identification of Acanthamoeba at the genetic and specific levels using the polymerase chain reaction. *J. Protozool.* 1992; 39:378-385.

[140] Ogilvie BM, Selkirk ME, Maisels RM: The molecular revolution and nematode parasitology: yesterday, today, and tomorrow. *J. Parasitol.* 1990; 67:607-618.

[141] Schad GS, Chowdhury AB, Dean CG et al: Arrested development in human hookworm infections: An adaptation to a seasonally unfavorable external environment. *Science.* 1973; 180:502-504.

[142] Selkirk ME, Maisels RM. Molecular and cellular biology of helminth parasites IV. *Int. J. Parasitol.* 2006;36(6):615-6

[143] Finkelmann FD, Pearce EJ, Urban JF Jr et al. Regulation and biological function of helminth-induce cytokine responses. *Parasitol. Today* 1991; 7:A62-A66.

[144] Behnke JM: Evasion of immunity by nematode parasites causing chronic infections. *Adv. Parasitol.* 1987; 26: 1-71

[145] Ephenson LS, Latham MC, Kinoti SN et al. Improvements in physical fitness of Kenyan schoolboys infected with hookworm, Trichuris trichiura and Ascaris lumbricoides following a single dose of albendazole. *Trans. R Soc. Trop. Med. Hyg.* 1990; 84:277-282.

[146] Haswell-Elkins MR, Elkins DB, Anderson RM: Evidence for predisposition of humans to infection with Ascaris, hookworm, Enterobius, and Trichuris in a South Indian fishing community. *Parasitology.* 1987; 95:323-37.

[147] Costa-Macedo LM, Costa M, Almeida LM. Ascaris lumbricoides in infants: a population-based study in Rio de Janeiro, Brasil. Cad Saude Publica. 1999 ; 15(1):173-8

[148] Sangkhathat S, Patrapinyokul S, Wudhisuthimethawee P, Chedphaopan J, Mitamun W. Massive gastrointestinal bleeding in infants with ascariasis. *J. Pediatr. Surg.* 2003; 38(11):1696-8.
[149] Thein Hlaing, Thane-Toe, Than-Saw et al. A controlled chemotherapeutic intervention trial on the relationship between Ascaris lumbricoides infection and malnutrition in children. *Trans. R. Soc. Trop. Med. Hyg.* 1991; 85:523-28.
[150] Jernigan J, Guerrant RL, Pearson RD. Parasitic infections of the small intestine. *Gut.* 1994; 35:289-93.
[151] Crompton DWT: The prevalence of ascariasis. *Parasitol. Today.* 1989: 4:162-9.
[152] Bundy DAP, Cooper ES: Trichiura and trichuriasis in humans. *Adv. Parasitol.* 28:107-173, 1989.
[153] Crompton DW How much human helminthiasis is there in the world? *J. Parasitol.* 1999; 85(3):397-403.
[154] Goodman D, Haji HJ, Bickle QD, Stoltzfus RJ, Tielsch JM, Ramsan M, Savioli L, Albonico M. A comparison of methods for detecting the eggs of Ascaris, Trichuris, and hookworm in infant stool, and the epidemiology of infection in Zanzibari infants. *Am. J. Trop. Med. Hyg.* 2007;76(4):725-31.
[155] Jeske J, Kamerys J, Ochecka-Szymańska A. Efficacy of mebendazole in treatment of selected parasitoses--a retrospective study. *Wiad. Parazytol.* 2000; 46(1):127-39.
[156] Bethony J, Brooker S, Albonico M, Geiger SM, Loukas A, Diemert D, Hotez PJ. Soil-transmitted helminth infections: ascariasis, trichuriasis, and hookworm. *Lancet.* 2006 May 6; 367(9521):1521-32.
[157] MacDonald TT, Spencer J, Murch SH et al. Immunoepidemology of intestinal helminthic infections. 3. Mucosal macrophages and cytokine production in the colon of children with Trichuris trichiura dysentery. *Trans. Roy. Soc. Trop. Med. Hyg.* 1994;88:265-268
[158] Anonymous. *Children's worms* [Editorial]. BMJ 1974; 4:3.
[159] Haswell-Elkins MR, Elkins DB, Manjula K, Michael E, Anderson RM. The distribution and abundance of Enterobius vermicularis in a South Indian fishing community. *Parasitology* 1987; 95:339-54.
[160] Gupta SC, Gupta AK, Keswani NK, Singh PA, Tripathi AK, Krishna V. Pathology of tropical appendicitis. *J. Clin. Pathol.* 1989; 42:1169-72.
[161] Magnaval J-F, Michault A, Calon N, et al. Epidemiology of human toxocariasis in La Reunion. *Trans. R Soc. Trop. Med. Hyg.* 1994; 88:531-533.
[162] Fenoy S, Cuellar C, Guiillen JL. Serological evidence of toxocariasis in patients from Spain with a clinical suspicion of visceral larva migrans. *J. Helminthol.* 1997; 71:9-12.
[163] Mirdha BR, Khokar SK. Ocular Toxocariasis in a North Indian Population. *J. Trop. Pediatrics* 2002; 48:328-330.
[164] Stoll NR. This wormy world. *J. parasitol.* 1947; 33:1-18.
[165] Banwell JG, Schad GA: Hookworm. *Clin. Gastroenterol.* 1978; 7:128-156
[166] Gilman RH: Hookworm disease: Host pathogen biology. *Rev. Infect Dis.* 1982; 4:824-829.
[167] Zimmerman HM. Fatal Hookworm Disease in infancy and childhood in Guam. *The Am. J. Pathol.* 1946; XXII (6):1081-1100.

[168] Liu Lx, Weller PF: Strongyloidiasis and other intestinal nematode infections. *Infect Dis. Clin. North Am.* 1993; 7(3):655-682.
[169] Liu Lx, Weller PF: Eosinophilic mengitis. *Seminar. Neurol.* 1993; 13(2):161-68.
[170] Burke JA. Strogyloidiasis inn childhood. *Am. J. Dis. Child* 1978; 132:1130-1136.
[171] Gam A, Neva FA, Krotoski WA. Comparative sensitivity and specificity of ELISA and IHA for serodiagnosis of strongyloidiasis with larval antigens. *Am. J. Trop. Med. and Hyg.* 1987; 37:157-161.
[172] Perera M, Whitehead M, Molyneux D, Weerasooriya M, Gunatilleke G. Neglected patients with a neglected disease? A qualitative study of lymphatic filariasis. *PLoS Negl. Trop. Dis.* 2007; 21:1(2):e128.
[173] Rwegoshora RT, Simonsen PE, Meyrowitsch DW, Malecela-Lazaro MN, Michael E, Pedersen EM. Bancroftian filariasis: house-to-house variation in the vectors and transmission -- and the relationship to human infection -- in an endemic community of coastal Tanzania. *Ann. Trop. Med. Parasitol.* 2007 ;101(1):51-60.
[174] Satapathy AK, Sartono E, Sahoo PK, Dentener MA, Michael E, Yazdanbakhsh M, Ravindran B. Human bancroftian filariasis: immunological markers of morbidity and infection. *Microbes. Infect.* 2006; 8(9-10): 2414-23.
[175] Shenoy RK, Suma TK, Kumaraswami V, Rahmah N, Dhananjayan G, Padma S, Abhilash G, Ramesh C. Preliminary findings from a cross-sectional study on lymphatic filariasis in children, in an area of India endemic for Brugia malayi infection. *Ann. Trop. Med. Parasitol.* 2007; 101(2):173-80.
[176] Lammie PJ, Lindo JF, Secor WE, Vasquez J, Ault SK, Eberhard ML. Eliminating lymphatic filariasis, onchocerciasis, and schistosomiasis from the Americas: breaking a historical legacy of slavery. *PLoS Negl. Trop. Dis.* 2007; 1(2):e71.
[177] Hodgkin C, Molyneux DH, Abiose A, Philippon B, Reich MR, Remme JH, Thylefors B, Traore M, Grepin K. The future of onchocerciasis control in Africa. *PLoS Negl. Trop. Dis.* 2007 31;1(1):e74.
[178] Boussinesq M. Loiasis. *Ann. Trop. Med. Parasitol.* 2006;100(8):715-31.
[179] Araya J, Kawabata Y, Tomichi N, Kaneko K, Hayashi K, Iwabuchi K, Terasaki Y, Kawashima T, Watanabe M. Allergic inflammatory reaction is involved in necrosis of human pulmonary dirofilariasis. *Histopathology* .2007;51(4):484-90.
[180] Hwang KP, Chen ER. Clinical studies on Angiostrongylus cantonensis infection among children in Taiwan. *SEA. J. Trop. Med. Pub. Health.* 1991; 22(suppl.):194-199.
[181] Punyagupta S, Juttijudata P, Bunnag T. Eosinophilic meningitis Thailand: clinical studies of 484 typical cases probably caused by *Angiostrongylus cantonensis. Am. J. Trop. Med. and Hyg.* 1975; 24:921-923.
[182] Sawanyawisuth K, Kitthaweesin K, Limpawattana P, Intapan PM, Tiamkao S, Jitpimolmard S, Chotmongkol V. Intraocular angiostrongyliasis: clinical findings, treatments and outcomes. *Trans. R Soc. Trop. Med. Hyg.* 2007 ;101(5):497-501
[183] Sawanyawisuth K, Sawanyawisuth K. Treatment of Angiostrongyliasis *Trans R Soc. Trop. Med. Hyg.* 2008;110(10):990-96.
[184] Wong MH. Multiple Infestation with Dipylidium Caninum in an Infant. *Can. M A J.* 1955; 72:453-455.

[185] Matsaniotis N, Karpathios T, Koutovzis J, Nicolaidou P. Fretzaayas A, Papadellis F. Thomaidis T. Hydatid disease in Greek Children. *Am. J. Trop. Med. Hyg.* 1983; 32 (5): 1075-78.

[186] The hydatid cyst of the lung in children: 54 cases *Tunis Med.* 2005; 83(1): 24-27.

[187] Sakamoto T, Gutierrez C. Pulmonary complications of cystic echinococcosis in children in Uruguay. *Pathol. Int.* 2005; 55(8):497-503.

[188] Rumana M, Mahadevan A, Navil KM, Kovoor JM, Yasta IC, Santhosh V, Indira B, Shankar SK. Cestode parasitic infestation: Intracranial and spinal hydatid disease – a clinicopathological study of 29 cases from South India. *Clin. Neuropathl.* 2006; 25 (2): 98-104.

[189] Garg RK. Childhood Neurocysticercosis: Issues in diagnosis and management. *Indian. Pediatr.* 1995; 32: 1023-29.

[190] Singhi P, Ray M, Singhi S et al. Clinical spectrum of 500 children with neurocysticercosis and response to albendazole therapy. *J. Child. Neurol.* 2000; 15: 207-213.

[191] Kalra V, Suri M, Jailkhani BL. A profile of childhood neurocysticercosis. *Indian. J. Pediatr.* 1994; 61: 33-42.

[192] Gupta RK, Kumar R, Chawla S et al. Demonstration of scolex within calcified cysticercus cyst: Its possible role in the pathogenesis of perilesional edema. *Epilepsia* 2002; 43: 1502-1508.

[193] Alarcon de Noya B, Ruiz R, Losada S, Colmenares C, Contreras R, Cesari IM, Noya O. Detection of schistosomiasis cases in low-transmission areas based on coprologic and serologic criteria The Venezuelan experience. *Acta. Trop.* 2007; 103(1):41-9.

[194] Schwartz E, Kazarsky P.Wilson M, Cetron M. Schistosoma infection among river rafter on Omo River Ethiopia. *J. Travel Med.*.2005,12:3-8

[195] Lun ZR, Gasser RB, Lai DH, Li AX, Zhu XQ, Yu XB. Clonorchiasis: a key food borne zoonosis in China. *Lancet. Infect. Dis*. 2005; 5:31-41.

[196] Haswell-Elins M, Levri E. Food-borne trematodes. In: Cook G, Zumla A, editors. Manson's tropical diseases. 21st ed. London: W.B. Saunders; 2003. p. 1471-86.

[197] Lee GS, Cho IS, Lee YH, Noh HJ et al. Epidemiology study of clonorchiasis and metagonimiasis along Geum-gang (River) in Okcheon –gun (county), Korea. *Korean J. Parasitol.* 2002; 40:9-16.

In: Topics in Prevalent Diseases
Editors: N. C. Chavez-Tapia and M. Uribe
ISBN 978-1-60456-959-9

Chapter 13

Gastrointestinal Viral Infections in Children

Gabriel Ignacio Parra,[1,*] Karin Bok[2] and José Paulo Gagliardi Leite[3]
[1] Molecular Biology Department, Research Institute of Health Science, National University of Asunción, Paraguay
[2] Laboratory of Infectious Diseases, National Institute of Allergy and Infectious Diseases, National Institutes of Health,
Bethesda, Maryland, USA
[3] Laboratory of Comparative Virology, Oswaldo Cruz Institute, Oswaldo Cruz Foundation, Ministry of Health, Rio de Janeiro, Brazil

Acute diarrheal disease is an important cause of morbidity and mortality worldwide, affecting mainly infants and young children.

It has been estimated that during the 1990s, approximately 1.4 billion diarrhea episodes occurred annually in children under 5 years of age, 9 million of whom required hospitalization, and 2.5 million of whom died from diarrhea (~20% of the total death). Although this number is below the ones published for the 1970s (4.6 million) and the 1980s (3.0 million), it is still a heavy burden to the global population [1].

Several etiologic agents, such as bacteria, parasites, viruses and/or food poisoning, can cause diarrhea; however, the main etiologic agent can vary depending on different factors such as demographic variables of the population under study, the origin of the samples, different geographical regions, etc.

In this chapter, we will focus our attention on the three main viral agents that cause gastroenteritis (i.e. rotaviruses, noroviruses and astroviruses), with special emphasis on virus diversity and epidemiology in developing countries.

* Present address: Department of Neurosciences, Lerner Research Institute, The Cleveland Clinic Foundation, 9500 Euclid Avenue, Cleveland, OH 44195, USA. E-mail: gabriel_parra@hotmail.com.

Rotaviruses

Overview

Rotavirus is considered the greatest worldwide viral cause of acute gastroenteritis in infants and young children, causing an average of 611,000 (454,000 – 705,000) deaths per year. Even though the global deaths from childhood diarrhea decreased during the last two decades, the number of diarrhea hospitalizations attributable to rotavirus has increased [2]. In addition, rotavirus incidence is similar in developed and developing countries, which suggests that its control could not be carried out by improving only the hygiene and water supply in the population [3]. Therefore, there is a general consensus that a vaccine would be the best strategy to prevent the severity of the diarrhea caused by rotaviruses.

Rotaviruses are spread through fecal-oral contact, and the incubation period is approximately two days. The symptoms of the disease are characterized by fever, vomiting, watery diarrhea, and abdominal pain. These symptoms could persist from three to ten days, and infected children may have profuse watery diarrhea up to several times per day. Since virtually every child is already infected by rotavirus during the two first years of age, repeated infections tend to be less severe due to the immunity acquired from previous infections [4].

The first description of rotavirus in humans was made by Ruth Bishop et al. in 1973, when they visualized virus particles by electron microscopy (EM) in the epithelial cells of duodenal mucosa from children with acute non-bacterial gastroenteritis; soon after, this observation was confirmed by others [5, 6]. The name (rotavirus) comes from the Latin "rota", meaning "wheel", due to the characteristic wheel-like appearance of the virus when viewed by EM.

Rotaviruses belong to the *Reoviridae* family, have an icosahedral, nonenveloped, triple-layered capsid (i.e. the core, inner and outer capsid), and a genome of 11 double-stranded RNA (dsRNA) segments. Each segment codes for one protein, except for the last one, which codes for two proteins. Thus, six structural proteins (VP1 – VP4, VP6, VP7), and six non-structural proteins (NSP1 - NSP6) have been detected [7].

Based on antigenic and genetic differences of the VP6 protein, seven groups (A – G) have been identified so far. Groups A, B and C have been detected in humans and animals; but groups D, E and F have been found only in animals so far [7, 8].

Each group presents a characteristic migration pattern (termed "electropherotype") of its eleven genomic segments. For instance, group A rotaviruses show four clusters of genes arranged as follows: 4-2-3-2. In addition, depending on the mobility of the segments from the last cluster, two main electropherotypes (i.e. long or short) can be found in humans [7]. The study of the different electropherotypes has been extensively used in epidemiology, especially during the 1980s (see also Diagnosis and Identification in this chapter).

Group A rotaviruses are by far the most prevalent in humans, and can be divided in at least two subgroups (SGI and SGII) based on differences in the VP6 protein.

The outermost capsid of group A rotaviruses is composed of VP4 and VP7 proteins, which specify the P (which stands for ***P***rotease sensitive protein) and G (which stands for ***G***lycoprotein) serotypes, respectively. Based on sequence differences of these two proteins,

28 [P] genotypes that do not correlate with VP4 serotypes and 16 G genotypes which correlate with VP7 serotypes have been described so far. Thus, a dual nomenclature based in the G and P types has been adopted to identify rotaviruses (e.g., the most prevalent human strain is named G1P[8]) [7, 9-11]. It is worth pointing out that the P genotypes are described using square brackets to differenciate from the P serotypes (e.g. the genotype P[8] correspond to the serotype P1A).

The great diversity of rotaviruses is created by the: (1) accumulation of point mutations; that can lead to the origin of new serotypes/genotypes and/or intragenotypes variants; (2) recombination and rearrangements of their genes; (3) ability of animal rotavirus to infect humans; and (4) ability of co-circulating rotavirus strains to reassort [12-14]. The latter is a property that allow rotavirus to generate different combination of genes, thus, after infection of one cell with two different rotaviruses, theoretically, 2^{11} new viruses can arise. Despite this theoretical number, a genetic link between different genes has been shown, and few combinations of genes are the most commonly detected. Thus, based on RNA hybridization and full-genome sequencing methods, three genogroups (or gene constellations) have been detected in rotavirus strains isolated from humans (i.e. genogroup "Wa", "DS-1" and "AU-1") [15, 16]. The strains from the "Wa" genogroup usually present the combinations G1P[8], G3P[8], G4P[8] or G9P[8] with SGII and long electropherotype; and the strains from genogroup "DS-1" usually present the combinations G2P[4] and G9P[6] with SGI and short electropherotype [14, 17, 18]; while strains from genogroup "AU-1" are from animal origin.

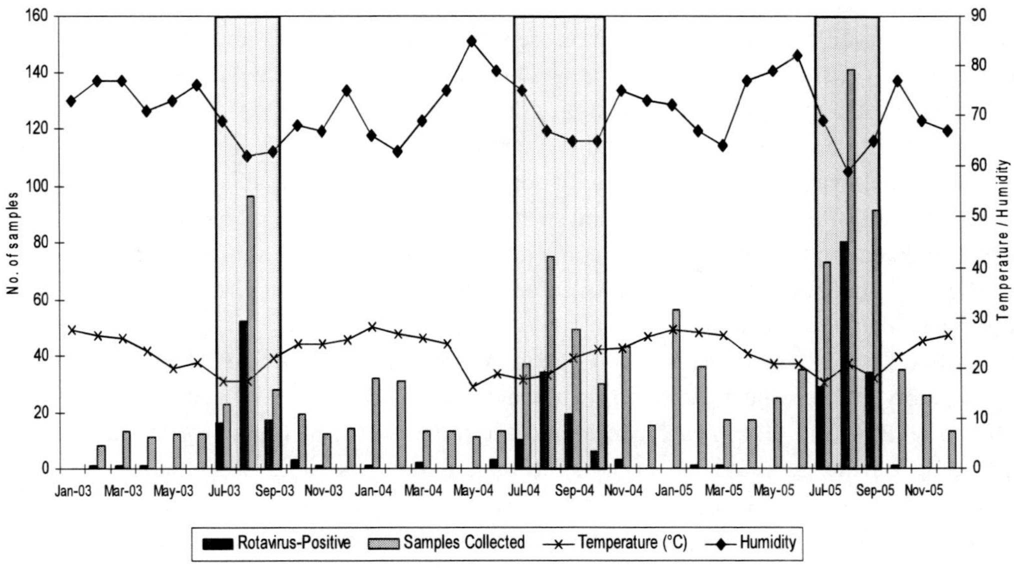

Figure 1. Monthly distribution of rotavirus infection in Paraguayan children with acute diarrhea, mean humidity and mean temperature, from January 2003 to December 2005. The periods with the highest incidence of rotavirus infections are highlighted.

Epidemiology

Rotavirus spreads through the fecal-oral route, is a highly contagious virus, and affects males and females, as well as different ethnic groups, equally [4].

Epidemiological studies have shown that rotavirus infections are the cause of approximately 30% of the gastroenteritis detected in children under 5 years old, showing the highest incidence in children between 6 and 24 months of age [19]. This age-group is at greatest risk for developing severe disease as well. Since the natural immunity acquired by previous infections is incomplete, adults also become infected, showing incidences that could range from 3% to 33%; however, the resulting illness is usually mild [20, 21].

Rotaviruses can be detected year-round, but a seasonal pattern of the infection showing the highest incidence during the coolest and driest months of the year has been shown in temperate zones (Figure 1); whereas in tropical zones the seasonality of the infection is not well defined [4, 22, 23]. For instance, seasonal patterns of rotavirus infections have been described in the south region of South-America, i.e. Argentina, Paraguay (Figure 1), Chile, and in the central and southern states of Brazil [24-26]. It is worth pointing out that slightly seasonal peaks during the coolest and driest months of the year in tropical countries [27], or the lack of seasonal patterns in temperate zones have been shown, therefore the influence of meteorological conditions in the incidence of rotavirus is not well understood yet [22, 25, 28].

Since the VP4 and VP7 proteins elicit neutralizing antibodies, they are the main targets for vaccine development (for the current vaccines characteristics see Table 1 in this chapter). Thus, the surveillance of the P and G serotypes circulating in the human and animal population is considered essential to understand the evolution of rotaviruses and, ultimately, evaluate the efficacy of the vaccination programs.

The first descriptions of the G and P types were carried out by using serological assays, but the limited availability of reagents for serotype detection made this task difficult, mainly in laboratories from developing countries. The introduction of molecular techniques for genotype detection has helped to overcome this [29], and, thus, the surveillance systems from developing countries have been improved and new data about rotavirus epidemiology have become available [13, 14, 30].

Although 28 P genotypes and 16 G genotypes have been described, 12 P genotypes and 11 G genotypes have been detected in humans so far. Of them, the combinations G1P[8], G2P[4], G3P[8] and G4P[8] are considered the most prevalent types worldwide. However, depending on the geographical region, the uncommon types and combinations have been detected at a high percentage of incidences (Figure 2) [13, 14, 30]. Thus, for example, in developed countries, the G1P[8] is the most prevalent combination, accounting for ≥ 70% of the characterized strains; whereas in developing countries, it accounts for less than 35% of the strains. The other three strains account for 17%-22% and 27%-34% in developed and developing countries respectively (Figure 2).

The lower percentages of G1P[8] strains in developing countries are mainly due to the high percentages (16%-43%) of unusual strains detected in those countries. The unusual strains are largely represented by G5P[8], G8P[4]/G8P[6], and G9P[11]/G10P[11] strains in South America, Africa and Asia, respectively. In this regard, strains bearing these types are mainly found in pigs (G5) and cows (G8, G10 and P[11]); therefore, it has been suggested that the emergence of these strains in the human population is the result of interspecies transmission, as a whole virus or just a few genes by reassortment, from animal to humans [13, 15]. The appearance of these strains in developing countries is explained by the close contact of the population with living animals.

Table 1. Details of the two new rotavirus vaccines (Rotarix® and RotaTeq®)

	Rotarix®	RotaTeq®
Manufacturer	Glaxo Smith Kline	Merck
Origin	Human strain (RIX 4414). Live attenuated vaccine.	Bovine/Human reassortant strains. Live vaccine.
Serotype/Genotype coverage	G1, P[8] (monovalent)	G1, G2, G3, G4, P[8] (pentavalent)
Vaccination Schedule	2 doses Dose 1: 6-14 weeks of age Dose 2: before 24 weeks of age	3 doses Dose 1: 6-14 weeks of age Last dose: before 32 weeks of age
Administration	Oral; applicator	Oral; squeeze tube
Presentation	Lyophilised powder that requires reconstitution	Ready-to-use liquid
Storage	Store either in a refrigerator or at room temperature (≤ 37°C). Do not freeze.	Store in a refrigerator (2 – 8°C)
Safety and efficacy trials	Randomized controlled trial (Phase III)	Randomized controlled trial (Phase III)
Participants	63 225 healthy infants from 12 countries. Eleven from Latin America and one from Europe.	68 038 healthy infants from 11 countries. Five from Europe, five from America, and one from Asia.
Outcomes of interest	The vaccine prevented: 85% of hospitalizations for rotavirus gastroenteritis (up to 1 year of age); 84.7% of severe gastroenteritis (1st season), 79% of severe gastroenteritis (2nd season); 42% of hospitalization for gastroenteritis of any cause.	The vaccine prevented: 95.8% of hospitalizations for rotavirus gastroenteritis; 98.2% of severe gastroenteritis (1st season), 88% of severe gastroenteritis (2nd season) 59% of hospitalization for gastroenteritis of any cause
Association with intussusception	None	None

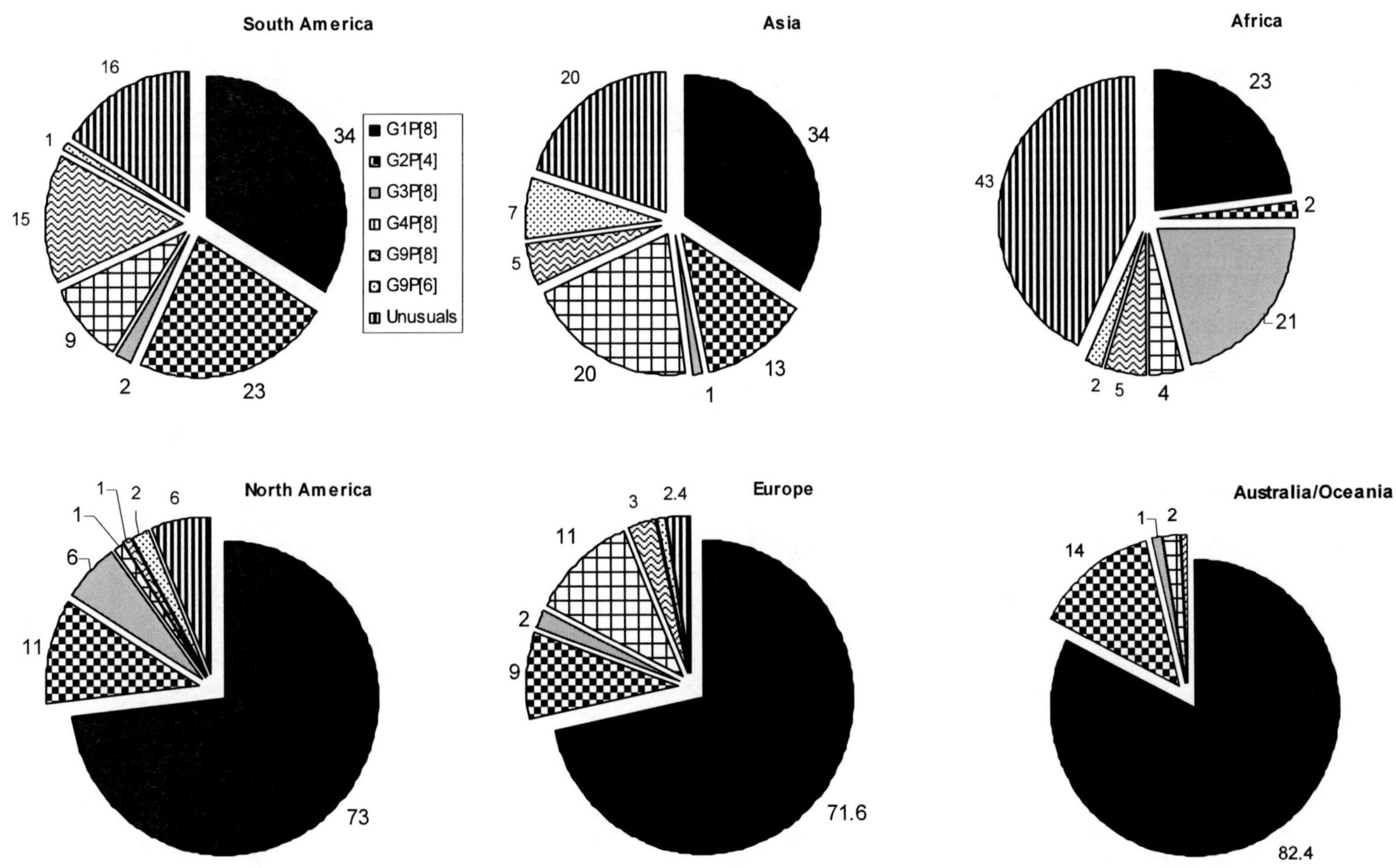

Figure 2. Worldwide distribution of G/P combinations of human group A rotavirus. Adapted from Santos et al. (2005).

During the last decade, the G9 strains were considered the most important unusual strains detected in humans, mainly because it is worldwide spread and because its prevalence has increased over the years. Currently, these strains are considered to be the fourth most prevalent G type in the human population, with incidences that range from 0.5 to 4% in developed countries, and from 7 to 16% in developing areas of the globe (Figure 2). Since at least three genetic lineages and many P genotypes (P[4], P[6], P[8]-P[11] and P[19]) have been detected in human G9 strains, the origin of the two G9 strains (G9P[6] and G9P[8]) detected at high frequencies worldwide is still unclear [30].

In South America, the G4P[8] strains have an overall incidence of less that 10%; however, this genotype has been extensively studied because its incidence increased up to ~40% in Argentina and Paraguay at the end of the 1990s and the early 2000s [25, 31, 32]. The study of the intragenotype diversity of the VP7 gene from the G4 strains has shown that the high incidences detected in these countries are attributable to the emergence of strains from two atypical sublineages (Ib and Ic) [33]. Strains from sublineage Ic have been recently found co-circulating in Uruguay and Brazil as well as in Italy, Ireland and Japan, thus showing the worldwide spread of this strain in the human population. Interestingly, a nation-wide outbreak of rotavirus associated with strains from sublineage Ic has been recently reported in Nicaragua, with incidences ≥ 80% [34].

Finally, it is worth mentioning that an association between the genotypes and the severity of the infection has been shown. For instance, children infected with strains showing the combination between G2P[4] and short electropherotype present more severe gastroenteritis than children infected with strains G1P[8] and G4P[8] with long electropherotype [35]. Similar results have been reported for Brazilian children infected with G9P[8] strains [36]. Different reasons to explain these observations include the introduction of new strains into a naïve population, differences in the virulence of the strains, and the lack of maternal antibodies [35-37]. Therefore, repeated infections with different viral strains are possible, and the seasonal shift of rotavirus strains could be a mechanism used by the virus to evade the herd immunity acquired by previous infections, and, thus, ultimately persist in a settled population.

Noroviruses

Overview

The family *Caliciviridae* is composed of four genera: *Norovirus, Sapovirus, Vesivirus* and *Lagovirus*, but only the first two cause disease in humans. Noroviruses are the most important cause of non-bacterial epidemic gastroenteritis in children and adults, and are the second important cause of sporadic endemic diarrhea after rotaviruses [38]. Sapoviruses on the other hand, have been detected in sporadic and outbreak cases involving younger age groups. However, the impact of Sapoviruses as an agent causing gastroenteritis in children has not yet been fully established [39].

These viruses are 27-35 nm, non-enveloped, and their positive-sense single- stranded RNA (ssRNA) is organized into three open reading frames (ORFs). ORF1 encodes a large polyprotein that is processed into mature nonstructural proteins, ORF2 encodes the major capsid protein, VP1, and ORF3 encodes a minor structural protein, VP2 [39].

Noroviruses segregate into five major phylogenetic groups [43]. Genogroup I (NvGI) and Genogroup II (NvGII) are the two main groups that affect humans. Early studies in volunteers showed that stool sample filtrates from patients infected with either genogroup did not cross-react against the sera of each patient [40].

Noroviruses infect humans through the fecal-oral route but they can also spread by several modes of transmission, such as person-to-person contact and food or water. The transmission of these viruses is very efficient because of their resistance to unfavorable conditions of the environment. These viruses are able to infect volunteers after exposing the stool filtrate to pH 2.7 for three hours at room temperature, treating it with 20% ether at 4°C for 18 hours and incubating at 60°C for 30 minutes. In addition, noroviruses have been found to be stable after incubation on mineral and tap water for over two months at room temperature [41]. The incubation period is of limited duration, from 10 to 51 hours, and acute illness generally lasts from 24 to 48 hours [39]. The efficient transmission of these viruses makes closed crowded settings the ideal opportunity for a norovirus outbreak. Thus, noroviruses are easily spread in hospitals, schools, military settings, cruise ships, nursing homes, and so on. The site of primary replication of noroviruses has not yet been established, but evidence points to its replication in the upper gastrointestinal tract. Biopsies of the jejunum of volunteers who develop gastrointestinal illness following oral administration of norovirus exhibit histopathological lesions, and broadening and blunting of the villi of the proximal small intestine [39]. In addition, norovirus causes diarrhea and intestinal lesions in the proximal small intestine of experimentally infected gnobiotic calves. The viral capsid antigen has also been detected in the jejunum of these animals [42].

Due to the unavailability of cell culture for these viruses, alternative approaches have been used to study noroviruses. Norovirus recombinant viral like particles (VLPs) produced by expression with VP1 and VP2 in the baculovirus expression system have been shown to present antigenic and biochemical properties similar to the virus. These recombinant VLPs have been used as virus surrogates in many applications, such as immunosorbent assays, potential vaccine candidates, and as tools to investigate norovirus antigenic relationships. The key antigens of sapoviruses are also associated with VP1 and evidence exists for antigenic diversity [39].

Because of the fastidious nature of these viruses, it has not been possible to establish a unified system of norovirus serotyping based on neutralization. The results of cross-challenge studies in volunteers suggested that several distinct norovirus serotypes would exist. Immuno electron microscopy initially showed evidence of at least four distinct antigenic serotypes, but sequence analysis of capsid sequence of field isolates showed a marked genetic diversity [39]. In 2006, Zheng et al. proposed a genomic norovirus classification and a strain nomenclature based on the phylogenetic analysis of the amino acid sequences of the capsid proteins of 164 norovirus strains. This system divides noroviruses into genogroups I to V, clusters and strains. The uncorrected pairwise distances between genogroups are unusually large among RNA viruses, ranging from 45 to 61%. Genogroups are then further subdivided into 8 and 17 clusters for NvGI and NvGII respectively [43].

Detection of the viral genome in stools has shown that shedding after norovirus infection can occur both before the onset and after the resolution of symptoms. During a study of norovirus gastroenteritis in children in Japan, Murata et al. (2007) found that the median duration of norovirus shedding was 16 days (5-47 days) [44]. This suggests that infected individuals recovering from a norovirus illness can continue to shed the virus after the symptoms dissapear, a finding that has implications in the management of outbreaks.

The immune response elicited by a norovirus infection in humans is still not clear. Challenge studies have established that there is short-term immunity as well as long-term immunity in norovirus-infected volunteers. Short-term immunity is apparently virus-specific. Thus, volunteers that became ill after a norovirus challenge are usually resistant to re-challenge with this virus. Long-term immunity presents several outcomes. Some volunteers become ill after the initial challenge and become ill again following a re-challenge 27 to 42 months later. Other volunteers were refractory to the initial challenge as well as to the re-challenge. The presence of norovirus-specific antibodies does not necessarily correlate with resistance to illness [39].

Recent studies have found evidence of genetically determined resistance to norovirus infection. Such a mechanism involves the ABH and Lewis carbohydrate antigens present on gut epithelial cells. Norwalk VLP's have been found to bind to histo-blood group antigens expressed on epithelial cells, suggesting that genetically determined host factors relating to histo-blood group antigens might play a role in mediating susceptibility to infection [45]. Non-secretor individuals (individuals that do not express these antigens on epithelial cells) have been found to be resistant to infection by some specific norovirus strains. In addition, a recent study has shown that non-secretor individuals had significantly lower antibody titers than secretor ones and that they were also antibody negative significantly more often [46]. Since then, numerous interaction patterns between ligand and virus have been described, and they all appear to be strain-specific.

Epidemiology

Noroviruses have been clearly established as the main cause of non-bacterial epidemic gastroenteritis and the second virus in importance in sporadic cases in developed countries. In the United States, this group of enteric viruses causes an estimated 23 million cases of acute gastroenteritis every year and more than 90% of the outbreaks of nonbacterial gastroenteritis [47]. However, their role as a cause of gastroenteritis in economically developing areas is unclear because little information is available. Noroviruses present a wide range of incidence rates (4.5 to 30%, Table 2) depending on the country studied and the diagnostic method used. Regardless of the location of the study, norovirus seems to be widespread in all the continents. In South America, Chile reported more than 70% norovirus seroprevalence and 8% incidence in acute sporadic cases of gastroenteritis in children [48, 49]. Victoria et al. reported that norovirus was present in 20% of samples from hospitalized children in Rio de Janeiro, Brazil [50]. A similar norovirus incidence was detected in children with acute gastroenteritis in Argentina [51] and Thailand [52]. However, only 1.2 % of the specimens were positive for sapoviruses in the latter study. A high prevalence (>90%) of antibodies to

Table 2. Incidence and Molecular Epidemiology of Norovirus in Developing Countries

Country Studied	Year of Study	Study Subjects	Number of Samples Tested	NV Incidence/ Prevalence	Genogroups and/or Genotypes Detected	**Reference**
Albania	N/A*	Children (outpatients and inpatients)	313	13%	GI and GII	(143)
Argentina	1997-1998	Children (outpatients)	66	24.2%	GI and GII	(51)
Bangladesh	2004-2005	Children	917	4.5%	GII.4	(144)
Brazil	1998-2005	Children	289	14.5%	GI and GII	(145)
Brazil	2004	Children (inpatients)	318	20%	GII.4	(50)
Guatemala	1999	Children	522	94% seroprevalence	N/A*	(146)
Ghana	2005-2006	Children	243	10%	N/A*	(147)
Indonesia	1997-1999	Children	102	30%	GII.1	(148)
Madagascar	2004-2005	Children	237	6%	GII, GI.1, GI.3 and GI.4	(149)
Malawi	1998-1999	Children (inpatients)	398	6.5%	GII.3, GII.4, GII.11, GII.13, GII.16, GII.20	(150)
Pakistan	1990-1994	Children (inpatients)	517	10%	GII	(151)
South India	2001-2004	Children (inpatients and sporadic)	350 (IP) 673 (S)	15% (IP) 10% (S)	GII.1, GII.2, GII.3, GII.4, GII.6, GII.7, GI.3	(54)
Thailand	2002-2004	Children (inpatients)	248	14%	GII.4, GII.3, GII.1, GII.7, GII.2, GII.16	(52)
Argentina	2004	Outbreak	100	39%	GI, GII and GIV	(55)
Chile**	2000-2003	Outbreak	55	45%	GI and GII	(56)

*N/A: Not available

** The studies based on gastroenteritis outbreaks are shaded.

both sapovirus and norovirus was observed in Mexican children involved in a birth cohort at 20 to 24 months of age [53]. Almost 20% of hospitalizations of children with gastroenteritis in South India were due to caliciviruses [54]. Noroviruses were also an important cause of the food-related gastroenteritis outbreaks reported in countries like Argentina and Chile [55, 56] (Table 2).

A wide variety of norovirus genotypes also circulates in developing areas. NvGII is the most commonly distributed norovirus genogroup, both in developed and developing areas. NvGI and NvGIV were also described as circulating genotypes in Brazil and Argentina. Within NvGII, cluster GII.4 seems to be by far the most common cause of outbreaks and sporadic diarrhea cases [57]. The mechanism by which this genotype is able to prevail since its discovery in the late 1980's is still unclear. Lindesmith et al. (2003) recently suggested that antigenic drift in response to protective herd immunity maintained GII.4 persistence in human populations, and that distinct evolutionary patterns were used to maintain less prevalent noroviruses [45].

Astroviruses

Overview

Applenton and Higgins (1975) analyzing fecal samples from an outbreak of gastroenteritis observed via EM small round non-enveloped structural viruses (SRSV) with diameters of 28-nm [58]. Madeley and Cosgrove (1975) also observed SRSV in diarrheic fecal samples in an EM; however 10% of them showed a morphological characteristic of a five- or six pointed star shape and they named these particles "astrovirus" ("astron" = star in Greek)[59]. In 1981 the isolation of human astroviruses has been achieved [60]; and almost eight years after that an enzyme immunoassay (EIA) and cell lines for human astrovirus were available [61-63]. After cloning and sequencing, human and animal astroviruses were classified into the *Astroviridae* family that is constituted by two genera: *Mamastrovirus* (mammalian) and *Aviastrovirus* (avian) [64, 65]. In mammalians, astroviruses are associated with acute gastroenteritis and have been described in humans and animals: lamb, calves, deer, piglets, kittens, mice, dogs, and minks. In avian, astroviruses are associated with gastroenteritis and have been described in turkeys, chickens and ducks. Astroviruses are also associated with a fulminant hepatitis in ducks.

Astroviruses are non-enveloped viruses and the intact particles show resistance to organic solvents, detergents, and at temperatures of 50°C and 60°C for 60 and 5 minutes, respectively. They are stable at pH 3.0 and are very persistent in the environment. The particles are stable at -70°C to -80°C for years; however, they lose their infectivity when submitted to repeated freezing and thawing [66, 67].

The astrovirus genome is composed of a positive-sense, ssRNA that varies in length from 6.4kb to 7.3kb, excluding the poly (A) tail at the 3' extremity and presents a subgenomic ssRNA that is responsible to translate the capsid proteins. The genome contains three open reading frames designated ORF1a, ORF1b, and ORF2, as well as terminal non-coding regions. ORF1a and 1b encode nonstructural proteins, including a serine protease and RNA-dependent RNA polymerase, respectively. The icosahedral capsid is formed by three proteins, which are generated by proteolytic cleavages of the primary translation product (VP90) of ORF2 that is located at the 3' end of the ssRNA. The 3' region is common to both genomic and subgenomic RNA and it shows the greatest sequence variability in the astrovirus genome [67, 68].

Epidemiology

Seroprevalence studies indicate that most children have antibodies to astroviruses, suggesting that the virus infection occurs during the first years of life. Early epidemiological studies in human astroviruses were based on EM and EIA, and the detection rates were very low and varied depending on the study. Improved surveillance and application of more sensitive molecular assays, such as reverse transcription-polymerase chain reaction (RT-PCR) and typing (sequencing), have increased awareness of the epidemiology of astroviruses in diarrheic diseases [69-72]. Currently, astroviruses are ubiquitous and are common causes of diarrhea in young children worldwide. The elderly and the immunocompromised patients are also included in the high-risk groups [71-75]. Outbreaks of gastroenteritis associated with astroviruses infections have been reported in children's day care centers and schools [71, 72, 76-79], as well as in homes for the elderly [80] and military academies [81].

Human astroviruses are classified in eight genotypes (HAstV-1 to -8) based on the nucleotide sequence analysis of ORF-2. These eight genotypes showed good correlation with the eight serotypes determined according to the reactivity of the capsid proteins with type-specific monoclonal antibodies [82-85].

Although astroviruses infections generally result in disease with low severity, they usually affect a large number of children. The severity of human astroviruses infections in relation to the genotype has not been fully elucidated. HAstV-1 is the most common genotype identified worldwide; however, with improved methodologies and the increase in the number of studies, mainly in developing countries, other genotypes have been detected at high incidences. Mixed infections involving other enteric viruses are often described, making the clinical evaluation of astrovirus infections more difficult [69, 86, 87].

In Latin America astrovirus infections have been well documented in different countries. In Cordoba, Argentina, Giordano et al. (2001) described astroviruses in 4.5% of hospitalized children with severe diarrhea. A similar rate (5% and 3.7%) has been described in children up to 3 years old from Buenos Aires and Mendoza, Argentina, respectively [51, 88]. Although Giordano et al. (2004) observed a higher incidence (12.4%) of astroviruses in outpatients from a Public Pediatric Hospital in Cordoba, Argentina [89]; Espul et al. (2004) observed the presence of astroviruses equally distributed between hospitalized and non-hospitalized children in Mendoza, Argentina. An association of human astroviruses with outbreaks was also reported in Argentina [55].

In Santiago, Chile, Gaggero et al. (1998) demonstrated an astrovirus prevalence of 16.5%, and 7% of mixed infection between astroviruses and group A rotaviruses. HAstV-1 (58%), -2 (20%), and -4 (8%) were characterized [90]. In Bogotá, Colombia, and Caracas,

Venezuela, human astroviruses have been reported in 5% and 10%, respectively, being HAstV-1 the most prevalent genotype [91].

The first descriptions of human astrovirus infections in Brazil were made using EM [92-94]. Recently, RT-PCR became the main methodology for diagnosis in surveillance studies to investigate outbreaks and sporadic cases of human astrovirus infections in different regions of Brazil [95-102]. Overall, the astrovirus incidence in Brazil range from 4.3% to 14%, and the genotypes detected were HAstV-1, -2, -3, -4, -5, -6 and -8, being the former the most prevalent.

An outbreak of acute gastroenteritis among Maxakali Indians with HAstV-2 as the etiologic agent was reported [103]. Of note is that three gastroenteritis outbreaks associated with HAstV-2 infection had been reported previously: i) in children who attended child care centers in Norfolk, USA [104]; ii) in a hospital in Melbourne, Australia [82]; iii) in an emergency room in Bogotá [91].

A prevalence of 61% of human astroviruses was observed by Maldonado et al. (1998) in rural Mayan infants living in the highlands of Chiapas, Mexico. In a prospective study carried out in México City, Guerrero et al. (1998) demonstrated the occurrence of human astroviruses in 5% of the children studied, with an incidence rate of 0.1 episode/child year. Co-infection with another pathogen was observed in 42% of cases. HAstV-2 was characterized in 35% of cases, followed by HAstV-4 (15%), -3 (11%), -1 (4%), -5 (4%).

In a multi-centric study conducted in México, astroviruses were observed in 5.4% of symptomatic and in 2.5% of asymptomatic children [87]. HAstV-1 (29%) and -3 (25%) were the most prevalent in children with diarrhea, followed by HAstV-8 (17%), -2 and -4 (13% each). In children without diarrhea, HAstV-3 (36%), -1 and -8 (18% each), -2, -4, - 7 (9% each) were also detected.

Overall, astrovirus infections are prevalent in children up to 1 year old and HastV-1 is the most prevalent in Latin America. However, other genotypes are also present and are responsible for sporadic outbreaks of acute gastroenteritis.

Considering the prevalence of human astroviruses and genotype diversity in developing countries on continents other than South America, in Bangkok, Thailand, Hermann et al. (1991) detected astroviruses in 8.6% of children with gastroenteritis compared with 2% of children without diarrhea [105]. Liu et al. (2004) detected a rate of 9% of astrovirus infections in hospitalized children in Beijing, China and co-infection with group A rotavirus represented 19.2% of the cases. The peak of infection occurred between October and March and HAstV-1 was the prevalent genotype [106].

Chen et al. (2007) observed astroviruses in 2.7% of hospitalized children in Northern Taiwan [107], and, in Bangladesh, Unicomb et al. (1998) found astroviruses in 15% of patients with persistent diarrhea, 4% of patients with acute diarrhea and 2% in healthy controls. In a study to determine the seasonal distribution and clinical characteristics of astrovirus infections in India, Bhattacharya et al. (2006) observed a rate of 5.8% in symptomatic cases; in 52% of the cases astrovirus was detected as the sole agent and mixed infections were observed with group A rotavirus (32%), picobirnavirus (2%), and group A rotavirus and picobirnavirus (2%). Of note is that astrovirus infections were detected throughout the year [108].

Regarding the African continent, Steele et al. (1998) described a rate of 7% in South Africa and the infections were more prevalent in the autumn and early winter [109]. Kiulia et al. (2007) described a rate of 6.3% of astrovirus infections in hospitalized Kenyan children [110].

Naficy et al. (2000) in Egypt observed the age-specific incidence rate of astrovirus diarrheic episodes and concluded that it was similar to that of group-A-rotavirus-diarrhea, 0.19 episodes per person-year. The most frequent serotypes were: HAstV-1 (43%), -5 (16%), -8 and -3 (12% each), -6 (7%), -4 (5%), -2 (4%), and mixed infection HAstV-6/-8 (1%) [111].

Most of the data on astrovirus infections and genotypes are provided by developed countries. In Finland, Pang and Vesikari (1999) observed a astrovirus infections in 9% of the children studied and Putzker et al. (2000) in Germany, 1.2% with a peak in the winter season [112, 113]. In Barcelona, Spain, an occurrence of 4.9% has been shown. HAstV-1 (38%), -4 (26%), -3 (19%), -8 (11%), and -2 (6%) were the genotypes characterized [114].

The presence of gastro enteric viruses was investigated in hospitalized children, in London, UK, by Simpson et al. (2003) [115]. Astroviruses and mixed infections corresponded to 2.3% and 8.9% of the cases, respectively. In Italian children, the presence of astroviruses was 3.1%, and most of the cases occurred between March and May. HAstV-1 (80%) and -3 (20%) were the two genotypes detected [116].

Sakamoto et al. (2000) investigating astrovirus infections in 5 regions of Japan reported an incidence of 5.9%. HAstV-1 represented 80% of the infections, followed by HAstV-3 (17%) and -4 (3%) [84]. Mustafa et al. (2000) in Melbourne, Australia, conducted a surveillance study and observed the presence of astrovirus in 4.4%, 2.2%, 3.9% and 1.4% in hospitalized children from 1995 to 1998, respectively. HAstV-1 was the most prevalent, followed by HAstV-2, -4, and – 8 [82].

Regarding astrovirus serotypes/genotypes distribution worldwide, studies show that HAstV-1 is the most common worldwide, although the predominant serotypes/genotypes may vary according to region and season. However, with the intensification of studies mostly in developing countries a new profile concerning the prevalent genotypes ought to be achieved.

The co-infection rates involving astroviruses with group A rotaviruses, human caliciviruses, and/or enteric adenoviruses are greater in developing countries, probably due to the poorer sanitation conditions. Barreto et al. (2006) showed that virus infections were more widespread than bacterial and parasitic infections in very low income communities of Salvador, Bahia, Northeast Brazil [117]. The results from improvements to the sanitary conditions of these communities have been reported recently [118].

The astroviruses seasonal distribution varies in different regions worldwide. In countries with temperate climates most astrovirus infections are noted during the winter-dry season and coincide with rotavirus seasonality. In tropical climates, the infections occur all year round or during the rainy season [82, 109, 114]. However in a continental country like Brazil, in the Southeast region astroviruses are more common in the dry season [101], in contrast with the Central west region when it is more widespread during the period with the highest relative air humidity [99].

Diagnosis and Identification of Viral Gastroenteritis

Rotaviruses, noroviruses and astroviruses were discovered using EM; therefore, this method played an important role in the early diagnosis of these viruses [6, 119, 120].

During infection, virus particles are excreted in the feces (e.g. $>10^{10}$ rotaviral particles/gram can be found in the stool of a child with diarrhea); therefore, viral proteins or genes can be easily detected in fecal samples from patients using enzyme immunoassays (EIA) and/or genomic detection techniques.

The development of monoclonal and polyclonal antibodies increased the sensitivity and specificity of EIA tests for rotavirus and astrovirus detection [29, 72]. On the other hand, real-time PCR detection-based assays are the most reliable and sensitive assays developed for noroviruses so far (i.e. NvGI and NvGII) [121, 122] Multiplex RT-PCR tests were also developed to detect different gastroenteric viruses; however, their sensitivity is lower than individual tests [123, 124].

Since rotaviruses present a dsRNA segmented genome, polyacrylamide gel electrophoresis (PAGE) has been widely used as a diagnostic tool and epidemiological studies. Although PAGE presents a lower sensitivity than EIA tests, it can detect rotaviruses from different groups and differences in the migration pattern of the segments, thus allowing a simple differentiation among strains circulating in a given geographical region.

Rotaviruses, noroviruses and astroviruses are serotyped/genotyped using numerous multiplex RT-PCR strategies. For rotaviruses, the VP4 and VP7 genes are the targets for P and G typing, respectively [29]. In astroviruses and noroviruses the most commonly used strategies are based on amplification of the capsid gene [84]. However, failure or incorrect characterization of field strains by these RT-PCR strategies has been reported worldwide, mainly due to both the accumulation of point mutations and the diversification on specific lineages. [125-127]. Alternatively, primers with degenerated nucleotides [125, 128, 129], microarrays [130-132], real-time based multiplex assays, and PCR-enzyme-linked immunosorbent assays [133] are some of the attempts to overcome the failure or incorrect characterization of field strains detected in surveillance programs.

Finally, an association between RT-PCR and virus isolation in cell culture techniques has been reported in order to improve the sensitivity of astrovirus detection in fecal and environmental samples as well as to investigate the infectiousness of virus particles [134-136].

Prevention, Control, and Treatment of Viral Gastroenteritis

Viral gastroenteritis is usually a self-limited illness in people with a healthy immune system. Treatment of the disease consists of oral rehydration and maintenance of the electrolyte balance. However, about one in 40 children with rotavirus infection requires hospitalization for intravenous rehydration, which is also recommended when vomiting and diarrhea are severe in norovirus and astrovirus infections [137].

Water and food contaminated with fecal material have been implicated as the cause of viral gastroenteritis outbreaks. Therefore, prevention must include personal hygiene and disinfection of contaminated surfaces with household chlorine bleach-based cleaners. Infected individuals can continue to shed virus in their feces for several days after the illness resolves and so should continue to take precautions after recovering from the symptoms. Children with diarrhea should be barred from child care facilities for as long as the duration of the disease.

Preventive vaccination is only currently available for rotavirus. Vaccines against this virus are being implemented in the public health systems of eight Latin American countries. The two types of vaccine available have shown to be safe and immunogenic, showing high levels of efficacy during large clinical trials in both developed and developing countries [138, 139] (Table 1). RotaShield was the first rotavirus vaccine licensed in August 1998; however, it was wthdrawn from the market one year later because of its association with intussusception. Further epidemiological studies showed that the risk of intussusception was higher in vaccinated children if the first dose of Rotashield was administered after the three months of age. In addition, the same study showed that no cases occurred in infants vaccinated before the first two months of age [140]. Therefore, the current available vaccines have a schedule of vaccination that begins at approximately two months of age and ends at six months of age, with a minimum of four weeks between doses (Table 1). The two rotavirus vaccines do not contain all the virus serotypes circulating in humans but are still able to prevent >85% of hospitalizations for rotavirus gastroenteritis, and provide 79-98% protection against severe rotavirus disease, depending on the schedule of administration and population evaluated during the clinical trials [138, 139].

Norovirus vaccine development has been challenging due to the lack of cell culture to study this virus and the poor understanding of the immunity. The unavailability of propagation techniques has been overcome by the synthesis of recombinant VLPs as previously stated. Norovirus VLPs have been proved to be immunogenic and safe when administered to volunteers in phase I studies. If the presence of norovirus-specific antibodies in humans is found to correlate with protection from the disease, recombinant VLP's may prove to have a potential as a vaccine [39]. In addition, a promising antiviral therapy specific for norovirus is being studied. This prevention strategy is based on administering virus-specific anti-sense drugs that appear inhibit virus protein translation inside the cell efficiently. Preliminary results indicate that this strategy could be applied to treat a wide variety of circulating strains [141].

Perspectives

The developing world seems to present an incresed prevalence of viral gastroenteritis and a wider range of genotype diversity of the three viruses mentioned in this chapter. This is probably due to the precarious sanitary conditions in these countries. Rotavirus surveillance programs are essential to study whether the epidemiological profile of viral gastroenteritis will change after the introduction of rotavirus vaccines in these countries. Also, alternative approaches should be considered in any prospective studies in order to account for newly discovered viruses that might be responsible for acute gastroenteritis [142]

References

[1] Kosek M, Bern C, Guerrant RL. The global burden of diarrhoeal disease, as estimated from studies published between 1992 and 2000. *Bull. World Health Organ.* 2003; 81(3):197-204.

[2] Parashar UD, Gibson CJ, Bresee JS, Glass RI. Rotavirus and severe childhood diarrhea. *Emerg. Infect Dis*. 2006;12(2):304-306.

[3] Parashar UD, Hummelman EG, Bresee JS, Miller MA, Glass RI. Global illness and deaths caused by rotavirus disease in children. *Emerg. Infect Dis.* 2003;9(5):565-72.

[4] Kapikian AZ, Hoshino Y, Chanock RM. Rotaviruses. In: Knipe DM, Howley PM, Griffin DE, Lamb RA, Martin MA, Roizman B, et al., editors. Fields virology. 4th ed. Philadelphia, Pa: Lippincott/Williams and Wilkins; 2001. p. 1787-1833.

[5] Kapikian AZ, Kim HW, Wyatt RG, Rodriguez WJ, Ross S, Cline WL, et al. Reoviruslike agent in stools: association with infantile diarrhea and development of serologic tests. *Science* 1974;185(156):1049-53.

[6] Bishop RF, Davidson GP, Holmes IH, Ruck BJ. Virus particles in epithelial cells of duodenal mucosa from children with acute non-bacterial gastroenteritis. *Lancet* 1973; 2 (7841): 1281-3.

[7] Estes M. Rotaviruses and their replication. In: Knipe DM, Howley PM, Griffin DE, Lamb RA, Martin MA, Roizman B, et al., editors. Fields virology. 4th ed. Philadelphia, Pa: Lippincott/Williams and Wilkins; 2001. p. 1747-1785.

[8] Iturriza Gomara M, Wong C, Blome S, Desselberger U, Gray J. Molecular characterization of VP6 genes of human rotavirus isolates: correlation of genogroups with subgroups and evidence of independent segregation. *J. Virol.* 2002; 76 (13):6596-601.

[9] Fukai K, Takahashi T, Tajima K, Koike S, Iwane K, Inoue K. Molecular characterization of a novel bovine group A rotavirus. *Vet. Microbiol.* 2007; 123 (1-3): 217-24.

[10] Steyer A, Poljsak-Prijatelj M, Barlic-Maganja D, Jamnikar U, Mijovski JZ, Marin J. Molecular characterization of a new porcine rotavirus P genotype found in an asymptomatic pig in Slovenia. *Virology* 2007;359(2):275-82.

[11] Parra GI, Galeano ME, Arbiza J. Genetic relationship between porcine rotavirus strains bearing a new P-type. *Vet. Microbiol.* 2007;125(1-2):193-5.

[12] Gouvea V, Brantly M. Is rotavirus a population of reassortants? *Trends Microbiol.* 1995;3 (4):159-62.

[13] Gentsch JR, Laird AR, Bielfelt B, Griffin DD, Banyai K, Ramachandran M, et al. Serotype diversity and reassortment between human and animal rotavirus strains: implications for rotavirus vaccine programs. *J. Infect Dis.* 2005;192 Suppl 1:S146-59.

[14] Desselberger U, Iturriza-Gomara M, Gray JJ. Rotavirus epidemiology and surveillance. *Novartis Found Symp*. 2001;238:125-47; discussion 147-52.

[15] Matthijnssens J, Rahman M, Yang X, Delbeke T, Arijs I, Kabue JP, et al. G8 rotavirus strains isolated in the Democratic Republic of Congo belong to the DS-1-like genogroup. *J. Clin. Microbiol.* 2006;44(5):1801-9.

[16] Nakagomi O, Nakagomi T, Akatani K, Ikegami N. Identification of rotavirus genogroups by RNA-RNA hybridization. *Mol. Cell Probes* 1989;3(3):251-61.

[17] Iturriza-Gomara M, Anderton E, Kang G, Gallimore C, Phillips W, Desselberger U, et al. Evidence for genetic linkage between the gene segments encoding NSP4 and VP6 proteins in common and reassortant human rotavirus strains. *J. Clin. Microbiol.* 2003; 41 (8): 3566-73.

[18] Ramachandran M, Kirkwood CD, Unicomb L, Cunliffe NA, Ward RL, Bhan MK, et al. Molecular characterization of serotype G9 rotavirus strains from a global collection. *Virology* 2000;278(2):436-44.

[19] Kane EM, Turcios RM, Arvay ML, Garcia S, Bresee JS, Glass RI. The epidemiology of rotavirus diarrhea in Latin America. Anticipating rotavirus vaccines. *Rev. Panam. Salud Publica* 2004;16(6):371-7.

[20] Anderson EJ, Weber SG. Rotavirus infection in adults. *Lancet Infect Dis.* 2004;4(2):91-9.

[21] Martínez M, Fariña N, Rodríguez M, Russomando G, Parra GI. Incidence of Rotavirus in adults with diarrhea in Asuncion, Paraguay. *Rev. Arg. de Microbiología* 2005;37:99-101.

[22] Cook SM, Glass RI, LeBaron CW, Ho MS. Global seasonality of rotavirus infections. *Bull. World Health Organ.* 1990;68(2):171-7.

[23] Ansari SA, Springthorpe VS, Sattar SA. Survival and vehicular spread of human rotaviruses: possible relation to seasonality of outbreaks. *Rev. Infect Dis.* 1991; 13 (3): 448-61.

[24] Pereira HG, Linhares AC, Candeias JA, Glass RI. National laboratory surveillance of viral agents of gastroenteritis in Brazil. *Bull. Pan. Am. Health Organ.* 1993;27(3):224-33.

[25] Bok K, Castagnaro N, Borsa A, Nates S, Espul C, Fay O, et al. Surveillance for rotavirus in Argentina. *J. Med. Virol.* 2001;65(1):190-8.

[26] Candia N, Parra GI, Chirico M, Velazquez G, Farina N, Laspina F, et al. Acute diarrhea in Paraguayan children population: detection of rotavirus electropherotypes. *Acta Virol.* 2003;47(3):137-40.

[27] Perez-Schael I, Gonzalez R, Fernandez R, Alfonzo E, Inaty D, Boher Y, et al. Epidemiological features of rotavirus infection in Caracas, Venezuela: implications for rotavirus immunization programs. *J. Med. Virol.* 1999;59(4):520-6.

[28] Callejas D, Estevez J, Porto-Espinoza L, Monsalve F, Costa-Leon L, Blitz L, et al. [Effect of climatic factors on the epidemiology of rotavirus infection in children under 5 years of age in the city of Maracaibo, Venezuela]. *Invest Clin.* 1999;40(2):81-94.

[29] Fischer TK, Gentsch JR. Rotavirus typing methods and algorithms. *Rev. Med. Virol.* 2004; 14 (2):71-82.

[30] Santos N, Hoshino Y. Global distribution of rotavirus serotypes/genotypes and its implication for the development and implementation of an effective rotavirus vaccine. *Rev. Med. Virol.* 2005;15(1):29-56.

[31] Parra GI, Espinola EE, Amarilla AA, Stupka J, Martinez M, Zunini M, et al. Diversity of group A rotavirus strains circulating in Paraguay from 2002 to 2005: detection of an atypical G1 in South America. *J. Clin. Virol.* 2007;40(2):135-41.

[32] Parra GI, Bok K, Martinez V, Russomando G, Gomez J. Molecular characterization and genetic variation of the VP7 gene of human rotaviruses isolated in Paraguay. *J. Med. Virol*. 2005;77(4):579-86.

[33] Bok K, Matson DO, Gomez JA. Genetic variation of capsid protein VP7 in genotype g4 human rotavirus strains: simultaneous emergence and spread of different lineages in Argentina. *J. Clin. Microbiol.* 2002;40(6):2016-22.

[34] Bucardo F, Karlsson B, Nordgren J, Paniagua M, Gonzalez A, Amador JJ, et al. Mutated G4P[8] rotavirus associated with a nationwide outbreak of gastroenteritis in Nicaragua in 2005. *J. Clin. Microbiol.* 2007;45(3):990-7.

[35] Cascio A, Vizzi E, Alaimo C, Arista S. Rotavirus gastroenteritis in Italian children: can severity of symptoms be related to the infecting virus? *Clin. Infect Dis*. 2001; 32 (8): 1126-32.

[36] Linhares AC, Verstraeten T, Wolleswinkel-van den Bosch J, Clemens R, Breuer T. Rotavirus serotype G9 is associated with more-severe disease in Latin America. *Clin. Infect Dis*. 2006;43(3):312-4.

[37] Kang G. Rotavirus genotypes and severity of diarrheal disease. *Clin. Infect Dis*. 2006; 43 (3): 315-6.

[38] Glass RI, Noel J, Ando T, Fankhauser R, Belliot G, Mounts A, et al. The epidemiology of enteric caliciviruses from humans: a reassessment using new diagnostics. *J. Infect Dis*. 2000;181 Suppl 2:S254-61.

[39] Green KY. Caliciviridae: The Noroviruses. In: Knipe DM, editor. Fields Virology. Fifth ed. Philadelphia: Lippincott Williams and Wilkins, a Wolters Kluwer Business; 2007. p. 949-979.

[40] Lew JF, Kapikian AZ, Valdesuso J, Green KY. Molecular characterization of Hawaii virus and other Norwalk-like viruses: evidence for genetic polymorphism among human caliciviruses. *J. Infect Dis.* 1994;170(3):535-42.

[41] Ngazoa ES, Fliss I, Jean J. Quantitative study of persistence of human norovirus genome in water using TaqMan real-time RT-PCR. *J. Appl. Microbiol.* 2007.

[42] Souza M, Azevedo MS, Jung K, Cheetham S, Saif LJ. Pathogenesis and immune responses in gnotobiotic calves after infection with human norovirus (HuNoV) genogroup II.4-HS66 strain. *J. Virol*. 2007.

[43] Zheng DP, Ando T, Fankhauser RL, Beard RS, Glass RI, Monroe SS. Norovirus classification and proposed strain nomenclature. *Virology* 2006;346(2):312-23.

[44] Murata T, Katsushima N, Mizuta K, Muraki Y, Hongo S, Matsuzaki Y. Prolonged norovirus shedding in infants <or=6 months of age with gastroenteritis. *Pediatr. Infect Dis. J.* 2007;26(1):46-9.

[45] Lindesmith L, Moe C, Marionneau S, Ruvoen N, Jiang X, Lindblad L, et al. Human susceptibility and resistance to Norwalk virus infection. *Nat. Med.* 2003;9(5):548-53.

[46] Larsson MM, Rydell GE, Grahn A, Rodriguez-Diaz J, Akerlind B, Hutson AM, et al. Antibody prevalence and titer to norovirus (genogroup II) correlate with secretor (FUT2) but not with ABO phenotype or Lewis (FUT3) genotype. *J. Infect Dis.* 2006; 194 (10):1422-7.

[47] Fankhauser RL, Monroe SS, Noel JS, Humphrey CD, Bresee JS, Parashar UD, et al. Epidemiologic and molecular trends of "Norwalk-like viruses" associated with outbreaks of gastroenteritis in the United States. *J. Infect Dis.* 2002;186(1):1-7.

[48] O'Ryan ML, Mamani N, Gaggero A, Avendano LF, Prieto S, Pena A, et al. Human caliciviruses are a significant pathogen of acute sporadic diarrhea in children of Santiago, Chile. *J. Infect Dis.* 2000;182(5):1519-22.

[49] O'Ryan ML, Vial PA, Mamani N, Jiang X, Estes MK, Ferrecio C, et al. Seroprevalence of Norwalk virus and Mexico virus in Chilean individuals: assessment of independent risk factors for antibody acquisition. *Clin. Infect Dis.* 1998;27(4):789-95.

[50] Victoria M, Carvalho-Costa FA, Heinemann MB, Leite JP, Miagostovich M. Prevalence and molecular epidemiology of noroviruses in hospitalized children with acute gastroenteritis in Rio de Janeiro, Brazil, 2004. *Pediatr. Infect Dis. J.* 2007; 26 (7): 602-6.

[51] Bereciartu A, Bok K, Gomez J. Identification of viral agents causing gastroenteritis among children in Buenos Aires, Argentina. *J. Clin. Virol.* 2002;25(2):197-203.

[52] Khamrin P, Maneekarn N, Peerakome S, Tonusin S, Malasao R, Mizuguchi M, et al. Genetic diversity of noroviruses and sapoviruses in children hospitalized with acute gastroenteritis in Chiang Mai, Thailand. *J. Med. Virol.* 2007;79(12):1921-6.

[53] Farkas T, Deng X, Ruiz-Palacios G, Morrow A, Jiang X. Development of an enzyme immunoassay for detection of sapovirus-specific antibodies and its application in a study of seroprevalence in children. *J. Clin. Microbiol.* 2006;44(10):3674-9.

[54] Monica B, Ramani S, Banerjee I, Primrose B, Iturriza-Gomara M, Gallimore CI, et al. Human caliciviruses in symptomatic and asymptomatic infections in children in Vellore, South India. *J. Med. Virol.* 2007;79(5):544-51.

[55] Gomes KA, Stupka JA, Gomez J, Parra GI. Molecular characterization of calicivirus strains detected in outbreaks of gastroenteritis in Argentina. *J. Med. Virol.* 2007; 79 (11): 1703-9.

[56] Vidal R, Solari V, Mamani N, Jiang X, Vollaire J, Roessler P, et al. Caliciviruses and foodborne gastroenteritis, Chile. *Emerg. Infect Dis.* 2005;11(7):1134-7.

[57] Tu ET, Bull RA, Greening GE, Hewitt J, Lyon MJ, Marshall JA, et al. Epidemics of gastroenteritis during 2006 were associated with the spread of norovirus GII.4 variants 2006a and 2006b. *Clin. Infect Dis.* 2008;46(3):413-20.

[58] Appleton H, Higgins PG. Letter: Viruses and gastroenteritis in infants. *Lancet* 1975; 1(7919): 1297.

[59] Madeley CR, Cosgrove BP. Letter: 28 nm particles in faeces in infantile gastroenteritis. *Lancet* 1975;2(7932):451-2.

[60] Lee TW, Kurtz JB. Serial propagation of astrovirus in tissue culture with the aid of trypsin. *J. Gen. Virol.* 1981;57(Pt 2):421-4.

[61] Herrmann JE, Hudson RW, Perron-Henry DM, Kurtz JB, Blacklow NR. Antigenic characterization of cell-cultivated astrovirus serotypes and development of astrovirus-specific monoclonal antibodies. *J. Infect Dis.* 1988;158(1):182-5.

[62] Brinker JP, Blacklow NR, Herrmann JE. Human astrovirus isolation and propagation in multiple cell lines. *Arch Virol.* 2000;145(9):1847-56.

[63] Willcocks MM, Carter MJ, Laidler FR, Madeley CR. Growth and characterisation of human faecal astrovirus in a continuous cell line. *Arch Virol.* 1990;113(1-2):73-81.

[64] Jiang B, Monroe SS, Koonin EV, Stine SE, Glass RI. RNA sequence of astrovirus: distinctive genomic organization and a putative retrovirus-like ribosomal frameshifting signal that directs the viral replicase synthesis. *Proc. Natl. Acad. Sci. USA* 1993; 90 (22): 10539-43.

[65] Monroe SS, Carter MJ, Herrmann JE, Mitchell DK, Sanchez-Fauquier A. Family Astroviridae. In: Fauquet CM, Mayo MA, Maniloff J, Desselberger U, Ball LA, editors. Virus taxonomy: Eighth Report of the International Committee on Taxonomy of Viruses. London: Elsevier/Academic Press; 2005. p. 859-864.

[66] Abad FX, Villena C, Guix S, Caballero S, Pinto RM, Bosch A. Potential role of fomites in the vehicular transmission of human astroviruses. *Appl. Environ. Microbiol.* 2001; 67(9): 3904-7.

[67] Mendez E, Arias CF. Astroviruses. In: Knipe DM, editor. Fields Virology. Fifth ed. Philadelphia: Lippincott Williams and Wilkins, a Wolters Kluwer Business; 2007. p. 982-1000.

[68] Matsui SM, Kiang D, Ginzton N, Chew T, Geigenmuller-Gnirke U. Molecular biology of astroviruses: selected highlights. *Novartis Found Symp.* 2001;238:219-33; discussion 233-6.

[69] Glass RI, Noel J, Mitchell D, Herrmann JE, Blacklow NR, Pickering LK, et al. The changing epidemiology of astrovirus-associated gastroenteritis: a review. *Arch Virol. Suppl.* 1996;12:287-300.

[70] Koopmans MP, Bijen MH, Monroe SS, Vinje J. Age-stratified seroprevalence of neutralizing antibodies to astrovirus types 1 to 7 in humans in The Netherlands. *Clin. Diagn. Lab. Immunol.* 1998;5(1):33-7.

[71] Walter JE, Mitchell DK. Role of astroviruses in childhood diarrhea. *Curr. Opin. Pediatr.* 2000; 12 (3):275-9.

[72] Walter JE, Mitchell DK. Astrovirus infection in children. Curr. Opin. Infect Dis. 2003; 16 (3):247-53.

[73] Cunliffe NA, Dove W, Gondwe JS, Thindwa BD, Greensill J, Holmes JL, et al. Detection and characterisation of human astroviruses in children with acute gastroenteritis in Blantyre, Malawi. *J. Med. Virol.* 2002;67(4):563-6.

[74] Dalton RM, Roman ER, Negredo AA, Wilhelmi ID, Glass RI, Sanchez-Fauquier A. Astrovirus acute gastroenteritis among children in Madrid, Spain. *Pediatr. Infect Dis. J.* 2002; 21(11):1038-41.

[75] Gallimore CI, Taylor C, Gennery AR, Cant AJ, Galloway A, Lewis D, et al. Use of a heminested reverse transcriptase PCR assay for detection of astrovirus in environmental swabs from an outbreak of gastroenteritis in a pediatric primary immunodeficiency unit. *J. Clin. Microbiol.* 2005;43(8):3890-4.

[76] Konno T, Suzuki H, Ishida N, Chiba R, Mochizuki K, Tsunoda A. Astrovirus-associated epidemic gastroenteritis in Japan. *J. Med. Virol.* 1982;9(1):11-7.

[77] Mitchell DK, Monroe SS, Jiang X, Matson DO, Glass RI, Pickering LK. Virologic features of an astrovirus diarrhea outbreak in a day care center revealed by reverse transcriptase-polymerase chain reaction. *J. Infect Dis.* 1995;172(6):1437-44.

[78] Oishi I, Yamazaki K, Kimoto T, Minekawa Y, Utagawa E, Yamazaki S, et al. A large outbreak of acute gastroenteritis associated with astrovirus among students and teachers in Osaka, Japan. *J. Infect Dis.* 1994;170(2):439-43.

[79] Svraka S, Duizer E, Vennema H, de Bruin E, van der Veer B, Dorresteijn B, et al. Etiological role of viruses in outbreaks of acute gastroenteritis in The Netherlands from 1994 through 2005. *J. Clin. Microbiol.* 2007;45(5):1389-94.

[80] Gray JJ, Wreghitt TG, Cubitt WD, Elliot PR. An outbreak of gastroenteritis in a home for the elderly associated with astrovirus type 1 and human calicivirus. *J. Med. Virol.* 1987; 23(4):377-81.

[81] Belliot G, Laveran H, Monroe SS. Outbreak of gastroenteritis in military recruits associated with serotype 3 astrovirus infection. *J. Med. Virol.* 1997;51(2):101-6.

[82] Mustafa H, Palombo EA, Bishop RF. Epidemiology of astrovirus infection in young children hospitalized with acute gastroenteritis in Melbourne, Australia, over a period of four consecutive years, 1995 to 1998. *J. Clin. Microbiol.* 2000;38(3):1058-62.

[83] Noel JS, Lee TW, Kurtz JB, Glass RI, Monroe SS. Typing of human astroviruses from clinical isolates by enzyme immunoassay and nucleotide sequencing. *J. Clin. Microbiol.* 1995; 33(4):797-801.

[84] Sakamoto T, Negishi H, Wang QH, Akihara S, Kim B, Nishimura S, et al. Molecular epidemiology of astroviruses in Japan from 1995 to 1998 by reverse transcription-polymerase chain reaction with serotype-specific primers (1 to 8). *J. Med. Virol.* 2000; 61 (3):326-31.

[85] Taylor MB, Cox N, Vrey MA, Grabow WO. The occurrence of hepatitis A and astroviruses in selected river and dam waters in South Africa. *Water Res.* 2001;35(11):2653-60.

[86] Marie-Cardine A, Gourlain K, Mouterde O, Castignolles N, Hellot MF, Mallet E, et al. Epidemiology of acute viral gastroenteritis in children hospitalized in Rouen, France. *Clin. Infect Dis.* 2002;34(9):1170-8.

[87] Mendez-Toss M, Griffin DD, Calva J, Contreras JF, Puerto FI, Mota F, et al. Prevalence and genetic diversity of human astroviruses in Mexican children with symptomatic and asymptomatic infections. *J. Clin. Microbiol.* 2004;42(1):151-7.

[88] Espul C, Martinez N, Noel JS, Cuello H, Abrile C, Grucci S, et al. Prevalence and characterization of astroviruses in Argentinean children with acute gastroenteritis. *J. Med. Virol.* 2004;72(1):75-82.

[89] Giordano MO, Martinez LC, Isa MB, Paez Rearte M, Nates SV. Childhood astrovirus-associated diarrhea in the ambulatory setting in a Public Hospital in Cordoba city, Argentina. *Rev. Inst. Med. Trop. Sao Paulo* 2004;46(2):93-6.

[90] Gaggero A, O'Ryan M, Noel JS, Glass RI, Monroe SS, Mamani N, et al. Prevalence of astrovirus infection among Chilean children with acute gastroenteritis. *J. Clin. Microbiol.* 1998; 36(12):3691-3.

[91] Medina SM, Gutierrez MF, Liprandi F, Ludert JE. Identification and type distribution of astroviruses among children with gastroenteritis in Colombia and Venezuela. J. Clin. Microbiol. 2000;38(9):3481-3.

[92] Leite JP, Barth OM, Schatzmayr HG. Astrovirus in faeces of children with acute gastroenteritis in Rio de Janeiro, Brazil. *Mem. Inst. Oswaldo Cruz* 1991;86(4):489-90.

[93] Nozawa CM, Vaz MG, Guimaraes MA. Detection of astrovirus-like in diarrhoeic stool and its coexistence with rotavirus. *Rev. Inst. Med. Trop. Sao Paulo* 1985;27(5):238-41.

[94] Tanaka H, Kisielius JJ, Ueda M, Glass RI, Joazeiro PP. Intrafamilial outbreak of astrovirus gastroenteritis in Sao Paulo, Brazil. *J. Diarrhoeal Dis. Res.* 1994;12(3):219-21.

[95] Soares CC, Maciel de Albuquerque MC, Maranhao AG, Rocha LN, Ramirez ML, Benati FJ, et al. Astrovirus detection in sporadic cases of diarrhea among hospitalized and non-hospitalized children in Rio De Janeiro, Brazil, from 1998 to 2004. *J. Med. Virol.* 2008;80(1):113-7.

[96] Gabbay YB, Linhares AC, Cavalcante-Pepino EL, Nakamura LS, Oliveira DS, da Silva LD, et al. Prevalence of human astrovirus genotypes associated with acute gastroenteritis among children in Belem, Brazil. J. Med. Virol. 2007;79(5):530-8.

[97] Gabbay YB, Linhares AC, Oliveira DS, Nakamura LS, Mascarenhas JD, Gusmao RH, et al. First detection of a human astrovirus type 8 in a child with diarrhea in Belem, Brazil: comparison with other strains worldwide and identification of possible three lineages. *Mem. Inst. Oswaldo Cruz* 2007;102(4):531-4.

[98] Gabbay YB, Luz CR, Costa IV, Cavalcante-Pepino EL, Sousa MS, Oliveira KK, et al. Prevalence and genetic diversity of astroviruses in children with and without diarrhea in Sao Luis, Maranhao, Brazil. *Mem. Inst. Oswaldo Cruz* 2005;100(7):709-14.

[99] Santos RA, Borges AM, da Costa PS, Teixeira JM, Giugliano LG, Leite JP, et al. Astrovirus infection in children living in the Central West region of Brazil. *Mem. Inst. Oswaldo Cruz* 2007;102(2):209-13.

[100] Silva AM, Leite EG, Assis RM, Majerowicz S, Leite JP. An outbreak of gastroenteritis associated with astrovirus serotype 1 in a day care center, in Rio de Janeiro, Brazil. *Mem. Inst. Oswaldo Cruz* 2001;96(8):1069-73.

[101] Victoria M, Carvalho-Costa FA, Heinemann MB, Leite JP, Miagostovich MP. Genotypes and molecular epidemiology of human astroviruses in hospitalized children with acute gastroenteritis in Rio de Janeiro, Brazil. *J. Med. Virol.* 2007;79(7):939-44.

[102] Silva PA, Cardoso DD, Schreier E. Molecular characterization of human astroviruses isolated in Brazil, including the complete sequences of astrovirus genotypes 4 and 5. *Arch Virol.* 2006;151(7):1405-17.

[103] Gabbay YB, Chamone CB, Nakamura LS, Oliveira DS, Abreu SF, Cavalcante-Pepino EL, et al. Characterization of an astrovirus genotype 2 strain causing an extensive outbreak of gastroenteritis among Maxakali Indians, Southeast Brazil. *J. Clin. Virol.* 2006; 37(4):287-92.

[104] Mitchell DK, Matson DO, Jiang X, Berke T, Monroe SS, Carter MJ, et al. Molecular epidemiology of childhood astrovirus infection in child care centers. *J. Infect Dis.* 1999; 180(2):514-7.

[105] Herrmann JE, Taylor DN, Echeverria P, Blacklow NR. Astroviruses as a cause of gastroenteritis in children. *N Engl. J. Med.* 1991;324(25):1757-60.

[106] Liu CY, Shen KL, Wang SX, Liu YY, Zhaori GT. Astrovirus infection in young children with diarrhea hospitalized at Beijing Children's Hospital. *Chin. Med. J.* (Engl) 2004; 117(3):353-6.

[107] Chen SY, Chang YC, Lee YS, Chao HC, Tsao KC, Lin TY, et al. Molecular epidemiology and clinical manifestations of viral gastroenteritis in hospitalized pediatric patients in Northern Taiwan. *J. Clin. Microbiol.* 2007;45(6):2054-7.

[108] Bhattacharya R, Sahoo GC, Nayak MK, Ghosh S, Dutta P, Bhattacharya MK, et al. Molecular epidemiology of human astrovirus infections in Kolkata, India. *Infect Genet. Evol.* 2006;6(6):425-35.

[109] Steele AD, Basetse HR, Blacklow NR, Herrmann JE. Astrovirus infection in South Africa: a pilot study. *Ann. Trop. Paediatr.* 1998;18(4):315-9.

[110] Kiulia NM, Mwenda JM, Nyachieo A, Nyaundi JK, Steele AD, Taylor MB. Astrovirus infection in young Kenyan children with diarrhoea. *J. Trop. Pediatr.* 2007;53(3):206-9.

[111] Naficy AB, Rao MR, Holmes JL, Abu-Elyazeed R, Savarino SJ, Wierzba TF, et al. Astrovirus diarrhea in Egyptian children. *J. Infect Dis.* 2000;182(3):685-90.

[112] Pang XL, Vesikari T. Human astrovirus-associated gastroenteritis in children under 2 years of age followed prospectively during a rotavirus vaccine trial. *Acta Paediatr.* 1999; 88(5):532-6.

[113] Putzker M, Sauer H, Kirchner G, Keksel O, Malic A. Community acquired diarrhea--the incidence of Astrovirus infections in Germany. *Clin. Lab.* 2000;46(5-6):269-73.

[114] Guix S, Caballero S, Villena C, Bartolome R, Latorre C, Rabella N, et al. Molecular epidemiology of astrovirus infection in Barcelona, Spain. *J. Clin. Microbiol.* 2002; 40 (1): 133-9.

[115] Simpson R, Aliyu S, Iturriza-Gomara M, Desselberger U, Gray J. Infantile viral gastroenteritis: on the way to closing the diagnostic gap. *J. Med. Virol.* 2003;70(2):258-62.

[116] De Grazia S, Giammanco GM, Colomba C, Cascio A, Arista S. Molecular epidemiology of astrovirus infection in Italian children with gastroenteritis. *Clin. Microbiol. Infect* 2004;10(11):1025-9.

[117] Barreto ML, Milroy CA, Strina A, Prado MS, Leite JP, Ramos EA, et al. Community-based monitoring of diarrhea in urban Brazilian children: incidence and associated pathogens. *Trans R Soc. Trop. Med. Hyg.* 2006;100(3):234-42.

[118] Barreto ML, Genser B, Strina A, Teixeira MG, Assis AM, Rego RF, et al. Effect of city-wide sanitation programme on reduction in rate of childhood diarrhoea in northeast Brazil: assessment by two cohort studies. *Lancet* 2007;370(9599):1622-8.

[119] Ashley CR, Caul EO, Paver WK. Astrovirus-associated gastroenteritis in children. *J Clin. Pathol.* 1978;31(10):939-43.

[120] Kapikian AZ, Wyatt RG, Dolin R, Thornhill TS, Kalica AR, Chanock RM. Visualization by immune electron microscopy of a 27-nm particle associated with acute infectious nonbacterial gastroenteritis. *J. Virol.* 1972;10(5):1075-81.

[121] Hoehne M, Schreier E. Detection of Norovirus genogroup I and II by multiplex real-time RT- PCR using a 3'-minor groove binder-DNA probe. *BMC Infect Dis.* 2006;6:69.

[122] Trujillo AA, McCaustland KA, Zheng DP, Hadley LA, Vaughn G, Adams SM, et al. Use of TaqMan real-time reverse transcription-PCR for rapid detection, quantification, and typing of norovirus. *J. Clin. Microbiol.* 2006;44(4):1405-12.

[123] Rohayem J, Berger S, Juretzek T, Herchenroder O, Mogel M, Poppe M, et al. A simple and rapid single-step multiplex RT-PCR to detect Norovirus, Astrovirus and Adenovirus in clinical stool samples. *J. Virol. Methods* 2004;118(1):49-59.

[124] Yan H, Yagyu F, Okitsu S, Nishio O, Ushijima H. Detection of norovirus (GI, GII), Sapovirus and astrovirus in fecal samples using reverse transcription single-round multiplex PCR. *J. Virol. Methods* 2003;114(1):37-44.

[125] Iturriza-Gomara M, Green J, Brown DW, Desselberger U, Gray JJ. Diversity within the VP4 gene of rotavirus P[8] strains: implications for reverse transcription-PCR genotyping. *J. Clin. Microbiol.* 2000;38(2):898-901.

[126] Parra GI, Espinola EE. Nucleotide mismatches between the VP7 gene and the primer are associated with genotyping failure of a specific lineage from G1 rotavirus strains. *Virol. J.* 2006;3:35.

[127] Espinola EE, Parra GI, Russomando G, Arbiza J. Genetic diversity of the VP4 and VP7 genes affects the genotyping of rotaviruses: Analysis of Paraguayan strains. *Infect Genet Evol.* 2008;8(1):94-9.

[128] Martella V, Terio V, Arista S, Elia G, Corrente M, Madio A, et al. Nucleotide variation in the VP7 gene affects PCR genotyping of G9 rotaviruses identified in Italy. *J. Med. Virol.* 2004;72(1):143-8.

[129] Zintz C, Bok K, Parada E, Barnes-Eley M, Berke T, Staat MA, et al. Prevalence and genetic characterization of caliciviruses among children hospitalized for acute gastroenteritis in the United States. *Infect Genet Evol.* 2005;5(3):281-90.

[130] Brown DW, Gunning KB, Henry DM, Awdeh ZL, Brinker JP, Tzipori S, et al. A DNA oligonucleotide microarray for detecting human astrovirus serotypes. *J. Virol. Methods* 2008; 147(1):86-92.

[131] Chizhikov V, Wagner M, Ivshina A, Hoshino Y, Kapikian AZ, Chumakov K. Detection and genotyping of human group A rotaviruses by oligonucleotide microarray hybridization. *J. Clin. Microbiol.* 2002;40(7):2398-407.

[132] Lovmar L, Fock C, Espinoza F, Bucardo F, Syvanen AC, Bondeson K. Microarrays for genotyping human group a rotavirus by multiplex capture and type-specific primer extension. *J. Clin. Microbiol.* 2003;41(11):5153-8.

[133] Santos N, Honma S, Timenetsky MD, Linhares AC, Ushijima H, Armah GE, et al. Development of a Microtiter Plate Hybridization-based PCR-enzyme-linked Immunosorbent Assay (PCR-ELISA) for Identification of Clinically Relevant Human Group A Rotavirus G and P Genotypes. *J. Clin. Microbiol.* 2007.

[134] Grimm AC, Cashdollar JL, Williams FP, Fout GS. Development of an astrovirus RT-PCR detection assay for use with conventional, real-time, and integrated cell culture/RT-PCR. *Can. J. Microbiol.* 2004;50(4):269-78.

[135] Chapron CD, Ballester NA, Margolin AB. The detection of astrovirus in sludge biosolids using an integrated cell culture nested PCR technique. *J. Appl. Microbiol.* 2000; 89(1):11-5.

[136] Mustafa H, Palombo EA, Bishop RF. Improved sensitivity of astrovirus-specific RT-PCR following culture of stool samples in CaCo-2 cells. *J. Clin. Virol.* 1998;11(2):103-7.

[137] ESPGAN Working Group on Acute Diarrhoea. Recommendations for feeding in childhood gastroenteritis. *Pediatr. Gastroenterol. Nutr.* 1997;24:619-620.

[138] Vesikari T, Matson DO, Dennehy P, Van Damme P, Santosham M, Rodriguez Z, et al. Safety and efficacy of a pentavalent human-bovine (WC3) reassortant rotavirus vaccine. *N Engl. J. Med.* 2006;354(1):23-33.

[139] Ruiz-Palacios GM, Perez-Schael I, Velazquez FR, Abate H, Breuer T, Clemens SC, et al. Safety and efficacy of an attenuated vaccine against severe rotavirus gastroenteritis. *N Engl. J. Med.* 2006;354(1):11-22.

[140] Simonsen L, Viboud C, Elixhauser A, Taylor RJ, Kapikian AZ. More on RotaShield and intussusception: the role of age at the time of vaccination. *J. Infect Dis.* 2005;192 Suppl 1:S36-43.

[141] Smith AW, Iversen PL, O'Hanley PD, Skilling DE, Christensen JR, Weaver SS, et al. Virus-specific antiviral treatment for controlling severe and fatal outbreaks of feline calicivirus infection. *Am. J. Vet. Res.* 2008;69(1):23-32.

[142] Vicente D, Cilla G, Montes M, Perez-Yarza EG, Perez-Trallero E. Human bocavirus, a respiratory and enteric virus. *Emerg. Infect Dis.* 2007;13(4):636-7.

[143] Fabiana A, Donia D, Gabrieli R, Petrinca AR, Cenko F, Bebeci D, et al. Influence of enteric viruses on gastroenteritis in Albania: epidemiological and molecular analysis. *J. Med. Virol.* 2007;79(12):1844-9.

[144] Dey SK, Nguyen TA, Phan TG, Nishio O, Salim AF, Rahman M, et al. Molecular and epidemiological trend of norovirus associated gastroenteritis in Dhaka City, Bangladesh. *J. Clin. Virol.* 2007;40(3):218-23.

[145] Soares CC, Santos N, Beard RS, Albuquerque MC, Maranhao AG, Rocha LN, et al. Norovirus detection and genotyping for children with gastroenteritis, Brazil. *Emerg. Infect Dis.* 2007;13(8):1244-6.

[146] Steinberg EB, Mendoza CE, Glass R, Arana B, Lopez MB, Mejia M, et al. Prevalence of infection with waterborne pathogens: a seroepidemiologic study in children 6-36 months old in San Juan Sacatepequez, Guatemala. *Am. J. Trop. Med. Hyg.* 2004; 70 (1): 83-8.

[147] Reither K, Ignatius R, Weitzel T, Seidu-Korkor A, Anyidoho L, Saad E, et al. Acute childhood diarrhoea in northern Ghana: epidemiological, clinical and microbiological characteristics. *BMC Infect Dis.* 2007;7:104.

[148] Subekti DS, Tjaniadi P, Lesmana M, Simanjuntak C, Komalarini S, Digdowirogo H, et al. Characterization of Norwalk-like virus associated with gastroenteritis in Indonesia. *J. Med. Virol.* 2002;67(2):253-8.

[149] Papaventsis DC, Dove W, Cunliffe NA, Nakagomi O, Combe P, Grosjean P, et al. Norovirus infection in children with acute gastroenteritis, Madagascar, 2004-2005. *Emerg. Infect Dis.* 2007;13(6):908-11.

[150] Dove W, Cunliffe NA, Gondwe JS, Broadhead RL, Molyneux ME, Nakagomi O, et al. Detection and characterization of human caliciviruses in hospitalized children with acute gastroenteritis in Blantyre, Malawi. *J. Med. Virol.* 2005;77(4):522-7.

[151] Phan TG, Okame M, Nguyen TA, Maneekarn N, Nishio O, Okitsu S, et al. Human astrovirus, norovirus (GI, GII), and sapovirus infections in Pakistani children with diarrhea. *J. Med. Virol.* 2004;73(2):256-61.

In: Topics in Prevalent Diseases
Editors: N. C. Chavez-Tapia and M. Uribe

ISBN 978-1-60456-959-9

Chapter 14

Asthma among Rural Bangladeshi Children: Prevalence and Risk Factors

K. Zaman*, Haruko Takeuchi[2] and Shams El Arifeen[1]

[1] International Centre for Diarrhoeal Disease Research, Bangladesh (ICDDR, B)
[2] Tokyo University Graduate School of Public Health, Japan

Introduction

Asthma is a chronic obstructive lung disease characterized by intermittent dry cough, expiratory wheeze, chest tightness, shortness of breath and dyspnoea; the signs and symptoms are exacerbated by physical exercise and triggered by allergens (dust, pollen, etc.) and irritants (cold, dry air, etc.). The management of asthma has dramatically improved; however, the prevalence of asthma has increased worldwide. Approximately 300 million people worldwide currently have asthma and about 180,000 annual deaths (Braman, 2006).

Studies have shown an increase prevalence of asthma in the developed countries in the UK, USA, Australia and New Zealand (ISAAC, 1998; Robertson, 1991). Lower prevalence has been reported from Asian countries, e.g., India (7%) and Pakistan (8%) (ISAAC, 1998). Asthma causes a great deal of morbidity and mortality among children in rural Bangladesh. According to Bangladesh Bureau of Statistics Asthma and respiratory diseases ranked as the second leading cause of death in Bangladesh in 2003 (BBS, 2007). Estimates of current and lifetime prevalence of wheeze and asthma of children in tropical countries in the 1990s showed an increasing trend and there was an observed association between urbanization and prevalence of exercise-induced bronchospasm (Barbin and Kelly, 1998).

Hospital admissions rates for asthma have been increased in different countries including in the United Kingdom, New Zealand, Australia and the United States (Hyndman et al., 1994). The reasons for this increase may be due to increase in severity of cases, changes

* email: kzaman@icddrb.org.

in delivery of care, asthma treatment, admission and readmission policies or due to environmental factors.

It has been estimated that economic costs associated with asthma exceed those of TB and HIV/AIDS. The direct medical treatment cost and indirect costs (wage loss, loss of school days, early retirement, etc.) related to asthma are enormous (Braman, 2006).

Differences exist in the prevalence of asthma between countries and within the countries. These are more within the developing countries than the developed countries and more pronounced among young children. These variations are probably attributable to the differences in the prevalence of atopy and the changes in environment (Karunasekera et al.,, 2001).

Risk Factors

Several risk factors for the development of asthma have been identified. These are hereditary atopy, recurrent respiratory tract infections, indoor and outdoor environmental factors (tobacco and smoke exposure), attacks of pneumonia during their infancy, maternal and paternal asthma, low family income and early exposure to protein antigens such as cow's milk and egg white (ISAAC, 1998; Host, 2002; Zaman et al., 2007). Respiratory syncytial virus (RSV) is a common cause of severe bronchiolitis and pneumonia among children <2 years of age. Studies documented that bronchiolitis during the first year of life is a risk factor for the development of asthma and sensitization to common allergens during the subsequent 2 years (Sigurs et al., 1995). Although the relationship between RSV infection and later development of atopy and asthma in later life is not straightforward but this association is important from public heath perspective since under-diagnosis and under-treatment exacerbates asthma.

There are reports that respiratory infections e.g. pneumonia has been associated with asthma (Busse, 1993). Acute lower respiratory infections (ALRI) caused by RSV was associated with increased risk of subsequent allergic sensitization (Sigurs et al., 1995). RSV bronchiolitis during the first year of life apparently is an important risk factor for the development of asthma and sensitization to common allergens during the subsequent 2 years (Martinez et al., 1995; Stein et al., 1999).

Asthma in Bangladesh

Few epidemiological studies have been conducted in Bangladesh to understand the burden of asthma and its risk factors. A nationwide survey was done in 1999 among populations aged 5 years and above in urban and rural areas to understand the magnitude of asthma problem. Face to face interviews were conducted. The prevalence of recent wheeze (within last 12 months) was 6.9% (Hassan et al, 2002). It was revealed that the prevalence of asthma was higher among children aged 5-14 years compared to adults (15-44 years) (7.3% versus 5.3%). Asthma was more common in families with ≤ 3 people than in larger households (OR 2.20, 95% CI: 1.24-3.20) and in poor (OR = 1.41, 95% CI: 1.04-1.92) and illiterate groups (OR = 1.51, 95% CI: 1.01-2.24). The risk of asthma was greater among active smokers compared to non-smokers. The authors explained that children in less crowded household might have less respiratory infections compared to larger household and certain viral infections in early life may be protective in subsequent development of allergic disease (Strachan, 1989). The findings of higher prevalence of asthma among poor and illiterate groups were consistent with findings from other studies (Martinez, 1995; Lin et al., 1999).

ISAAC (International Studies of Asthma and Allergies in Childhood) questionnaire was used to conduct a survey among urban and rural schools in Dhaka district in Bangladesh in 2000. The prevalence of recent wheeze was 9.1% among 6-7 year old and 6.1% among 13-14 year old children (Kabir et al., 2005). It was higher among male children compared to females (9.0% vs. 5.9%).

A study conducted in rural Bangladesh at Matlab in 2001 to determine the prevalence of asthma and also used an adopted questionnaire of the ISAAC. A total 50 villages was randomly selected from 67 villages from the intervention area of Matlab Health Demographic Surveillance System (HDSS) area of the International Centre for Diarrhoeal Disease Research, Bangladesh (ICDDR,B). All children aged 60-71 months were eligible and 1587 children were included in the study. The prevalence of wheezing in the last 12 months prior to the survey was 16.1% and it was significantly higher among children who had attacks of pneumonia during their infancy compared to children who did not (23.0% vs. 14.6%). Risk factors identified in the study were maternal asthma (OR=3.01, 95% CI 2.02-4.47), paternal asthma (OR= 3.12, 95% CI 1.85, 5.26), maternal eczema (OR= 1.81, 95% CI 1.14-2.87) and family income $\leq$ 100 US$ (OR for US$ 51-99=1.63, 95% CI 1.05, 2.53; OR for US $ $\leq$ 50= 2.12, 95% CI 1.31, 3.44) (Zaman et al., 2007). The same study also investigated the association between Ascaris infection, serum level of anti-Ascaris IgE and wheezing. The results revealed that a high titre of anti-Ascaris E was associated with an increased risk of asthma symptoms (Takeuchi et al., 2007).

The results of these studies should be interpreted cautiously considering the differences in methodology, population and time periods. Results revealed that asthma is a major cause of morbidity and mortality in Bangladesh and the wheezing was more common among low income population and parents with low education levels (Hassan et al, 2002). The prevalence of asthma was similar to neighbouring countries but lower than in the developed countries. It has been estimated that about 7 million people including 4 million children suffer from asthma related symptoms in Bangladesh.

Whereas the "hygiene hypothesis" states that unclean and lower socio-economic environment protect against asthma and allergy and studies have shown the inverse associations between asthma and early infectious diseases (Strachan, 1989; Ball, 2000; Alm, 1999; Matricardi et al., 2000, Yazdanbakhsh M et al., 2002), the results of Bangladesh studies contradict these hypothesis. These conflicting findings between the developed and developing countries suggest that there may be other contributing factors which are linked to lower socio-economic environment. In addition, the association between ALRI and asthma requires additional studies because many children suffered from ALRI/pneumonia in Bangladesh.

ALRI is the leading cause of mortality among children in Bangladesh. Effective management of pneumonia is critical since most of these deaths can be averted with proper use of antibiotics. Since the risk of asthma is higher among children who had suffered pneumonia during their childhood, greater efforts are needed to prevent pneumonia during their infancy to reduce subsequent development of asthma.

Despite improvement in management of asthma, barriers remain for its effective treatment in the developing countries. These include limited access to health care facilities, lack of proper diagnosis, cost of treatment, poor compliance etc.

Acknowledgement

This research study was funded by the ICDDR,B and its donors who provide unrestricted support to the Centre for its operations and research. Current donors providing unrestricted support include: Australian International Development Agency (AusAID), Government of Bangladesh, Canadian International Development Agency (CIDA), Government of Japan, Government of the Netherlands, Swedish International Development Cooperative Agency (SIDA), Swiss Development Cooperation (SDC) and Department for International Development, UK (DFID). We gratefully acknowledge these donors for their support and commitment to the Centre's research efforts.

References

Alm JS, Swartz J, Lilja G et al. Atopy in children of families with an anthroposophic lifestyle. *Lancet* 1999; 353: 1485-8.

Ball TM, Castro-Rodriguez JA, Griffith KA et al. Siblings, day-care attendance, and the risk of asthma and wheezing during childhood. *N Engl. J. Med.* 2000; 343: 538-43.

Bangladesh Bureau of Statistics (BBS). Statistical Yearbook of Bangladesh 2005. Government of the peoples Republic of Bangladesh; 2007.p.814.

Brabin BJ, Kelly Y. Prevalence of childhood asthma in the tropics. *Ann. Trop. Paediatr.* 1998; 18 Suppl: S33-39.

Braman SS. The global burden of asthma. *Chest* 2006; 130: $S-12S.

Busse WW. Role and contribution of viral respiratory infections to asthma. *Allergy* 1993; 48: 57-61.

Hassan MR, Kabir AR, Mahmud AM, et al. Self-reported asthma symptoms in children and adults of Bangladesh: findings of the National Asthma Prevalence Study. *Int. J. Epidemiol.* 2002; 31: 483-8.

Host A. Frequency of cows milk allergy in childhood. *Ann. Allergy Asthma Immunol.* 2002 (suppl); 89: 33-37.

Hyndman SJ, Williams DRR, Merrill SL, Lipscombe JM, Palmer CR. Rates of admission to hospital for asthma *BMJ* 1994; 308: 1596-1600.

The International Study of Asthma and Allergies in Childhood (ISAAC) Steering Committee. Worldwide variation in prevalence of symptoms of asthma, allergic rhinoconjunctivitis, and atopic eczema: ISAAC. *Lancet* 1998; 351: 1225-32

Kabir ML, Rahman F, Hassan MQ et al. Asthma, atopic eczema and allergic rhino-conjunctivitis in school children. *Mymensingh Med. J.* 2005;14: 41-5.

Karunasekera KAW, Jayasibghe JACT, Alwis WGR. Risk factors of childhood asthma: A Sri Lankan study. *J. Trop. Pediatr.* 2001; 47: 142-145

Lin S, Fitegerald E, Hwang SA, Munsie JP, Stark A. Asthma hospitalization rates and socio-economic status in New York State (1987-1993). *J. Asthma* 1999; 36: 239-251.

Martinez FD, Wright AL, Taussig LM, Holberg CJ, Halonen M, Morgan WJ, and the Group Health Medical Associates. Asthma and wheezing in the first six years of life. *N Engl. J. Med.* 1995; 332: 133-138.

Matricardi PM, Rosmini F, Riondino S, et al. Exposure to foodborne and orofecal microbes versus airborne viruses in relation to atopy and allergic asthma: epidemiological study. *BMJ* 2000; 320:412-7.

Robertson CF, Heycock E, Bishop J, Nolan T, Olinsky A. Phelan PD. Prevalence of asthma in Melbourne schoolchildren: changes over 26 years. *BMJ.* 1991; 302: 1116-1118.

Sigurs N, Bjarnason R, Sigurbergsson F, Kjellman B, Bjorksten B. Asthma and immunoglobulin E antibodies after respiratory syncytial virus bronchiolitis: a prospective cohort study with matched controls. *Pediatrics* 1995; 95:500-5.

Stein RT, Sherrill D, Morgan WJ, Holberg CJ, Halonen M, Taussig LM, Wright AL, Martinez FD. Respiratory syncytial virus in early life and risk of wheeze and allergy by age 13 years. *Lancet* 1999; 354: 541-45.

Strachan DP. Hay fever, hygiene, and household size. *BMJ* 1989; 299: 1259-60.

Takeuchi H, Zaman K, Takahashi J, Yunus M, Chowdhury HR, Arifeen SE, Baqui AH, Wakai S, Iwata T. High titre of anti-Ascaris immunoglobin E associated with bronchial asthma symptoms in 5-yaer-old rural Bangladeshi children. *Clinical and Experimental Allergy* 2007; 38: 276-282.

Yazdanbakhsh M, Kremsner PG, van Ree R. Allergy, parasites and the hygiene hypothesis. *Science* 2002; 296: 490-494.

Zaman K, Takeuchi H, Yunus M, Arifeen SE, Chowdhury HR, Baqui AH, Wakai S, Iwata T. Asthma in rural Bangladesh. *Indian J. Pediatr.* 2007; 74: 539-543.

In: Topics in Prevalent Diseases
Editors: N. C. Chavez-Tapia and M. Uribe
ISBN 978-1-60456-959-9

Chapter 15

Maternal Mortality in Minorities

***Abha Aggarwal*[1], *Arvind Pandey*[1], *Rohini Sehgal*[2] *and Suneeta Mittal*[2]**

[1]National Institute of Medical Statistics, Indian Council of Medical Research, Ansari Nagar, New Delhi, India

[2]Department of Obstetrics and Gynecology, All India Institute of Medical Sciences, Ansari Nagar, New Delhi, India

Introduction

In developing countries including India, reduction in maternal mortality has been the key developmental goal for monitoring the progress of reproductive and child health in the population. The need of setting such goals is discussed and documented in various national and international deliberations. The commitment was reiterated in many health policy documents and country reports and National Plans of Action developed on the aftermath of many UN summits and conferences including the World Summit for children, New York, the International Conference on Population and Development (Cario, 1994) and World Conference on Women (Beijing 1995), and the Millennium Declaration (New York 2000) [1] Although various safe motherhood initiatives have been taken globally for reduction in maternal deaths, yet decline in Maternal Mortality Ratio based on the available data suggests that very little progress has been achieved over the last decade. The dimensions of the problem and associated factors which contribute to high maternal mortality also show that the pace of decline in reduction of MMR committed in Millennium Development Goals (MDG) adopted at the Millennium Summit is far from the desired level in developing countries especially in poor population. Concerned over the continued high maternal mortality rates in developing countries, WHO Headquarters had organized a series of inter-regional meetings for monitoring maternal deaths. Participants emphasized while the efforts might begin with measuring number of maternal deaths, these should progress towards the underlying causes of maternal deaths and its preventive measures [2]. Maternal deaths being preventable represent a larger tragedy than deaths from other diseases.

Time is overdue for epidemiologists to turn their attention to the areas of the world where the neglected tragedy of high maternal mortality is persisting and examine the causes and factors associated with maternal deaths. The causal factors are known, most of them related to lack of provision of appropriate health care. It is a tragic situation as deaths follow or occur during a natural process.

In spite of growing concern about reproductive health, information on levels, trends and differentials in maternal mortality remains fragmentary in most developing countries. In addition abortion and stillbirth related deaths are often not accounted. At the community level in the low resource areas there is no perception about severity of obstetric complications. Even when efforts are made for attention, there is lack of means or knowledge. Poverty, low literacy and overall low status of women prevent women from taking antenatal care even if services are available. [3-7]

To bring down maternal mortality, numbers of issues have to be settled like the methods of data collection and their quality, standardization of techniques, recognition of causal factors including near-miss cases in clinical audits, strengthening of preventive measures and above all attitudinal change of policymakers and health care professionals. Further, to improve the quality of maternal health care services, a number of issues regarding maternal deaths need to be standardized and made universal all over the world.

This chapter reviews the definition of maternal mortality and 'Near miss mortality', a description of the dimensions of the problem and issues in measuring maternal mortality. The next section of the chapter will be a brief discussion on methodologies and data collection systems for measuring maternal mortality. Lastly the chapter reviews the 'causes of maternal deaths', 'Role of Health Services', 'Importance of Preventive measures' and Strategies to reduce maternal mortality. In this chapter Minority Perspective indicates the poor population in developing countries with special reference to India.

What Is Maternal Death?

A maternal death is the outcome of a chain of events and disadvantages throughout a woman's life. WHO defined a maternal death as "the death of a woman while pregnant or within 42 days of termination of pregnancy, irrespective of the duration and site of pregnancy from any cause related to or aggravated by the pregnancy or its management but not from accidental or incidental causes". Maternal deaths may be direct or indirect. Direct maternal death is result of complications of pregnancy, delivery or their management or a chain of events resulting from any of them. Indirect maternal death is death resulting from previous existing disease or disease that developed during pregnancy, not related to direct obstetric cause and aggravated by physiological effects of pregnancy. Other fatalities during pregnancy but unrelated to pregnancy are accidental, incidental or non obstetric maternal deaths. Cases with incidental maternal deaths include maternal deaths secondary to domestic violence against woman especially in poor population which may be related to pregnancy and may be affected by the socio-economic and cultural environment. The concept of late maternal deaths has been introduced in ICD-10 and is defined as the death of a women from direct or indirect obstetric causes more than 42 days but less than one year after termination of pregnancy [3].

Near Miss Mortality and Morbidity

A *"near miss"* refers to any pregnant or "recently-delivered" woman in whom immediate survival was threatened and who survived by chance or because of the hospital care that she received. Severe maternal morbidity or "near misses" occur in larger numbers than maternal deaths. Larger numbers provide stronger evidence and more robust conclusions. It is also possible to speak to the woman to obtain her views about what happened and the care she received. Since this can also be regarded as a "great save", it is less threatening to staff. However, case definition can be difficult and requires local agreement. Case ascertainment involves time and resources. There is no right or wrong definition of a "near miss". What is important is that the definitions used in any review are appropriate to local circumstances to enable local improvements to be made in maternal care [8-11].

Near miss mortality may be defined as women who nearly died with severe life threatening conditions but, with good luck or good intensive care, survived.

Further, maternal morbidity also represents a huge burden of disease for women and their families. The prevention efforts against maternal deaths need to be broadened to include efforts to curb near miss morbidity that is the life threatening morbidity. A scoring system for near miss morbidity needs to be incorporated into clinical case reviews and epidemiological studies to enhance monitoring of obstetric care [8]. Standardization of inclusion criteria and of methods for case assessment would facilitate comparisons over time and among countries [11-12]. The criteria currently used to identify a *near miss* vary greatly. However, areas with similar health care facilities, medical records and personnel should be able to agree on suitable criteria, making their incorporation into maternal death enquiries feasible. There is a trend towards higher incidence of near miss morbidity in developing countries [12]. Studies on severe maternal morbidity worldwide may provide a valuable contribution to the reduction in maternal mortality. In this way an effort should be directed for the development of a common set of criteria to allow the comparison of data across the globe. Additional studies are still needed, but the adoption of a two levels screening strategy may be appropriate. The first level should be based in comprehensive criteria of severe maternal morbidity, followed by the application of restrictive criteria such as organ dysfunction or failure. This approach may be effective for the development of a consistent severe maternal morbidity surveillance system.

In developed countries where maternal death is rare, the factors surrounding the death are often peculiar to the event and are not generalizable, making analysis of maternal deaths less useful. Confidential enquiries into maternal deaths have been associated with decreases in maternal deaths, but since in developed countries, maternal deaths are rare, the relevance of the information gleaned from the occasional maternal death to the general population is becoming distant. The incorporation of *near misses* into the confidential enquiry systems might allow for more relevant data on maternal care being made applicable [10].

Hall [11] listed several reasons for their inclusion.

1. Larger numbers lead to more robust conclusions.
2. More rapid reporting on maternal care issues (because of the larger number of cases).
3. Useful lessons learnt from *near misses* will reinforce the lessons learnt when these cases previously died.
4. *Near misses* will provide relevant controls for maternal deaths, since presumably most women who die pass through a phase of organ dysfunction before dying.
5. Provided an ethical solution can be found to the confidentiality problem, the *near misses* can be interviewed providing valuable information on the risk factors and substandard care.
6. Obstetric requirements for intensive care can be quantified.
7. Comparative ratios/indices can be calculated.

However, before such a system is introduced, consensus will need to be attained on the criteria used to identify a *near miss*

Dimensions of the Problem

Each year around 536,000 women die from complications of pregnancy and childbirth of which more than 99 percent of these deaths occur in less developed regions [3].

For every woman who dies approximately 15-30 women suffer from serious injuries, infection and disabilities [2-4]. Maternal mortality is one health statistical tool showing largest difference between developed and developing countries. Current estimates of maternal mortality ratio varies more than 1000 per 100,000 live births in some African countries to around 500 in many countries in Asia, 200-400 in several countries in South Asia and less than 10 per 100,000 in European countries. By the broad MDG regions, the maternal mortality ratio (MMR) in 2005 was highest in developing regions (at 450 maternal deaths per 100 000 live births), in stark contrast to developed regions (at 9 maternal deaths per 100,000 live births) and countries of the Commonwealth of independent states (at 51 maternal deaths per 100,000 live births). Among the developing regions sub-Saharan Africa had the highest MMR at 900 followed by south Asia (490) [3].

South East Asia accounts for 170,000 maternal deaths per year. World Health Organization (WHO) indirect estimation for India was about 120,000 –140,000 maternal deaths in 2002. About 270,000 maternal deaths occurred in the sub Saharan Africa region alone, followed by South Asia (188000)[3]. Thus, Sub-Saharan Africa and South Asia accounted for 86% of global maternal deaths. According to WHO estimates in 2005 India was the country with highest number of maternal deaths (117,000). It was followed by Nigeria (59,000), Congo (32,000) and Afghanistan (26,000) [3].

India with population of more than 1 billion accounts for 20-24% all maternal deaths in the world [5] while along with the 10 other countries, accounted for almost 65% of global maternal deaths in 2005.

India is a vast country, having a per capita gross national income of only US $460, and 86 percent of the population with an income below US $2 per day, making the public health challenges in India great. [13] Although various safe motherhood initiatives have been taken, yet decline in maternal mortality ratio in India is far from the desired level of 100 by 2012, a goal set by the National Rural Health Mission (NRHM) and 109 by 2015 as per millennium development goals (MDG). Two national health surveys carried out in 1992-1993 and 1998-1999 reported maternal mortality ratios of 437 and 540 per 100000 live births, respectively [14-15]. The past estimates for India which used indirect methods, (such as those using age-specific mortality rates among women) suggested that maternal mortality ratio had declined from 750 in 1960s to about 400 in the 1990s.and was 407 per 100,000 live births in the nineties [1]. The maternal mortality declined by 24 percent during 1997 to 2003 to 301 per 100,000 livebirths [16]. A recent study conducted in India for estimation of MMR on pilot basis gives MMR of 356 per hundred thousand live births with standard error of 37 maternal deaths[17]. This indicates that India is still far behind the goal set by health planners. The fact that the poor people are both more likely to become ill and less likely to get appropriate treatment has not changed resulting in highest maternal deaths in poor population.

MMR can be translated into women's lifetime chances of maternal deaths globally as a whole is about 1 in 74 varying from 1 in 4000 in developed countries to 1 in 61 in developing to 1 in 17 in underdeveloped countries [5]. The International Conference on Population and Development in 1994 had recommended reduction in maternal mortality by at least 50% of the 1990 levels by the year 2000 and further one half by the year 2015. Within the MDG monitoring framework, the international community committed itself to reducing the maternal mortality ratio (MMR) by three quarters between 1990 and 2015. [3]

While an annual decline of 5.5% in MMR between 1990 and 2015 is required to achieve Million Development Goals 5, figures released show an annual decline of less than 1%. [18]

These estimates provide an up-to-date indication of the extent of the maternal mortality problem globally. To bring down maternal deaths, it is essential to go beyond just measuring the numbers and rates, find the causes of death, and ensure that none of these women have died in vain, by making necessary tools available to prevent future maternal deaths. [19]

WhyIt Is Important to Measure Maternal Mortality

The goals set for reducing maternal mortality in various international deliberations reflects its importance of measuring estimates which not only indicates the health status of women in a country but is also required for planning health interventions for further reducing maternal deaths. Maternal mortality is a sentinel event to assess quality of a health care system, access to health care and the adequacy of the health care system in responding to their needs. The information about the levels and trends of maternal mortality is needed as not only it tells about the risks in pregnancy and child birth, but also it implies about woman's health, their social and economic status. (Source: WHO Revised estimates 1990)

Measuring Maternal Mortality

There are three distinct measures of maternal mortality which are used to measures the maternal mortality ratio, maternal mortality rate and life time risk of maternal death. The most commonly used measure is the maternal mortality ratio that is the number of maternal deaths during a given time period per 100,000 live births during the same time period. Mathematically it can be estimated as follows:

Maternal Mortality Ratio (MMR)	=	Number of maternal deaths to women (15-49 years) / Number of live births to women (15-49 years)	X 100000
Maternal Mortality Rate (MM_rate)	=	Number of maternal deaths to women (15-49 years) / Number of living women (15-49 years)	X 100000
Lifetime Risk of Maternal Death	=	$1 - (1\text{-MM\_rate}/1{,}00{,}000)^{35}$	

(Source Ref. 16)

Issues in Measuring Maternal Mortality

It is extremely difficult to assess levels of maternal mortality at National Level as it requires the information on the deaths of women of reproductive age, cause of death as well as the number of new born which are generally under reported. The correct figures are difficult to get as only few countries keep records for such events, in addition where records are available cause of death is not adequately classified. Even in countries with complete vital registration system and good cause of death attribution, misclassification of maternal deaths arises due to various other reasons.

In developing countries where vital registration system are absent or inadequate it is possible to estimate maternal mortality using survey techniques but these have a number of disadvantages including cost. For conducting the survey sample size required to estimate maternal mortality at national level is a major issue beside the methodology to be used for collection of such sensitive data. Further, in poor population, the number of maternal deaths as well as the number of births is generally under reported as most of the deliveries are conducted at home by untrained dais.

Approaches for Measuring Maternal Mortality

There are various approaches for obtaining data on levels of maternal mortality. These are considerately varied in terms of methodology. The main approaches are described briefly below.

Vital Registration

In developed countries, a well defined system for registration of vital events like birth, death and deaths by cause exist for periodic surveillance. The information on maternal mortality derives from the system for implementing program. In India, the Indian Census is the largest single source of a variety of statistical information on different characteristics of the people of India. It is also entrusted with the responsibility of registration of Births and Deaths through Sample Registration System (SRS) under the office of Registrar General, India under the Ministry of Home Affairs .The Government evaluates programs on fertility and mortality using the Sample Registration System (SRS) data. Sample registration System gives trends in maternal mortality in recent years, examines the major cause of maternal mortality and provides estimates of current and future burden from maternal deaths. The estimates provided by this system had large standard errors and for some states in India, the sample size was inadequate to give reliable estimates. For such a situation direct household survey, though expensive, could be the best alternative with suitable survey technique [16, 17].

Direct Household Survey Methods

Household survey provides an alternative method where vital registration data are not appropriate for the assessment of cause –specific mortality. However, household survey using direct estimation is expensive and complex to implement because large sample sizes are needed to provide statistically reliable estimate using effective survey methodologies and proper sample size determination. The details are provided in the next section. In a vast country like India, maternal mortality varies greatly across the states and in the past even indirect estimates could not generate maternal mortality trends in various regions. The data collection systems and guidelines prepared by WHO, Geneva, 2004 are examples for developing countries to develop their own maternal death review process, forms, audit sheets and questionnaires [7,19].

Sisterhood Method

The sisterhood method is a survey-based measurement technique that in high-fertility populations substantially reduces sample size requirements because it obtains information by interviewing respondents about the survival of all their adult sisters. Although sample size requirements may be reduced, the problem of wide confidence intervals remains. Furthermore, the method provides a retrospective rather than a current estimate, averaging experience over a lengthy time period (some 35 years, with a mid point around 12 years before the survey) [20]. For methodological reasons, the indirect method is not appropriate for use in setting where fertility level are low [(Total Fertility Rate (TFR) <4)] or where there has been substantial migration, civil strife, war or other causes of social dislocation. The only advantage of this method is small sample size and hence is less expensive and time consuming than a prospective community based survey. (Source: WHO Revised estimates 1990)

Verbal Autopsy Method

A verbal autopsy is a newly developed technique in which relatives of the deceased person are interviewed regarding the circumstances leading to the death. Information on the signs and symptoms preceding the death is used to reconstruct the illness leading to death and to assign the most probable cause of death (Garenne and Fontaine 1986; Zimicki 1986).

The verbal autopsy method has been widely used to assess the causes of maternal deaths effectively in many studies [17, 21]. Verbal autopsies are the attractive method in countries where vital registration system is weak. The accuracy of these estimations, however, is very dependent on having access to information on the persons who died. This technique can be useful in poor settings where large numbers of maternal deaths are occurring outside health facilities. From the family and the community it is possible to find out the house where a maternal death occurred. Also information may be obtained about the awareness regarding the health care. It is a valuable tool for identifying areas that require immediate intervention ranging from improving awareness and transport to health facilities.

Census

Census is a complete enumeration of the population conducted every ten year. It is also called decennial censuses. These are conducted by a system developed in a country. This method of data collection uses a high quality questionnaire which include question on deaths in the household in a defined reference period, often one or two years, followed by more detailed questions which would permit the identification of maternal deaths on the basis of time of death relative to pregnancy (verbal autopsy). The advantages of such an approach are that it would generate both national and sub national figure and that it would be possible to undertake analysis according to the characteristics of the household. Trend analysis would be possible because sampling errors would be eliminated or greatly reduced. However, data obtained from enquiries into recent deaths in the household in a census require careful evaluation, and often adjustment. A number of countries have used the census to generate maternal mortality figures and work is under way to assess the extent to which such approaches may prove of value in measuring maternal mortality. [19, 22]

Determination of Sample Size for Estimating MMR

To arrive at the decision on the minimum sample size for estimating MMR at National or sub National level we need to estimate the number of births(n) to be estimated at said level. Calculation for estimating the number of births is based on the following formula

Sample size (n) = $(Z_\alpha)^2 pq/d^2$ (1)

where, Z_α = value of the standard normal deviate corresponding to α level of significance,

P = proportion (MMR),

and d = permissible relative margin of error.

The above sample size when multiplied by the design effect of the sampling design gives the estimated number of births to be covered in a survey. The required population corresponding to these many numbers of births could further be estimated using the birth rate. Depending upon the available infrastructure in a country the total population can be covered. It is illustrated with the following example.

Example:

Suppose a sample size is to be estimated for estimating MMR for India at country level. Assuming MMR to be as 400 per hundred thousand live births, birth rate as 28.5 per thousand population with 95% confidence level and 5% relative margin of error.

Solution: Here p= 0.004,

q= 0.996

t 5% level Z_α = 1.96

relative margin of error = 5% of p

or d = 0.0002

By putting these values in the mentioned formula (1) and solving, it gives

n = 382623

Using birth rate of 28.5 for thousand populations, this would amount to about 1.3 year population to be covered for estimating MMR.

Snowball Sampling for Capturing Maternal Deaths

Snowball sampling is a special non probability method for developing a research sample where existing study subjects recruit future subjects from among their acquaintances. The first subject is identified through some key person who knows about the community in poor settings. Thus the sample group appears to grow like a rolling snowball. This sampling technique is often used in hidden populations or rare events which are extremely difficult to locate respondents or are cost prohibitive, for example, maternal death, drug users or commercial sex workers in a community [21, 23].

While this technique can dramatically lower search costs, it comes at the expense of introducing bias because the technique itself reduces the likelihood that the sample will represent a good cross section from the population. In estimating the number of events by the snowball method, the capture-recapture method must be used: how many of the events named were already in the sample, and how many are genuine new names?

The method of snowball sampling also provides the possibility of estimating the total number of events i.e. maternal deaths. Besides providing an estimate of the MMR, the snowball method gives, just as other sampling methods, information about the composition of the maternal deaths. It should be noted here that the snowball sample is in itself not a representative group of events since better-known events have a much greater chance of being included in the sample than less well-known events. This bias will need to be taken into account when interpreting the data on the composition of the snowball sample it has been found to be feasible and cost effective technique in capturing maternal deaths in one of the study in India wherein a few households where a maternal death occurred were identified through some key-informants in the village (geographically smallest unit in India). The households where maternal deaths have occurred are then asked to provide name of other households where similar event has occurred and so on. Thereafter, the household named additional are asked to name any more they know with maternal death [21]. By this method of snowball sampling, all the maternal deaths could be covered in less time and cost. It also gives the composition of the maternal deaths.

Causes of Maternal Deaths

Causes for maternal deaths are almost similar in all countries, only distributions of causes differ somewhat from region to region [7]. The causes of maternal death can be classified into three categories: direct, indirect and coincidental. Direct causes of maternal deaths refer to diseases or complications that occur only during pregnancy, including abortion, ectopic pregnancy (a pregnancy that develops outside the uterus), hypertensive diseases of pregnancy, ante partum and post partum hemorrhage, obstructed labor and puerperal sepsis. Indirect causes are diseases that may be present before pregnancy but are aggravated during pregnancy; examples include anemia, cardiovascular disease, malaria, tuberculosis, hepatitis and other infections. Coincidental causes are unexpected in nature; like suicide, deaths from road traffic accidents, besides others.

In fact the reasons the mothers die are many layered. Besides the medical causes, there are logistic causes like inadequate health care facilities, lack of transport and behind these, are all the social, cultural factors, child bearing and health seeking behavior. Generally the poor population in rural areas or in slums does not believe in institutional deliveries and the deliveries are usually conducted at home through untrained dais [21].

The Global Scenario

Direct causes: The maternal mortality is the result of any number of complications that beset pregnant women worldwide. About 80 percent of maternal deaths are following direct obstetric complications The most common direct causes of maternal deaths is obstetric hemorrhage (25 percent) generally occurring postpartum. Postpartum hemorrhage can lead to deaths very rapidly in the absence of prompt life saving care. Infections are responsible for 15 percent of maternal deaths. The other direct causes include unsafe abortion (13 percent), eclampsia (pregnancy induced hypertension, often accompanied by seizures) (12 percent) obstructed labour (8 percent) and other direct causes (8 percent) [18]. The other direct causes include ectopic pregnancy, embolism and anesthesia related deaths. Many of the direct causes mentioned above are preventable like puerperal infections resulting from poor hygiene during delivery and untreated reproductive infections. Hypertensive disorders of pregnancy, a common direct cause can be carefully monitored during pregnancy preventing 12 percent maternal deaths resulting from eclampsia. More than 18 million induced abortions are performed by untrained people or in unsafe environment or both, amounting 68000 maternal deaths each year [4].South America has the highest rate with 34 unsafe abortions per 1000 women, closely followed by Eastern Africa (31 unsafe abortions per 1000 women), Western Africa (25 unsafe abortions per 1000 women) and Central Africa (22 unsafe abortions per 1000 women). In contrast when termination of pregnancy is performed in ideal conditions the case fatality is no more than 1 per 100,000 procedures which is less than the risk of pregnancy carried term in best circumstances. [2] The global burden of diseases estimates for South Asia suggests major causes in order: hemorrhage (31%), sepsis (14%), hypertension (14%), abortion (14%) and obstruction (10%) (Figure 1). [16, 24]

Indirect causes: Among the 20 percent of maternal deaths which occur due to indirect causes are diseases of endocrine and metabolic system, anemia, cardiovascular diseases and infections like tuberculosis, malaria, viral hepatitis and increasingly HIV/AIDS [21, 25]. The relative frequency of the different indirect causes varies somewhat between areas. Studies in developing countries including rural northern Tanzania found 44% of maternal deaths due to cerebral malaria. The most common indirect cause for maternal death in poor population is found to be viral hepatitis, TB and respiratory disorder, anemia and post operative complications [21].

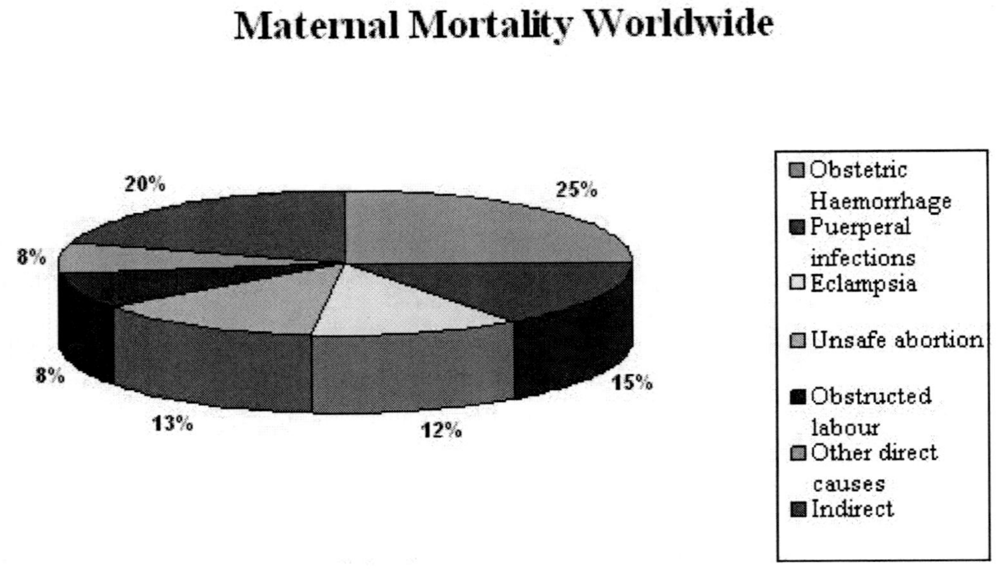

Figure 1. Worlwide maternal mortality.

Table 1. Causes of maternal deaths (n=70)

Causes of Maternal Death	(%)
Direct Causes	
PPH	21.4
Retain Placenta	17.2
Sepsis	11.4
Obstructed Labor	1.4
Embolism	1.4
Indirect Causes	
Anemia	21.4
Post Operative	8.6
Other Cause*	17.2
Total	100.0

*Other causes include jaundice, TB, respiratory disorder and suicide.

An Indian Experience

In India, the major causes of maternal deaths reported by Sample Registration System (SRS 2001-03) are: hemorrhage (38 percent), sepsis (11percent), hypertension(5 percent), obstructed labor (5 percent), abortion (8 percent), and other conditions (34 percent). Anemia which is a reduction of the concentration of hemoglobin in blood indirectly contributes to 19-22 percent of maternal deaths by aggravating hemorrhage, sepsis and toxemia [16].

A study conducted in Indian slums (a thickly populated area with no planned structure for toilets facilities, drinking water and electricity) found the major causes of maternal death as anemia (21.4 percent), postpartum hemorrhage (21,4 percent), followed by retained placenta (17.2 percent), and sepsis (11.4 percent) [21] (Table 1). Retained placenta leading to postpartum hemorrhage was a significant cause for maternal death and marginally higher than reported elsewhere by researchers in rural India, where retained placenta was found to be a cause of death in 12.5 % of cases [26-27]. Retained placenta is potentially life-threatening not only because of retention *per se*, but because of associated hemorrhage and infection as well as complications related to its removal. The data in poor population revealed that more than sixty percent of maternal deaths occurred due to direct causes and about 39 percent due to indirect causes. Of all indirect causes, anemia was found to be the major cause of deaths. Other indirect causes include jaundice, tuberculosis, respiratory disorders and suicide [21]. The reason for jaundice and tuberculosis in the pregnancy may be due to unhygienic conditions in slum population. Contrary to reported literature [16], where hypertensive disorders are one of the causes of maternal mortality; this study did not find any case of hypertensive disorder, may be because of the fact that slum population, where a large section of the pregnant women do not utilize the facility of ante natal services. Further, the cause of death was elicited by the gynecologist based on the information collected from family members after death of woman through verbal autopsy, who may not have been aware of any hypertensive disease [21].

In another descriptive, cross-sectional study conducted during 1989-90 in eight districts of Uttar Pradesh (U.P), which is one of the state of India having highest maternal mortality ratios found the most prevalent direct obstetric cause to be post partum haemorrhage (26.4%). The most prevalent indirect cause of maternal deaths was anemia and jaundice (17.4%). If timely medical care was available most of the maternal deaths could have been prevented [28].

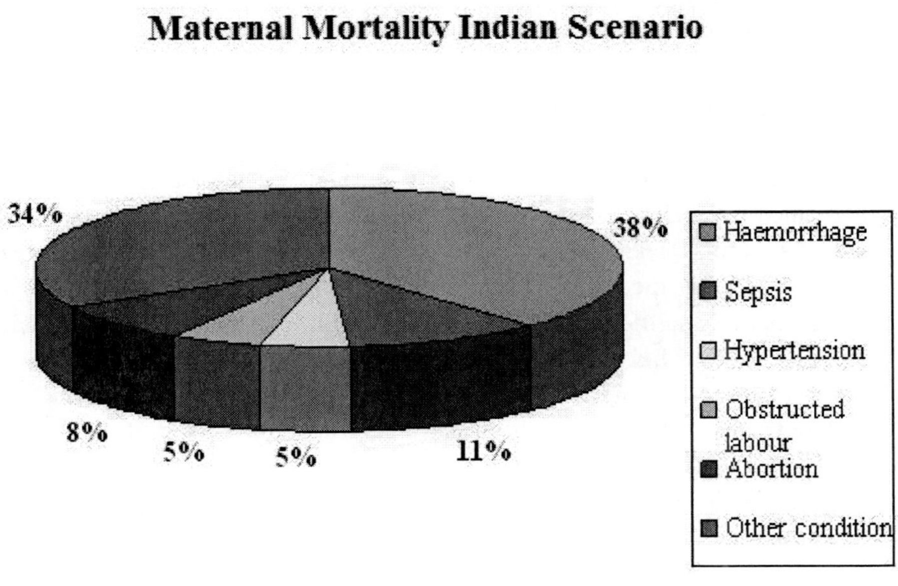

Figure 2. Indian Maternal Mortality.

Besides the medical causes there are logistic causes i.e. inadequate health care facilities, lack of transport, etc. and behind these, are all the social, cultural factors, child bearing and health seeking behavior. Due to poor living condition and low income most women in slum areas suffer from nutritional deficiencies and can not meet the need of required nutrients and thereby become anemic which is the most common cause for maternal deaths in India. Illegal abortions continue to be cause despite MTP facilities pointing towards a large unmet need of contraception. Also in rural areas or in slums, people do not believe in conducting delivery at hospital (Figure 2).

Role of Health Services

Maternal mortality is a disheartening public health problem especially in poor settings and its reduction is the key goal for developing countries. The health services in a country play an important role in reduction of maternal mortality. But in poor settings Health care policies restrict access to life saving emergency obstetric care (EmOC) and act as a barrier. Removing these barriers does not require many resources, but rather an administrative will and understanding of how to improve access to care in rural areas. The following is an example for such situation in rural India.

Policy Situations Affecting Emergency Obstetric Care in Developing Countries

In developing countries especially India a wide spectrum of policy situations affect emergency obstetric care [29]. Policy interventions aimed at improving access to emergency obstetrics care can incorporate the use of process indicators to both highlight problem areas and monitor the effects of policy change in terms of utilization and quality of services.

a. Obstetrics only by obstetricians. In low resource areas 70% people live in more than 550,000 villages. It is impossible for every health facility to have an obstetrician. In theory, medical officer can perform all medical emergency obstetric care procedures as defined by WHO, such as manual removal of placenta, assisted vaginal delivery. However, India lacks specific policies to promote provision of basic emergency obstetric care by medical officers. Most women arrive at facilities very late. The availability of qualified personnel at health facilities closer to home can help reduce delays in seeking and receiving needed care.
b. Anesthesia only by anesthetists. General duty doctors previously giving anesthesia decline to do so fearing litigation and cognizant of the lack of clear government policy. The government has to broaden their policies in resource poor settings so that more can be done in small rural hospitals and health center settings.
c. Traditional birth attendants live in their communities, which are usually the poorest of population. Training them about safe delivery, immediate basic care of newborn infants and instructing them to refer to the nearest essential obstetric care unit if any

danger signs become obvious, may prove to be an important cost effective strategy to reduce maternal and neonatal mortality in communities. They can also contribute in terms of health education and encouraging breast feeding. The advantage of such training is sustainability. A trained attendant will train the next family member that takes her position where she retires. Investing in such training should be considered by policy makers and donor agencies. [30]

Preventive Measures

To attain the goal set for reduction in maternal mortality needs attention on preventive measures to reduce maternal mortality at community level as well as hospital level in developing countries especially in poor population. Currently in India many Maternal and Child Health Programs are in vogue. Intervention strategies have been started by government to bring down maternal mortality a) The RCH program in 1997 made an effort to ensure that women have access to information and services for reproductive health care, b) Adoption of contraceptive practices by women could save 1, 00,000 maternal deaths. [31] c) Development of EOC facilities means hospital with well equipped trained staff and with minimal facilities of anesthesia, surgery and blood transfusion together with laboratory to provide 24 hrs emergency services. This calls not only for attitudinal change of policy makers and health care professionals but community involvement. d) Launching of "Twelve by Twelve (12 by 12) Initiative [32] – Making Pregnancy Safer- Targeting Anemia Eradication during Adolescence, could prevent one fourth of the maternal deaths occurring due to anemia in poor population.

Strategies for Change

Improvement in the maternal health status requires a strong and sustained government commitment, well targeted resources and increased awareness in the poor community regarding access to health care facilities provided in their areas.

The unacceptably high maternal mortality rate in India can be reduced by making concerted efforts along the following lines:

- Initiative from the government would be of paramount importance in this effort. This would include allocation of sufficient funds to all the health institutions including Primary Health Centers. Even more important is to ensure that the funds actually reach the users.
- Construction of better roads and transport facilities especially in the rural areas.
- Local dais and female health workers should be imparted periodic training and be incorporated as an integral part of health care system.
- Early registration of antenatal cases and at least three antenatal visits.
- Health education of couples to make them understand the importance of antenatal check ups, hospital deliveries and small family norms.

- Wide spread availability of Iron-Folic acid tablets and fortified food to the remotest of remote area
- Prevention of obstetric complications-eclampsia, obstructed labor etc
- Prevention and early treatment of infection, antepartum and post partum haemorrhage.
- Treatment of concomitant illnesses like diabetes, tuberculosis and malaria.
- Emphasizing the importance of observing proper aseptic measures while conducting deliveries.
- Providing facilities for hospital deliveries for high risk cases like severe anemia, diabetes and heart disease.
- Accountability in case of the unfortunate event of any maternal death. Taking appropriate remedial measures for preventing lapses noted in the management of theses cases will be of immense value in reducing the maternal mortality.
- Promotion of family planning.

(source: Reference 33)

Determinants of Maternal Deaths in a Poor Community: A Case Study in India

India is a country of more than one billion populations consisting of 593 administrative districts with about 80% of the population living in rural areas and the remaining 20% population in urban areas. Among the urban population a large section of population live in slum area (defined in earlier section). Delhi being the capital city of India has about 929 slums covering approximately 1.25 million populations. This population is catered by 21 health centers, 6 maternal homes and 105 health post created under the India Population Programme-VIII (IPP-VII) which aims to reduce fertility level in slum population thereby reducing MMR [21]. According to a recent study conducted in slum population of India, about sixty five percent of the population belongs to Scheduled Caste/Tribe and more than sixty percent were illiterate (Table 2).

In India, despite many Maternal and Child Health Care program in vogue about one fourth of women in poor population do not avail antenatal care services and these programs do not reach the poorest households. The study in Delhi slums found the various risk factors associated with maternal deaths as education, family type, current age of woman, age of marriage, parity, and various complications during pregnancy. The various complications include anemia, fever, jaundice, excessive bleeding and abnormal presentation of child. Jaundice during the pregnancy appears to be an important risk factor, which might have occurred due to poor sanitary conditions in and around the house. The other environmental factors found were utilization of health facilities that consist of antenatal care (ANC), delivery care and distance of residence from place of delivery and lack of transport to reach health facility [21].

National Family Health Survey (NFHS-3) conducted in India during 2005-06, about 40 percent of births took place in health facilities [34]. Most of the deliveries are taken place at home by either untrained dais or elderly ladies in the poor community. The most prevalent reason for not conducted the delivery at health facility is 'not essential' in their opinion. About 26 percent reported that it cost too much for conducting the delivery at health facility. Only 15 percent received recommended antenatal care, although 76 percent did receive some form of antenatal care. Only 44 percent received antenatal care in first trimester 58 percent of women did not receive any postnatal care [34].

The findings suggest that more focus should be required on mass education about the importance of antenatal registration and regular check ups, and on training of dais. As Institutional facilities and transport are more easily available in urban than the rural areas, women should be encouraged to go for institutional deliveries to reduce maternal mortality at the community level [21].

Table 2. Characteristics of the study population

Characteristics	**Percent (%)**	**Characteristics**	**Percent (%)**
*Type of house		*Caste*	
Kutcha	19.82	SC/ST¶	64.98
Pucca	31.72	General	35.02
Semi Pucca	48.46		
Number of rooms in the house		*Education level*	
1	62.33	Illiterate	63.44
2	22.91	Literate	36.56
3	14.32		
Separate kitchen		*Type of Family*	
No	78.19	Joint	33.48
Type of toilet		*Parity*	
open area	36.12	1	18.06
own flush toilet	11.01	2	25.55
own pit toilet	13.22	3	22.25
**others	12.78	4+	34.14
Electricity in the house			
No	2.86		

*Kutcha house- is a hut or built of bricks with temporary roof.

*Pucca house is a permanent structure

*Semi Pucca is a temporary house built of brick, cement with asbestos roof.

** Other includes sulabh system, which is a combined flush toilet system provided for a slum. This facility is provided by Municipal Corporation of Delhi. SC/ST indicates Schedule Caste and Schedule Tribe

The tragedy of maternal deaths in developing countries cannot be tackled in isolation Reproductive health of the women has to be a major health agenda in developing countries. Even today domestic violence, an important risk factor for incidental maternal deaths is experienced by 33.5 percent of women in reproductive age group in the recent NFHS-3 survey. Improving the status and empowering the women in society and within their households is critical to promote change in reproductive attitudes and behaviors, especially in patriarchal societies. The National Population policy 2000, specifically identified the low status of women in India as an important barrier to the achievement of population and maternal and child welfare goals. Reproductive health improves if women are empowered, have the ability to access information, take decisions and act effectively in their own interests or interest of those dependent on them [34].

Summary

Differences in maternal mortality are more than differences among rich and poor. Acknowledgement of the magnitude of maternal mortality and a strong political will is needed to reduce maternal mortality. The pace of decline is insufficient to achieve the major development goals for maternal deaths. The pattern of causes of death reinforces the key finding that rapid expansion of institutional and skilled birth attendance, especially in developing countries is needed to further reduce maternal mortality. Evidence is growing that community based interventions are effective in reducing maternal and neonatal deaths in countries with high mortality. Few major problems need to be addressed a) absence of links between communities, subcentre and referral facilities b)Shortage of equipment and trained staff at referral facilities and lack of emergency transport c)Improved accessibility and quality of EOC services d)social and cultural factors These are necessary steps if maternal deaths are to be prevented. A substantial increase in the resources for reproductive health care services is needed and the human resource crises in the health care system must be urgently addressed.

References

[1] Rawal A. Trends in maternal mortality and some policy concerns. *Indian Journal of Commun. Med.*. 2003 ;28:43-6.

[2] WHO. World Health Report 2005 Make every mother and child count. Geneva.

[3] WHO, UNICEF and UNFPA Maternal Mortality in 2005. Estimates developed by WHO, UNICEF and UNFPA.Geneva.;2006.

[4] WHO , Regional Health Forum 2005 ; Vol 9, No.1.

[5] AbouZahr C, Wardlaw T. Maternal Mortality in 1995: Estimates Developed by WHO, UNICEF, UNFPA. Geneva, Switzerland: World Health Organization.

[6] WHO, UNICEF and UNFPA, Maternal Mortality in 2000. Estimates Developed by WHO, UNICEF and UNFPA, Geneva. Last Updated 2006 May. Available from: http://www.childinfo.org/areas/maternalmortality.(accessed on June 6, 2007).

[7] World Health Organization: Beyond the Numbers: Reviewing maternal deaths and complications to make pregnancy safer. World Health Organization 2004, Geneva.

[8] Geller SE,Rosenberg D,Cox S,Brown M,Simonson L,Kipatrick S. A scoring system identified near miss maternal morbidity during pregnancy. *J. Clin. Epidemiol.* 2005 Sept 58(9):962.

[9] Pattinso RC and Hall M. Near misses: a useful adjunct to maternal death enquiries. *British Medical Bulletin* 67:231-243 (2003)

[10] Penney G.,Brace V. Near miss audit in Obstetrics.*Curr. Opin. Obstet. Gyneco.*l 2007 Apr;19(2):145-50.

[11] Hall MH.: Near misses and severe maternal morbidity. In: *Why Mothers Die 1997–1999: The Confidential Enquiries into Maternal Deaths in the United Kingdom.* Department of Health, Welsh Office, Scottish Home and Health Department, Department of Heath and Social Sciences, Northern Ireland. London: RCOG Press, 2001; 323–5.

[12] McClure EM, Goldenberg RL, Bann CM. Maternal mortality, stillbirth and measures of obstetric care in developing and developed countries. *Int. J. Gynaecol. Obstet.* 2007 Feb;96(2):139-46.

[13] World Bank, World Development Report 2002. Building Institutions for Markets. New York, NY: Oxford University Press; 2002:234. .

[14] International Institute for Population Sciences and Macro International. National Family Health Survey (MCH and Family Planning),India 1992-93, Mumbai,India;IIPS;1995:226

[15] International Institute for Population Sciences and Macro International. National Family Health Survey (NFHS-2), India 1998-99, Mumbai,India;IIPS;2000:196, 247-251

[16] Govt of India, Maternal mortality in India:1997-2003, Trends, Causes and Risk factors, Registrar General India, New Delhi in collaboration with Centre for Global Health Research University of Toronto, Canada.

[17] Singh P, Pandey A, Aggarwal A. House to house Survey vs snowball technique for capturing maternal deaths in India: A search for a cost effective method. *Indian J. Med. Res.* 125,April 2007: 350-556.

[18] http://news.xinhuanet.com/english/2007-10/13/content_6873207.htm.

[19] Ramacharandran Prema. Book Review; Beyond the numbers-Reviewing maternal deaths and complications to make pregnancy safer. *Indian J. Med. Res.* 122, July 2005, 87-90

[20] Graham W, Brass W, Snow RW. Indirect estimation of maternal mortality: sisterhood method. Studies in Family Planning, 1989; 20;125-35.

[21] Aggarwal Abha, Pandey A, Bhattacharya BN. Risk factors for maternal mortality in Delhi slums.A community based case-controlled study. *Indian J. Med. Sci*, Sep 2007; 61(9):517-26.

[22] Stanton C et al. Every death counts: measurement of maternal mortality via a census. Bulletin of the World Health Organization, 2001; 79 (7): 657-64

[23] Snijders, T. Estimation on the basis of snowball samples: how to weight, *Bulletin Methodologie Sociologique*, 1992; vol. 36; 59-70.

[24] "Maternal mortality: A Global Review." Women's International Network News" 24, no.3. 1998.:15-18. (http://www.deathreference.com/Me-Nu/Mortality-Childbirth.html)

[25] Gunnar Kvale, Bjorg Oslen, Hinderaker S.G etal (2005); Maternal Deaths in Developing Countries: A preventable tragedy Norsk. *Epidemiology; 5*(2):141-149.

[26] Chhabra S, Dhorey M: Retained placenta continues to be fatal but frequency can be reduced. *J.Obstet Gynaecol.* Nov 2002; 22(6):630-3.

[27] Chhabra S, Sirohi R.Trends in maternal mortality due to haemorrhage.Two decades of Indian Rural observation. *J. Obstet Gynaecol.* 2004; 24;40-3.

[28] Gupta N, Kumar S, Saxena NC, Nandan D, Saxena BN. Maternal mortality in seven districts of Uttar Pradesh--an ICMR task force study. : *Indian J. Public Health* 2006 Jul-Sep;50(3):173-8

[29] Mavalankar and Rosenfield: Maternal mortality in resource-poor setting: Policy Barriers to care . *Am. J. of Public Health* Feb 2005, Vol 95,No.2.

[30] Costello Anthony, Osrin David and Manandhar☹2004) Reducing maternal and neonatal mortality in the poorest communities *BMJ*; 329:1166-1168 (13 November)

[31] WHO (1998). Life in the 21st Century. A vision for all. Report of the Director-General.

[32] Suneeta Mittal. Launching Twelve by Twelve Initiative- Making Pregnancies Safer- Targeting Anemia Eradiction during Adolescence. http://pib.nic.in/release/rel_print_ page.asp?relid=27107(accessed on 6/15/2007 and 1/31/2008.)

[33] Surg Vadm Punit Arora. Maternal mortality: Indian scenario. *MJAFI* 2005;61:214-5.

[34] International Institute for Population Sciences. National Family Health Survey (NFHS-3) India, Vol. 1, 2005-06, IIPS, Mumbai, India; September 2007:208-210.

In: Topics in Prevalent Diseases
Editors: N. C. Chavez-Tapia and M. Uribe
ISBN 978-1-60456-959-9

Chapter 16

Depression in Minorities

Asae Oura and Mitsuru Mori
Department of Public Health, School of Medicine, Sapporo Medical University, Sapporo, Japan

Introduction

Depression is a frequent health problem which is growing at an alarming rate. It has been suggested that if the trend persists, by 2020, depression will be the second biggest health care problem after heart disease worldwide [1]. The prevalence of depression is increasing not only among adults, but also among adolescents [2]. This increase is mostly related to moderate forms of depressions without psychomotor and physical symptoms [3]. Nevertheless, this form of depression is still strongly affecting health and quality of life of the patients. Population based studies show that at any one time between 10 to 15 % of the child and adolescent population exhibit some symptoms of depression [4].

Many previous studies in various samples reported ethnic differences in depression. For example, several risk factors for depression among adolescents have been identified, including female gender, increasing age, lower socio-economic status, and Latino ethnic background [5, 6]. On the other hand, current literature reviews [7, 8] reported ethnic minority caregivers experience less psychological distress than their non Hispanic white counterparts.

In this chapter, we will discuss studies of depression among minorities. The main targets of the studies were Latin American, African American, and Asian American people. Table 1 shows a comparison of the different types of depression that exist between races of the studies in this chapter.

First, we describe the different types of depression between two or more races. Some evidence indicate [9], that the white, black, and Hispanic subjects constituted a probability sample of married and cohabiting couples 18 years of age and older living in households in the 48 contiguous United States. A total of 1635 couples participated in this study with a response rate of 85%. This is because the Center for Epidemiologic Studies Depression Scale

(CES-D) [10] was given only to one of the partners. Among men, the results show that black (OR=0.29, 95%CI= (0.13, 0.65)) and Hispanic (OR=0.40, 95%CI= (0.20, 0.81)) ethnicities are protective factors against depression. But among women, the results did not show significantly related. Other interesting study [11] examines the cross-sectional and longitudinal associations among the cognitive variables and depression symptoms among African American (n=79), Caucasian (n=273), and Hispanic (n=98) adolescents in the United States. Community adolescents (n=450), aged 14-18 years (mean age =15.7 years, SD=1.2) provided information regarding their depressive symptoms and cognitions at two surveys, 6 months apart. Depressive symptoms were measured by the BDI-II [12] at baseline and follow up. There were significant main effects on depressive symptoms at a baseline for ethnic groups ($p<0.05$), gender ($p<0.05$), and for the interaction between ethnic groups and gender ($p<0.05$). Hispanic youth scored higher than African American and Caucasian adolescents. The main effects for follow up depressive symptoms were also reassessed, controlling for parental education. The main effect for ethnic groups did not remain significant, whereas the main effects for gender and the interaction between ethnic groups and gender were significant. Again the gender difference in depressive symptoms was greater in the African American and Caucasian groups than the gender difference in the Hispanic group. For one cross sectional study [13], it used a random sample (n=3,310), female only of the Wave I database of the National Longitudinal Study of Adolescent Health. The data included Latinas (11.63%, n=385), African Americans (24.95%, n=826), Asian Americans (3.80%, n=126), Native Americans (2.02%, n=67), and Euro Americans (57.73%, n=1911). They ranged from 12 to 19 years old, with a mean age of 16 years (SD=1.77). Interviews for the study were conducted between April and December 1995, and depression was measured using a 19-item scale of CES-D. Euro-American females reported statistically significantly less adolescent depression ($p<0.01$) than did Latinas. Ethnic differences in perfectionism were examined among 59 of Asian American, 65 of African American, and 65 of Caucasian American college students in one study [14]. The subjects were minority students in seven existing datasets, collected from 1994 to 2000. A total of 189 students from two public universities in the north central region of the United States were participants in the study. The CES-D was used to measure emotional distress. Regression analysis revealed that perfectionism explained a significantly variance in depression symptoms for Asian Americans and Caucasians.

Secondly, we looked at studies with a focus on Hispanics. The study [15] examined the contribution of individual and family variables to depression symptoms among youths in a family-centered culture. The participants in the study were 262 adolescents from a high school in Mexico City from an approximately middle-class population. The mean age of participants was 15.9 years, and 60% of participants were females. Depression symptoms were assessed by the 20-item CES-D. As predicted, an analysis by F-test indicated significant gender differences in depressed mood, with females reporting a significant gender frequency of depressive symptoms. One study [16] showed depressive symptoms among 3,118 Mexican American adults who participated in the Hispanic Health and Nutrition Examination Survey (HHANES) in 1982–1984. Depression symptoms were assessed using diagnostic interviews and the CES-D. The rate of depression was 13.3%. Factors associated with increased risk of high levels of depression symptoms were as follows; female sex (OR=2.28), low educational achievement (0-6 years of education, OR=2.32: 7-11 years, OR=1.56 vs. up to 13 years), low income (OR=1.52–2.02), and US birth combined with Anglo-oriented acculturation. In other study [17] perform an analysis of the adolescent sample of the 2003 California Health Interview Survey, which included 3,196 telephone-interviews with Latino and non-Latino White adolescents using the CES-D. Unadjusted analysis suggested that the risk of depressive symptoms was twice as high among Latinos as compared to non-Latino Whites (10.5% vs. 5.5%). The Project Salud Bienestar y Envejecimiento (SABE) is a multiethnic cross-sectional study [18] of 10,661 men and women aged 60 and older from the following seven Latin American and Caribbean cities during 1999/2000. Study organizers used the Geriatric Depression Scale (GDS) to assess the presence of depression symptoms. The prevalence of depressive symptoms was higher among women than men in Buenos Aires, Havana, Mexico City, Montevideo, Santiago, and Sao Paulo. The prevalence of depression in the urban population of Latin America was relatively low, ranging across cities from 0.4 to 5.2 % in men and 0.3 to 9.5% women. Women were more exposed to social and material disadvantages during their life course than men but were not more vulnerable to them than men. Additional information from [19] Hispanic and non Hispanic white women with dementia caregivers and non-caregivers. Total of eighty-three women caregivers (20 Hispanic and 24 non-Hispanic white) and non-caregivers (19 Hispanic and 20 non-Hispanic white) completed the CES-D. Non-Hispanic white caregivers had higher depression scores than non-caregivers, but there was no significant difference for Hispanics. Multivariate regression analysis showed that both ethnicity and depression symptoms independently predicted daytime cortisol slope.

Thirdly, we discussed the depressive symptoms of African Americans. The subjects of representative African American and White samples of 22,957 deceased individuals aged 15 years or older (1993 US National Mortality Followback Survey (NMFS)) [20]. A matched case-control study was constructed for suicide decedents aged 15 to 64 years, with natural death controls frequency matched to case by age and gender. Respondents were asked to report on the frequency of a number of behavioral problems exhibited by the decedent in the last month of life. From the 10 items available that reflected depression symptoms, two items were determined to have sufficient numbers of responses and comparable factor loadings in factor analyses of all depressive symptoms. When compared with natural causes of death, white decedents were associated with depression symptoms (white: often OR=1.278, 95%CI= (1.132, 1.442), vs. not often; combined race: often OR=1.142, 95%CI= (1.015, 1.286), vs. not often). A sample in one study [21] of care workers who provide care to others outside of the home was drawn from a 1992 - 1994 National Survey of Families and Households. The final sample included 275 (11%) Blacks, and 2,218 (89%) Whites (not of Hispanic origin). Depressive symptoms were measured using a modified version of the CES-D. Black caregivers reported greater depressive symptoms than Whites.

Finally, we discussed the results from Asian American and Japanese subjects. Participants were a total of 173 early adolescents, included 84 European American, 59 Chinese American, and 30 Korean American, and there were a total of 297 college students, including 168 European Americans, 75 Chinese Americans, and 54 Korean Americans in one study [22]. Depression was assessed by a mean of a 16-item abbreviation [23] of CES-D. Ethnic differences in depressed mood emerged in the college sample with Asian Americans

Table 1. Comparison between races in depression

Study	Target	Race	Scale	Results
Caetano R et al.[9]	married and cohabiting couples 18 years of the age and older living in households	white, black, Hispanic	CES-D	Among men, black (OR=0.29) Hispanic(OR=0.40) (v.s. white)
Kennard BD et al. [11]	N=450 of Community adolescents aged 14-18 years	African American, Caucasian, Hispanic	BDI-II	Hispanic youth scored higher than African American and Caucasian adolescent.
Guiao IZ et al. [13]	N=3,310 (only female) of the Wave I database of the National Longitudinal Study of Adolescent Health.	Latinas, African Americans, Asian Americans, Native Americans, Euro Americans	CES-D	Euro-American females reported statistically significant less adolescent depression than did Latinas.
Castro JR[14]	college students	59 of Asian American, 65 of African American, 65 of Caucasian American	CES-D	Perfectionism explained significantly variance in depression symptoms for Asian Americans and Caucasians.
Mikolajczyk RT et al. [17]	2003 California Health Interview Survey	Latino non-Latino White (total was 3,196)	CES-D	The risk of depressive symptoms was twice as high among Latinos as compared to non-Latino Whites (10.5% vs. 5.5%).
Thompson DG [19]	dementia caregivers and non-caregivers	Hispanic women non Hispanic white women	CES-D	Non-Hispanic whites had higher depression scores than non-caregivers.
Drentea P et al. [21]	care workers who provide care to others outside of the home	275 (11%) Blacks, 2,218 (89%) Whites	CES-D	Black caregivers reported greater depressive symptomatology than Whites.
Jose PE et al. [24]	Children from a suburban area of a large Midwestern city	Chinese American European	CES-D	Chinese American adolescents reported more depression value than European American.
Kanazawa A et al.[25]	their elementary school teachers 40 years ago	176 European American, 209 Native Hawaiians, and 357 Japanese Americans	CES-D	Native Hawaiians reported suggesting generally higher levels of depressive symptoms.

reporting more symptoms. Ethnic differences in depressed mood were reduced to no significance when the quality of parent-adolescent relationships was statistically controlled.

The magnitude of associations between measures of parent-adolescent relationships and depressed mood was strikingly similar for European and Asian Americans in the same phase of adolescence. As anticipated, perceived parent-adolescent relationships accounted for more of the variance in depressed mood in early adolescence than in late adolescence: The numbers ranged from 44% to 51% for the junior high samples and about 10% for the college students. The participants of the study [24] were 55 second-generation Chinese American adolescents (27 girls, 28 boys) and 58 European American adolescents (29 girls, 29 boys) from a suburban area of a large Midwestern city. These participants were retained from the first wave of a longitudinal study begun 5 years earlier with 60 each of Chinese American and European American children. The mean age for the two groups at the second time of measurement was 16.8 years and 17.0 years, respectively. Depression was assessed by using the CES-D scale. Chinese American adolescents reported more depression value than European American. A community sample in one study [25] used 176 European Americans, 209 Native Hawaiians, and 357 Japanese Americans. Depression was measured using the CES-D. Native Hawaiians results suggest generally higher levels of depressive symptoms. The three ethnic groups varied in mental care usage with differing associations between depressive symptoms and experiences of stressful events.

Our study [26] reported depression among Japanese caregivers for the frail elderly in Japan. The study has measured Japanese version of CES-D for depression. One of our cross sectional study was conducted in 5 towns in Japan before and after the introduction of the Long term Care Insurance System (LTCIS), in order to evaluate the factors relating to depression among family caregivers for the frail elderly. Before LTCIS, 94 (50.3%) of 187 caregivers were depressed. And after the introduction of LTCIS, 75 (48.4%) of 155 caregivers were depressed. Depressed caregivers were more likely to consult with their doctors (before LTCIS: OR=2.99, after LTCIS: OR=4.01), to be in poor health (before LTCIS: OR=5.17, after LTCIS: OR=6.19) and to care for demented elderly with behavioral disturbances (before LTCIS: OR=2.75, after LTCIS: OR=2.35) than non-depressive caregivers both before and after the LTCIS. Before LTCIS, depressive caregivers were more likely to attend to the elderly for more than 16 hours per day (OR=2.77) than their counterparts. After the LTCIS, depressive caregivers were more likely to be a spouse (OR=2.92), to care for a frail elderly male (OR=2.79), and less likely to be able to go out without accompanying the elderly (OR=0.36), than their counterparts.

References

[1] Ustun TB; Chatterji S. Global burden of depressive disorders and future projections. In: Dawson A, Tylee A, editor. depression: Social and economic timebomb. London *BMJ* Books 2001.

[2] The changing rate of major depression. Cross-national comparisons. Cross-national Collaborative Group. *JAMA* 1992;268:3098-3105

[3] Birmaher B, Ryan ND, Williamson DE, Brent DA, Kaufman J, Dahl RE, Perel J, Nelson B. Childhood and adolescent depression: a review of the past 10 years. Part I. *J. Am. Acad. Child Adolesc Psychiatry* 1996;35:1427-1439.

[4] U.S. department of Health and Human Services Mental Health. A report of the surgeon General. Rockville MD, U.S. Department of Health and Human Services, Substance Abuse and Mental Health Services Administration, Center for Mental Health Services, National Institutes of Health, National Institute of Mental Health; 1999.

[5] Saluja G, Iachan R, Scheidt PC, Overpeck MD, Sun W, Giedd JN. Prevalence of and risk factors for depressive symptoms among adolescents. *Arch Pediatr. Adolesc. Med.* 2004;158:760-765.

[6] Roberts RE, Chen YR, Roberts CR. Ethnocultural differences in prevalence of adolescent suicidal behaviors. *Suicide Life Threat Behav.* 1997;27:208-217.

[7] Pinquart M, Soerensen S. Differences between caregivers and noncaregivers in psychological health and physical health: a meta-analysis. *Psychol. Aging* 2003; 18: 250-267.

[8] Irwin M, Brown M, Patterson T, et al. Neuropeptide Y and natural killer cell activity: findings in depression and Alzheimer caregiver stress. *FASEB J.* 1991;5:3100-3107

[9] Caetano R, Cunradi C. Intimate partner violence and depression among white, blacks, and Hispanics. *AEP* 2003;13:661-665.

[10] Radloff, LS. The CES-D scale: A self report depression scale for research in the general population. *Applied psychological measurement* 1997, 1, 385-401.

[11] Kennard BD, Stewart SM, Hughes JL, et al. Cognitions and depressive symptoms among ethnic minority adolescents. *Cultural Diversity and ethnic minority psychology* 2006;12:578-591.

[12] Beck A, Steer R, Brown G. BDI-III manual. New York: *Psychological corporation.* 1996.

[13] Guiao IZ, Thompson EA. Ethnicity and problem behaviors among adolescent females in the United States. *Health care for woman international* 2004; 25:296-310.

[14] Castro JR, Rice KG. Perfectionism and Ethnicity: Implication for depressive symptoms and self-reported academic achievement. *Cultural Diversity and Ethnic Minority Psychology* 2003;9:64-78.

[15] Gil-Rivas V, Greenberger E, Chen C, et al. Understanding depressed mood in the context of a family-oriented culture. *Adolescence* 2003; 38:93-109.

[16] Moscicki EK, Locke BZ, Rae DS, et al. Depressive symptoms among Mexican Americans: The Hispanic health and nutrition examination survey. *American Journal of Epidemiology* 1989; 130:348-360.

[17] Mikolajczyk RT, Bredehorset M, Khelaifat N, et al. Correlates of depressive symptoms among Latino and non-Latino white adolescents: findings from the 2003 California health interview survey. BMC Public Health 2007; 7:21.

[18] Alvarado BE, Zunzunegui MV, Beland F, et al. Social and gender inequalities in depressive symptoms among urban older adults of Latin America and the Caribbean. *Journal of Gerontology: social sciences* 2007; 62B:S226-S237.

[19] Thompson DG, Shurgot GR, Rider K, et al. Ethnicity, stress, and cortisol function in Hispanic and non-Hispanic white women: a preliminary study of family dementia caregivers and noncaregivers. *Am. J. Geriatr. Psychiatry* 2006;14:334-342.
[20] Kung HC, Pearson JL, Wei R. Substance use, firearm availability, depressive symptoms, and mental health service utilization among white and African American suicide decedents aged 15 to 64 years. *Ann. Epidemiol.* 2005; 15:614-621.
[21] Drentea P, Golder MA. Caregiving outside of the home: the effects of race on depression. *Ethnicity and health* 2006;11:41-57.
[22] Greenberger E, Chen C. Perceived family relationships and depressed mood in early and late adolescence: a comparison of European and Asian Americans. *Developmental Psychology* 1996; 32:707-716.
[23] Lin N. Measuring depressive symptomatology in China. *Journal of Nervous and mental diseases* 1989;177:121-131.
[24] Jose PE, Huntsinger CS. Moderation and mediation effects of coping by Chinese American and European American Adolescents. *The Journal of Geriatric Psychology* 2005; 166:16-43.
[25] Kanazawa A, White PM, Hampson SE. Ethnic variation in depressive symptoms in a community sample in Hawaii. *Cultural Diversity and ethnic minority psychology* 2007;13:35-44.
[26] Oura A, Washio M, Arai Y, et al. Depression among Caregivers of the Frail Elderly in Japan before and after the introduction of the Public Long Term Care Insurance System.. *Z Gerontol. Geriat.* 2007; 40:112-118.

In: Topics in Prevalent Diseases
Editors: N. C. Chavez-Tapia and M. Uribe

ISBN 978-1-60456-959-9

Chapter 17

Osteoporosis in Minorities

***Marta Pentek,*[1] *Ildiko Kaposi*[2], *Laszlo Gulacsi*[3] *and Gyula Poor*[4]**
[1]Rheumatology, Flor Ferenc County Hospital, Kistarcsa, Hungary
[2]College of Arts and Sciences, American University of Kuwait, Kuwait City, Kuwait
[3]Health Economics and Technology Assessment Research Centre, Corvinus University of Budapest, Budapest, Hungary
[4]First Department of Rheumatology, National Institute of Rheumatology and Physiotherapy, Budapest, Hungary

Abbreviations

BMD	bone mineral density
DXA	dual energy x-ray absorptiometry
EFC	extended-care facilities
EMEA	European Medicines Agency
FDA	Food and Drug Administration
OP	osteoporosis
ODM	osteodensitometry
RA	rheumatoid arthritis
WHO	World Health Organisation

Osteoporosis (OP) is defined as a systemic skeletal disease characterized by low bone mass and microarchitectural deterioration of bone tissue with a consequent increase of bone fragility and susceptibility to fractures. [1]

The clinical consequence of OP is a fracture. The classic osteoporotic fractures are hip, vertebral, wrist fractures but some other sites (e.g., proximal humerus, clavicula, rib, pelvic and tibial fractures) were also considered osteoporotic in epidemiologic studies. [2]

OP is one of the most important public health concerns due to the significant morbidity and mortality associated with osteoporotic fractures. Osteoporosis affects an estimated 75 million people in Europe, US and Japan. The lifetime risk in the US for a hip, spine, or forearm fracture at the age of 50 years has been estimated to be 40% in women and 13% in men. A woman's risk of hip fracture is equal to her combined risk of breast, uterine and ovarian cancer, according to the National Osteoporosis Foundation. Twenty percent of women die within 1 year after hip fracture, another 20% become permanently disabled and only one third of patients regain their previous level of function.

There is a geographic difference in fracture incidence, e.g. age- and sex-adjusted hip fracture rates are higher in northern Europe than in southern Europe. [2, 3] Osteoporosis has been shown to have a large genetic component but physical inactivity and impaired neuromuscular function also play role for developing fragility fractures. Aging, low bone mineral density and history of a fracture are major risk factors but also history of fragility fractures in a first degree relative is determinant which undercurves the importance of genetics in the etiology of the disease.

Racial and ethnic differences in risk and incidence of OP have been estalished. Approximately 20% of non-Hispanic White and Asian women aged 50 years and older have osteoporosis, compared with 5% to 10% of non-Hispanic Black women and 10% to 15% of Hispanic women of the same age in the US. It is estimated that an additional 50% to 65% of non-Hispanic White and Asian women have osteopenia (generalized reduction in bone mas but less severe than in OP), compared with 35% to 38% of Black women and another 49% of Hispanic women. Hip fractures are increasing at a greater rate than previously was estimated among Hispanic women. [4]

In 1995, health care expenditures attributable to osteoporotic fractures in the US were estimated at $13.8 billion, of which $10.3 billion (75.1%) was for the treatment of white women, $2.5 billion (18.4%) for white men, $0.7 billion (5.3%) for nonwhite women, and $0.2 billion (1.3%) for nonwhite men, i.e. one-fourth of the total was borne by other than white women population subgroups. [5]

Thus, disease burden of osteoporosis and related fractures is significant. Due to its partially racial and ethnic related character, studies on OP in minorities are especially worthwhile.

In this Chapter, first we present some basic diagnostic and treatment issues of OP which are crucial to understand the topic. Then we review the available medical literature on osteoporosis with especial relevance on minorities.

Table 1. Diagnosis of osteoporosis by bone mineral density measurement (WHO)

Definition*	T-score (bone mineral density, BMD)
Normal	no more than -1 SD below the young adult mean
Osteopenia	between -1.0 and -2.5
Osteoporosis	equal to or less than -2.5
Severe osteoporosis	below -2.5 for patients with a fragility fracture

*Other diagnostic measurements (radiographs, laboratory tests) are also required for the establishment of the diagnosis.

Basic Concerns on Osteoporosis

Diagnosis

Osteoporosis is often called a "silent disease" because bone loss occurs without symptoms. Bone Mineral Density (BMD) measurement using dual energy X-ray absorptiometry (DXA) has been the "gold-standard" for diagnosing osteoporosis and evaluating fracture risk.

The World Health Organization (WHO) has standardized the interpretation of BMD results, based on a comparison of a patient's BMD with the mean for a normal young adult population of the same sex and race. The patient's BMD is calculated as a T-score, which is the number of standard deviations above or below the mean BMD for normal young adults as presented in Table 1.

The tendency to fracture is inversely correlated with BMD, confirming the importance of BMD measurement. However, the WHO criteria were derived from European and North American postmenopausal women and may not be applicable to other races.

Risk Factors

Factors that increase the likelihood of developing osteoporosis and fractures are called "risk factors". Risk factors for osteoporosis suggested by the National Osteoporosis Foundation (http://www.nof.org) are presented in Table 2.

Therapy

There is range of drug treatment available for postmenopausal osteoporosis usually refered as "antiosteoporotic" therapy.

Antiresorptive and bone forming medications (bisphosphonates, selective estrogen receptor modulators, calcitonin, hormone replacement therapy, parathyroid hormone, strontium renalate) has been approved by the Food and Drug Administration (FDA) and the European Medicines Agency (EMEA) for postmenopausal women to prevent and/or treat osteoporosis. Different studies have consistently shown that, depending on the drug and the patient population, treatment reduces the risk of vertebral fracture by between 30-65% and of nonvertebral fractures by between 16-53%.

Vitamin D deficiency is common in many countries especially in older ages. Sunlight exposure can increase the BMD of vitamin D deficient bone and lead to the prevention of nonvertebral fractures.

Nutrition and supplementation (especially calcium and vitamin D) play important role but also fall prevention techniques, exercise, psychological support and rehabilitation following fractures are relevant.

Fewer therapies are available for men however the burden of osteoporosis in males should not be underestimated.

Table 2. Risk factors for osteoporosis

Characteristics	Risk factor
Age	Advanced age
Gender	Being female
Race	Being Caucasian or Asian, although African Americans and Hispanic Americans are at significant risk as well
Physical status	Being thin and/or having a small frame
	Current low bone mass
	Anorexia nervosa
Fracture history	Personal history of fracture after age 50
Family history	History of fracture in a 1° relative
	A family history of osteoporosis
Hormonal status	Estrogen deficiency as a result of menopause, especially early or surgically induced
	Abnormal absence of menstrual periods (amenorrhea)
	Low testosterone levels in men
Nutrition	Vitamin D deficiency
	Low lifetime calcium intake
Medications	Use of corticosteroids, chemotherapy, anticonvulsants, GnRH agonists, chronic heparin therapy, T4 in excessive doses, chemotherapy, lithium, aromatase inhibitors
Chronic medical conditions	Presence of chronic obstructive pulmonary disease, gastrectomy, hyperparathyroidism, hyperthyroidism, hypercortisolismh, vitamin D deficiency, hypogonadism, malignancy including multiple myeloma, renal disease, liver disease, malabsorptive states including celiac disease, rheumatoid arthritis)
Lifestyle	An inactive lifestyle
	Excessive use of alcohol
	Current cigarette smoking

Source: http://www.nof.org

Osteoporosis Care and Access to Therapy

Idetifying people for treatment are a key issue. Due to its "silent" character, OP is often underdiagnosed and undertreated in most of the countries. [6] Also poor compliance by patients with drug therapies for osteoporosis over a year leaves them at risk for fractures and higher healthcare costs.

Osteoporosis from the Point of View of Minorities

Epidemiology of Fractures

Researches on fracture incidence among minorities face several methodological difficulties (Table 3).

Hospitalization data either do not report on patient ethnicity or have just started recently. Somewhat different race and ethnicity categories were used previously and in the present.

Estimation of annual population by race or ethnicity for incidence calculation is usually based on intercensal population ratings. Furthermore, race/ethnicity categories have to be arranged to correspond to hospital discharge data.

Good quality data on the general population is essential for studies on minorities. The rate of fractures differs significantly by gender (more common in women) and age (more often in the elderly) and also by geographic regions. There is a general increase of fracture incidence by time worldwide. Therefore, recent gender and age matched data are required from the relevant geographic region for comparisons between general population and minorities.

However, such data are often not available. In Central Europe, there were no data on fractures from the past years and only some partial data were published in the previous decades either. A health insurance database analysis (covering the whole population) was performed in Hungary between 1999-2003 and results were compared with literature data. Hip fracture incidence was much higher in Sweden (695 versus 1689 / 100 000 female inhabitants aged 75-79 in Hungary and Sweden, respectively) but comparison with France, Spain and Serbia was less precise as these presented their data by larger age groups. [3]

Type of datasource can be decisive as well. A study in Finland detected an increase of proximal humerus fractures in a hospital database analysis among 1970-2002. However, due to the introduction of new orthopaedic techniques, patients are more likely to be admitted to hospital for proximal humerus fracture treatment in the recent years. Analysis of hospital registries can indicate a false increase.

Table 3. Challenges in estimating the occurrence of fractures in minorities

Factors to be considered	
–	Lack of data on race or ethnicity in hospital discharge and fracture databases
–	Use of various race and ethnicity categories in different registers and studies
–	Intercensal population estimates are used for annual population assessment by race or ethnicity
–	Uncertainities or abscense of fracture incidence data of the general population
–	Comparison of incidence should be matched by gender and age
–	Previous incidence data are not necessarily relevant to the present
–	Outpatient databases are not comparable with hospital registers

The insurance database analysis in Hungary (involving both inpatient and outpatient data) did not detect increase of humerus fractures in the 5 years period but much higher rates were found than in publications based on hospital registires. These findings highlight the importance of matching also the datasource to compare accurately the incidence of fractures.

Although the health insurance database is an excellent source for epidemiological studies of fractures and osteoporosis care on the national level, it does not contain data on ethnicity or race. Therefore, data on osteoporosis of minorities is still missing in the region.

The majority of fracture incidence data are available from the United States. Hip fracture incidence is generally held to be lower in the Black, Asian, and Hispanic populations in the United States, but some data suggest that individuals of Mexican ancestry may have a higher risk of hip fracture now than they did in earlier years.

Hospitalization data from California over the 18-year period (1983-2000) were evaluated by Zigmond et al., comparing secular trends in hip fracture incidence and repair for Hispanic women and men, with those for other racial/ethnic groups (non-Hispanic whites, blacks and Asians). [7] The number of patients increased from 20,108 in 1983 to 25,943 in 2000, comorbidity and age increased also in both genders. The overall age-adjusted annual incidence of hip fractures declined by 0.74%/year among California women (from 655 to 568 / 100,000 inhabitants), but was essentially unchanged among California men (from 247 to 238 / 100,000 inhabitants) due to the increase of the older population. The standardized annual hip fracture rates for non-Hispanic women aged ≥55 have fallen by 0.6%/year whilst no significant change occurred among Black or Asian women and a substantial increase (4.9%) was observed among Hispanic women. A similar difference was observed among Hispanic and non-Hispanic men (age group ≥ 55 years: 4.2% versus 0.5%/year).

Although the majority of patients continue to be non-Hispanic whites and ethnic minorities are an increasing proportion of all cases encountered these data support that the racial distribution of patients treated for hip fracture has changed in the past decades.

Kuwait is a fancy example to present the challenges of studying health issues among ethnic minorities. First of all, the total population in 1995 was about 1.88 million of whom the Kuwaiti nationals constituted a minority, 37%. The vast majority (88%) of non-Kuwaitis were from Southeast Asian and Arab countries (southeast Asians represented 51% and Arabs 37% of the non-Kuwaiti population). Furthermore, age-distribution of the population in Kuwait shows an uncommon pattern. It has a relatively young population structure compared with Europe and North-America: about 91% of Kuwaitis and 94% of non-Kuwaitis are aged <50 years. Since age is a major risk factor for fractures, such differences can have significant impact on the overall results.

A study was conducted in an Orthopaedic Hospital in Kuwait (providing services to residents about 70% of the total population) among 1992-1995. [8] A total of 513 new cases of hip fracture were recorded during the 4 years (female/male: 0.67; mean age women 68.7±16.3 and men 63.0±21.1). More cases occurred among Kuwaitis than non-Kuwaitis (57.1% versus 42.9%). The median age was lower in both genders among non-Kuwaiti patients (females: 70 versus 60 years; males: 68 versus 42 years). The incidence of hip fracture was higher than that reported from other countries in Asia and was comparable to some of the western European and North American populations. Although this analysis included also hip fractures not related to osteoporosis (no age limit, traffic accidents were not excluded), results highlight the importance of considering the racial/ethnic composition of a population in fracture epidemiology studies.

Bone Mineral Density

Previously only few longitudinal data were available on BMD and fractures in other than White postmenopausal populations and it was unknown whether a T score obtained by BMD measurement in nonwhite women has the same meaning in terms of fracture prediction.

The National Osteoporosis Risk Assessment (NORA) observational study of postmenopausal women in the United States (started in late 1997) involved a total of 197,848 women: Whites 90.7%, Blacks 3.9%, Hispanic Americans 3.5%, Asian Americans 1.0% and Native Americans 0.9%. [9] Baseline BMD and fractures of hip, rib, spine, wrist and arm were detected. Asian women had the lowest and Black women had the highest mean T score (–1.22 versus −0.39), in White women the mean Tscore was −0.89. Hispanic and Native American women had intermediate T scores (−1.13 and –1.11, respectively). Based on WHO criteria, 11.9% of Native American women, 10% of Asians, 9.8% of Hispanics, 7.2% of Whites, and 4.2% of Blacks were osteoporotic, whereas osteopenia was identified in 50.1% of Asians, 46.5% of Hispanics, 44.5% of Native Americans, 39.6% of Whites, and 28.1% of Black women. Age-adjusted estimates of osteoporosis of the hip, defined by T-score for BMD, are 17% for postmenopausal White women, 14% for Mexican American women, and 6% for black women.

The clinically relevant question is whether the unadjusted differences require the use of ethnic-specific T score equivalents for fracture prediction. [10] After adjustment for body weight and other risk factor covariates, Black women had the highest average BMD followed by Hispanic women, whereas Asians and Native Americans had BMD values differing little from those of Whites. Regarding the predictive power of BMD on fractures, in models adjusted for weight and other variables, BMD predicted 1-year fracture risk equally well in Whites, Blacks, and Hispanics, with similar patterns. Wider confidence intervals were observed in Native Americans and Asians due to smaller samples.

This large study showed that women present a similar pattern of increasing fracture risk with decreasing BMD levels, regardless of race or ethnicity. NORA women who were found to have osteopenia or osteoporosis had an increased risk of fracture in every ethnic group.

However, the NORA study examined solely postmenopausal women. In the National Health and Nutrition Examination Survey (NHANES) III, multiethnic data of femoral BMD in both genders were analyzed and the highest prevalence of osteoporosis was revealed among Mexican American and White women. [11]

Risk factors were also analyzed in the NHANES III study. Data analysis of 2,590 women and 2,391 men 50–79 years of age (involving African–American, Mexican–American and White women and men) established that low body-mass index, low calcium intake, current cigarette smoking, and physical inactivity were independent risk factors. The presence of one or more risk factors was associated with having osteoporosis and low BMD in all groups. The strength of these associations was greater when two or more risk factors were present but varied with race/ethnicity, gender, and age. Within gender groups, African-American women and White men had the greatest risk of OP when two or more risk factors were present. In the presence of one or more risk factors, African-American and White women aged 65–79 years were less likely to have osteoporosis than their younger counterparts. No increased risk for osteoporosis was found in younger Mexican-American women. However, the likelihood of having osteoporosis in 65 to 79-year-old Mexican-American women was greater than in African-American or White women in the same age group. When adjustment was made for age within each group, there were only minor changes in the results. [12]

A study by Araujo et al focussed on men: BMD of males from different race or ethnic groups has been analyzed. [13] White men aged 30–79 years were randomly sampled from Boston, MA: 367 Black, 401 Hispanic, and 451 White. Analyses on 1,209 men with available data confirmed that Black men had greater BMD than Hispanic or White men, differences between Hispanic and White subjects were restricted to the hip. Age-related declines in BMD were significantly steeper among Hispanic than Black or White men. These results underscore the differences by ethnic groups in men.

Recent African immigrants were studied by Gong et al. Bone mineral density of 143 (55 men and 88 premenopausal women) of Sub-Daharan Sudanese immigrants was measured in the US. Results (BMD) in the spine but not total body or hip was significantly lower compared with the normative values of African Americans and Caucasians. Total body and hip BMD was positively correlated with their length of stay in the United States suggesting potential environmental factors in the ethnic diversity of BMD. [14]

Differences in bone mineral density between ethnic groups have highly significant clinical relevance since both the diagnosis and intervention thresholds are related to T score i.e. standard deviation of BMD above or below the mean of "normal" young adults.

Results of the NHANES III suggested that using gender-specific and race-specific T-scores would yield a higher prevalence of osteoporosis in nonwhite populations than when calculated using the white female normative data. [11]

Osteoporosis is clearly an important public health problem among Chinese women. The US Census Bureau estimates that by the year 2050, one-tenth of the US population will be of Asian descent, many of them, Chinese American. A referent BMD database for Chinese American women has been published by Walker et al. [15] Healthy Chinese American women (n=359), ages 20–90, were recruited (years 2002-2004), BMD was measured at the lumbar spine and total hip. Osteoporosis diagnosis rates calculated with the Caucasian and newly established Chinese American BMD referent values were compared. Chinese American women have significantly lower BMD at the lumbar spine, total hip, and femoral neck across a wide spectrum of age groups. As a consequence, more than onehalf of Chinese American women ≥50 years of age, who would be characterized as osteoporotic using a Caucasian referent, would not be diagnosed as such if a Chinese American referent were utilized.

Similarly, bone mass in the proximal femur of native Chinese women was significantly lower, and the bone loss rate greater, than those of non-Asian women in the United States, by Hou et al. However at the femoral neck, the BMD of Chinese women was similar to that of non-Hispanic White women. [16]

The importance of using appropriate reference data considering ethnicity was highlighted by Mikuls at all as well. [17] Rheumatoid arthritis (RA) is an inflammatory arhritis with increased risk for OP. Bone Mineral Density of the hip and spine of African Americans with early RA was assessed in a study enrolling patients from the Consortium for the longitudinal Evaluation of African Americans with Early RA (CLEAR). T-score were calculated using reference data from Caucasians and from age-matched African Americans separately. Less patiens were diagnosed to have osteopenia or worse BMD using the Caucasian referent data than the African-American reference (33% versus 55%) and the same trend was observed regarding establishing diagnosis of OP (5% versus 16%). Diagnosis of OP is especially noteworthy in RA since osteoporosis related fractures are one of the most prevalent co-morbidities in RA leading to substantal mortality and lowered quality of life.

The Middle East and North Africa consensus on osteoporosis has reviewed published data on BMD, risk factors and fracture prevalence in the region. Studies conducted mainly on female populations found lower BMD than the standard established for the US/European reference data, except Kuwait where the range was similar.[18] Consequently, using North American and European curves provided by the instrument manufacturer can lead to an overestimation of OP in these populations.

In conclusion, differences in bone mineral density among racial and ethnic populations have been established by several studies. Appropriate diagnosis of osteoporosis in minority groups requires reference databases considering ethnicity.

Risk Factors for Fractures

The Women's Health Initiative study enrolled 159,579 women (50-79 years of age) to identify risk factors for fractures across ethnic groups. Annualized rates of fracture in Whites, Blacks, Hispanics, Asians, and American Indians were 2.0, 0.9, 1.3, 1.2, and 2.0%, respectively. Positive fracture history and more than two falls were significant predictors in all ethnic groups. Irrespective of their ethnicity, women with multiple risk factors have a high risk of fracture. However, other predominant factors were somewhat diverse: Blacks - at least a high school education; Hispanics - height (>162 cm), arthritis, corticosteroid use and parental history of fracture; Asians - age (per 5 years), current hormone therapy, parity (at least five); American Indians: current hormone therapy. [19]

Results of this large study emphasises that risk factors of fractures are not entirely consistent among different ethnic groups thus should be considered in clinical practice and screening programs.

Risk of Falls

Falls are major risk factors for fractures. However the role of ethnicity has not been well established in this field, yet.

In a study by Fulkner no ethnic differences were found in fall rates in older Caucasian and African-American community dwelling women. [20] In a sample of 1,665 Caucasian and 156 African-American women (mean age 76±5, range 65–93) from the Study of Osteoporotic Fractures at the University of Pittsburgh clinical center were followed prospectively for falls between May 1993 and December 1998. Totally 4,547 falls were reported over 9,508 person-years (mean 0.48/person/year, 95% CI=0.43–0.53) among patients aged ≥70 years. Irrespectively of age and body mass index, African-American women had a 19% higher rate of chronic conditions and twice the prevalence of functional impairments as Caucasians (e.g. cognitive impairment, poor visual acuity, depression, and slow walking speed). Adjusting for age, the observed fall rates were approximately 30% higher in Caucasians than African Americans but the difference was not statistically significant which is consistent with other previously published studies. Interestingly, ethnic differences were identified in the fall circumstances (location, surface, fall direction) and in the likelihood of falling on the hand.

Important methodological issues were revealed in a systematic literature review on socio-demographic variables of falls by Todd et al. [21] Comparing across studies is problematic due to differences not only in defining ethnic groups and sites of data collection, but also considering life-style and socio-economic status. For example, much lower rates of falls were reported amongst native Japanese in USA and Europe (approximately half the risk) but rates for Japanese-Americans were similar to those living in Japan. However it was not clearly established whether the differences observed relate to ethnicity or to rurality. Nevertheless, some broad general trends can be found, i.e. Caucasians living in US generally have higher falls injury admission rates, than other groups but it is uncertain whether it is due to more falls or more access to health services. Similarly to many aspects of osteoporosis minority studies, almost all papers discussing ethnicty and falls are from the USA: comparing Whites or Caucasians, Blacks or African-Americans and Hispanics or Mexican-Americans and less data are available from other countries.

In conlcusion, the relationship between falls and ethnicity remains wide open for research.

Access to Osteoporosis Care

Osteoporosis screening is crucial for the identification of patients at risk for fractures. Some studies suggest that there is some disparity among population groups in receiving bone mineral density measurement and antiporotic therapy.

Alam et al. reviewed retrospectively the medical records at Howard University Hospital (years 1992-2002), an urban tertiary care teaching hospital with a predominantly African-American population. [22] Of 58,841 patients who were admitted during the study period, 1,248 patients (2.1%) had fractures, 323 patients had fractures secondary to low-impact falls. Only 29 of these had a diagnosis of osteoporosis, 5 patients were discharged on antiosteoporotic medications, and only 1 patient was discharged with a bisphosphonate therapy.

Mikuls et al. conducted a computer assisted telephone interview using a population based random sample aged >50 drawn from 6 counties in Alabama, US. Of eligible African American and Caucasian female respondents, 251 (25%) reported a history of fracture after 45 years of age. African American women with a fracture history were less likely than Caucasian women with a history of fracture to receive a DXA (osteodensitometry) or prescription osteoporosis medicines. [23]

Female Medicare recipients aged 65-89 years old with hip fractures were involved between January 2001 and June 2003. Among all 35,681 women with hip fractures, 20.7% underwent bone mineral density testing in the 2 years prior to fracture and another 6.2% underwent testing in the 6 months after fracture. Logistic regression model adjusted for age, state, and comorbidity revealed that women of black race were about half as likely and Hispanic women about 2/3 as likely as White women to undergo testing before their fracture. They remained less likely also to undergo testing after fracture. Racial, but not socioeconomic, differences in osteoporosis evaluation continued to occur even after Medicare patients had demonstrated their propensity to fracture. [24]

A retrospective chart review at an urban academic hospital and a suburban community hospital was performed to determine whether there is a difference in physician screening for OP. [25] Significantly fewer African-American than white women were referred for a DXA scan (odds ratio: 0.39%, 95%; confidence interval: 0.22 to 0.68). Physicians were also less likely to mention consideration of osteoporosis in medical records and to recommend calcium and vitamin D supplementation for this population. Neither patient factors nor physician characteristics were associated with signifcant differences in referral rates between African-Americans and Whites. If referred, African-American women had comparable DXA completion rates when compared with white women. Recommendation for osteoporosis screening of African-American women was lower than in Whites despite of similar risk in both groups.

These studies support the differences in the receipt of osteoporosis care among minorities. However there is lack of data whether these result in true differences in fracture related outcomes.

Vitamin D and Calcium

Studies from the US support that there is a difference among ethnic groups in taking dietary supplements. Blacks in the US use dietary supplements less frequently than do Whites. However, Blacks produce less vitamin D3 than do Whites in response to usual levels of sun exposure and have lower 25-hydroxyvitamin D concentrations in winter and summer. There are well established evidences that vitamin D supplements decrease parathormone and bone turnover marker concentrations among Blacks. These data suggest that improving vitamin D status would benefit Blacks as well as Whites. [26]

In Israel, serum level of Vitamin D and risk factors for hypovitaminosis D was analysed involving 296 consecutive inpatients in the Soroka University Medical Center, which is situated in a sunny region of the country. Hypovitaminosis was found in 77%. Multivariate analysis confirmed significant association not only with sun exposure, vitamin D intake, and stroke but also with ethnic origin i.e. patients of Beduin origin had lower rates. [27]

In Australia, risk of osteoporosis was assessed by self-reported questionnaires focussing also on dietary calcium intake. [28] Asian women had less osteoporosis knowledge and lower calcium intake than Caucasian women (mean 793±49 versus 1298±56 mg/day) and postmenopausal Asian women were at greater risk of being below the recommended daily intake (73%) than Caucasian women (31%).

These findings suggest that improving knowledge on osteoporosis and preventive activities optimizing the calcium and D vitamin intake should be especially considered in ethnic groups.

Rehabilitation after Hip Fractures

Fractures, especially hip fractures can lead to significant disability. Rehablitation after acut treatment can improve the restitution of function and quality of life.

Ganesan et al assessed 324,760 subjects from the California Hospital Discharge Data Program (acut care hospitals) among 1990-2000 to analyse the hospitalisation rates in extended-care facilities (ECFs) among ethnic groups. [29] Patients aged ≥65 years with hip fractures related to osteoporosis were involved: 87% were Whites (Black, Hispanic and Asian/Other groups were also analyized), 76% female and 86% had Medicare health insurance. Compared to Whites (72%) other ethnic groups had lower rates of ECF placement, rate of Hispanics were the lowest (64%) and also Asians/Others were more likely to be discharged home but not the African Americans. Older age, multiple comorbidities, the presence of Medicare insurance and shorter length of stay were also significantly associated with placement in EFCs. Functional and cognitive statuses which can have impact on ECF placement were not analyzed. However, this study highlights that Hispanic elderly patients with hip fracture are more likely to be discharged home than Whites.

Less data are available regarding mortality after hip fracture considering ethnicity. Orces et al assessed adjusted death rates after hip fracture in Texas by age, sex, and ethnic group in a 9-year period (1990-1998). [30] The highest mortality rates were observed in Whites, predominantly in persons 80 years and older, rates in men by ethnic group consistently exceeded those in women. Upward trends in mortality were observed for both sexes in Whites and Blacks but Hispanics showed trends toward decreasing mortality rates.

These preliminary results leave many questions backwards such as short term (1 week) and long term (1 year) mortality rates, analysis of many other factors (e.g. time between fracture and primary care) to highlight this matter on a wider level.

Representation of Minorities in Clinical Trials

Generalizability of all types of clinical studies (e.g. observational cohort, randomized clinical trials) drawing samples from geographic areas in which substantial numbers minority group reside require involvement of adequate number of the diverse populations.

Subgroup-specific data are needed when ethnicity could modify the outcome, and they are also useful to document convincingly that the results are applicable to diverse groups. Lack of inclusiveness in treatment trials may overestimate effects by creating a best-case scenario. However oversampling to produce proportions of minorities beyond their levels of representation in a population may be necessary to achieve adequate numbers. Furthermore, assessment of the reliability and validity of survey instruments measuring outcomes (e.g.

health status and quality of life questionnaires) in diverse populations is critical to the conduct of high-quality research, appropriate adaptations are required. [31]

Nevertheless, representation of minorities can have significant impact on the applicability of the results. In a review by Nicholson et al, >99% of study participants were White in the hormone replacement–therapy studies. Thus, women from racial/ethnic minority groups and their physicians may have less confidence in applying the findings in their decision-making processes. [32]

A study examined whether ethnicity or socioeconomic status influenced a group's ability to meet eligibility criteria and willingness to enroll in an estrogen and OP trial. The ethnic rates among screened patiens were: 59% White, 27% African Americans, 14% Hispanics; 57.6% patients were eligible of which 32% were enrolled. African-Americans were less likely to be eligible for medical reasons than non-African Americans. Eligible Hispanics were more likely to be enrolled than non-Hispanics. African Americans were equally willing to enroll as Whites. Minority residents of low-income areas were more likely to enroll than minority residents of high-income areas. [33]

Observational studies are often based on self-reported data. Chen et al studied the validity of, and factors associated with, the accuracy of self-report for fractures involving participants from the Women's Health Initiative Clinical Trial and Observational Study cohorts. The populations included American Indian, Asian/Pacific Islander, Black, Hispanic, and non-Hispanic White (n = 6,652). Substantial variations in validity of self-report by the fracture site were found compared to medical records (hip 78%, forearm/wrist 81%, clinical spine fractures 51%). Multivariate analysis indicated that among multiple factors ethnicity significantly related to the validity of self-report. [34]

However, some significant economic issues should be also considered in designing clinical studies that are supposed to be relevant on minorities as well.

In a trial of risk factors for age-related bone loss and fractures enrollment of 140 minority patients was required. Researchers encountered specific problems with respect to identification of potential subjects, recruitment, obtaining informed consent, transportation to the study site, and collecting study data. Successful enrolment was achieved by focussing on the especial needs: (1) understand the target population; (2) establish explicit recruitment goals; (3) agree on research plans between study staff and minority communities; (4) continuously evaluate the recruitment process; and (5) maintain lines of communication. Success depended especially on the recruitment of cultural advisors from the different ethnic groups. However these special efforts increased the recruitment cost substantially, almost 5-fold higher to enroll the group of Asians, Hispanic, and Somali subjects than the Whites who were contacted by mail. [35]

Summary

Osteoporosis and related fractures present significant burden on the individual and society. Evidences support that racial and ethnic differences exist regarding bone health. Gender and age matched data from the relevant geographic region on the incidence of osteoporosis and fractures of the general population are essential for adequate comparisons with minorities. Available data suggest that several especial aspects should be considered in the osteoporosis care of minorities. Due to substantial variability in bone mineral density between different racial and ethnic populations, applicability of diagnostic tools should be tested unless either patients at risk of fractures remain misdiagnosed or unneccesary treatments will be applied in minority populations. Medical decisions should consider the differencies in nutrition and intake of dietary supplements as vitamin D play important role in the treatment. Regarding antiporotic drugs, most of the clinical trials still involve white women, thus results are not neccessarily relevant on other ethnic groups. However adequate representation of minorities in clinical studies bear especial methodological issues which may have impact also on the budgeting of the research.

There are several questions open for further research. Most studies discussing aspects of bone screening, risk factors, access to treatments in osteoporosis in minorities are from the US and practically there are no data from Europe. Not all issues are based on high quality evidences. Identification of further patient, provider and decision makers factors leading to disparities in osteoporosis care are needed to implement and develop successful programs aimed at eliminating the differences.

References

[1] Consensus Development Conference. Prophylaxis and treatment of osteoporosis. *Am. J. Med.* 1991;90:107–10.

[2] Johnell O, Kanis J. Epidemiology of osteoporotic fractures. *Osteoporos Int.* 2005;16:S3–S7.

[3] Péntek M, Horváth C, Boncz I, Falusi Z, Tóth E, Sebestyén A, Májer I, Brodszky V, Gulácsi L. Epidemiology of osteoporosis related fractures in Hungary from the nationwide health insurance database, 1999-2003. *Osteoporos Int.* 2008;19:243-9.

[4] Thomas PA. Racial and ethnic differences in osteoporosis. *J. Am. Acad. Orthop. Surg.* 2007;15(suppl 1):S26-30.

[5] Ray NF, Chan JK, Thamer M, Melton LJ 3rd. Medical expenditures for the treatment of osteoporotic fractures in the United States in 1995: report from the National Osteoporosis Foundation. *J. Bone Miner. Res.* 1997;12:24-35.

[6] Gulácsi L, Boncz I, Péntek M, Falusi Zs, Sebestyén A, Tóth E, Horváth Cs. (2006) Osteoporosis related health care utilisation in Hungary by the nationwide health insurance database. *Value Health*, 9:6: A381.

[7] Zingmond DS, Melton III LJ, Stuart L. Silverman. Increasing hip fracture incidence in California Hispanics, 1983 to 2000. *Osteoporos Int.* 2004;15:603–10.

[8] Memon A, Pospula WM, Tantawy AY, Abdul-Ghafar S, Suresh A, Al-Rowaih A. Incidence of hip fracture in Kuwait. *Int. J. Epidemiol.* 1998;27:860-5.

[9] Barrett-Connor E, Siris ES, Wehren LE, Miller PD, Abbott TA, Berger ML, Santora AC, Sherwood5. Osteoporosis and Fracture Risk in Women of Different Ethnic Groups. *J. Bone Miner. Res.* 2005;20:185–94.

[10] Becker C, Crow S, Toman J, Lipton C, McMahon DJ, Macaulay W, Siris E. Characteristics of elderly patients admitted to an urban tertiary care hospital with

osteoporotic fractures: correlations with risk factors, fracture type, gender and ethnicity. *Osteoporos Int.* 2006;17:410-6.

[11] Pothiwala P, EVANS EM, Chapman-Novakofsi KM. Ethnic Variation in Risk for Osteoporosis among Women: A Review of Biological and Behavioral Factors. *J. Womens Health (Larchmt).* 2006;15:709-19.

[12] Broussard DL, Magnus JH. Risk assessment and screening for low bone mineral density in a multi-ethnic population of women and men: does one approach fit all? *Osteoporos Int.* 2004;15:349-60.

[13] Araujo AB, Travison TG, Harris SS, Holick MF, Turner AK, McKinlay JB. Race/ethnic differences in bone mineral density in men. *Osteoporos Int.* 2007;18:943-53.

[14] Gong G, Haynatzki G, Haynatzka V, Kosoko-Lasaki S, Howell R, Fu YX, Gallagher JC, Wilson MR. Bone mineral density of recent African immigrants in the United States. *J. Natl. Med. Assoc.* 2006;98:746-52.

[15] Walker MD, Babbar R, Opotowsky AR, Rohira A, Nabizadeh F, Badia MD, Chung W, Chiang J, Mediratta A, McMahon D, Liu G, Bilezikian JP. A referent bone mineral density database for Chinese American women. *Osteoporos Int.* 2006;17(6):878-87.

[16] Hou YL, Wu XP, Luo XH, Zhang H, Cao XZ, Jiang YB, Liao EY. Differences in age-related bone mass of proximal femur between Chinese women and different ethnic women in the United States. *J. Bone Miner. Metab.* 2007;25:243-52.

[17] Mikuls TR, Saag KG, Curtis J, Bridges SL Jr, Alarcon GS, Westfall AO, Lim SS, Smith EA, Jonas BL, Moreland LW; CLEAR Investigators. Prevalence of osteoporosis and osteopenia among African Americans with early rheumatoid arthritis: the impact of ethnic-specific normative data. *J. Natl. Med. Assoc.* 2005;97:1155-60.

[18] Maalouf G, Gannagé-Yared MH, Ezzedine J, Larijani B, Badawi S, Rached A, Zakroui L, Masri B, Azar E, Saba E, Nammari R, Adib G, Abou Samra H, Alrawi Z, Salman S, El Muntasser K, Tarseen R, El Kharousi W, Al-Lamki M, Alothman AN, Almarzook N, El Dessouki M, Sulaimani R, Saleh J, Suhaili AR, Khan A, Delmas P, Seeman E. Middle East and North Africa consensus on osteoporosis. J. Musculoskelet Neuronal Interact. 2007;7:131-43.

[19] Cauley JA, Wu L, Wampler NS, Barnhart JM, Allison M, Chen Z, Jackson R, Robbins J. Clinical risk factors for fractures in multi-ethnic women: the Women's Health Initiative. *J. Bone Miner. Res.* 2007;22:1816-26.

[20] Faulkner KA, Cauley JA, Zmuda JM, Landsittel DP, Nevitt MC, Newman AB, Studenski SA, Redfern MS. Ethnic Differences in the Frequency and Circumstances of Falling in Older Community-Dwelling Women. *J. Am. Geriatr. Soc.* 53:1774–1779, 2005.

[21] Todd C, Ballinge C, Whitehead S. Reviews of socio-demographic faqctios related to falls and environmental interventions to prevent falls amongst older people living int he community. http://www.who.int/ageing/projects/3.Environmental%20and%20 socioeconomic%20risk%20factors%20on%20falls.pdf (Downloaded: 5 January, 2008)

[22] Alam NM, Archer JA, Lee E. Osteoporotic fragility fractures in African Americans: under-recognized and undertreated. *J. Natl. Med. Assoc.* 2004;96:1640-5.

[23] Mikuls TR, Saag KG, George V, Mudano AS, Banerjee S. Racial disparities in the receipt of osteoporosis related healthcare among community-dwelling older women with arthritis and previous fracture. *J. Rheumatol.* 2005;32:870-5.

[24] Neuner JM, Zhang X, Sparapani R, Laud PW, Nattinger AB. Racial and socioeconomic disparities in bone density testing before and after hip fracture. *J. Gen. Intern. Med.* 2007;22:1239-45.

[25] Miller RG, Ashar BH, Cohen J, Camp M, Coombs C, Johnson E, Schneyer CR. Disparities in osteoporosis screening between at-risk African-American and white women. *J. Gen. Intern. Med.* 2005;20:847-51.

[26] Dawson-Hughes B. Racial/ethnic considerations in making recommendations for vitamin D for adult and elderly men and women. *Am. J. Clin. Nutr.* 2004; 80 (suppl): 1763S – 6S.

[27] Hochwald O, Harman-Boehm I, Castel H. Hypovitaminosis D among inpatients in a sunny country. *Isr. Med. Assoc. J.* 2004;6:82-7.

[28] Liew YL, Mann D, Piterman L. Osteoporosis risks. A comparative study of Asian Australian and Caucasian Australian women. *Aust. Fam. Physician.* 2002;31:291-3.

[29] Ganesan K, Pan D, Teklehaimenot S, Norris K. Racial differences in institutionalization after hip fractures: California hospital discharge data. *Ethn. Dis.* 2005;15(4 Suppl 5):S5-30-3.

[30] Orces CH, Lee S, Bradshaw B. Sex and ethnic differences in hip fracture-related mortality in Texas, 1990 through 1998. *Tex. Med.* 2002;98:56-8.

[31] Jancey J, Howat P, Lee A, Clarke A, Shilton T, Fisher J, Iredell H. Effective recruitment and retention of older adults in physical activity research: PALS study. *Am. J. Health Behav.* 2006;30:626-35.

[32] Nicholson WK, Brown AF, Gathe J, Grumbach K, Washington AE, Perez- Stable EJ. Hormone replacement therapy for African American women: missed opportunities for effective intervention. *Menopause;* 1999;6:147–55.

[33] Unson CG, Ohannessian C, Kenyon L, Case A, Reisine S, Prestwood. Barriers to Eligibility and Enrollment Among Older Women in a Clinical Trial on Osteoporosis. *Journal of Aging and Health,* 2004;Vol. 16, No. 3:426-43.

[34] Chen Z, Kooperberg C, Pettinger MB, Bassford T, Cauley JA, LaCroix AZ, Lewis CE, Kipersztok S, Borne C, Jackson RD. Validity of self-report for fractures among a multiethnic cohort of postmenopausal women: results from the Women's Health Initiative observational study and clinical trials. *Menopause.* 2004;11:264-74.

[35] Marquez MA, Muhs JM, Tosomeen A, Riggs BL, Melton LJ 3rd. Costs and strategies in minority recruitment for osteoporosis research. *J. Bone Miner. Res.* 2003;18(1):3-8.

In: Topics in Prevalent Diseases
Editors: N. C. Chavez-Tapia and M. Uribe

ISBN 978-1-60456-959-9

Chapter 18

Road Traffic Crashes and Injury Prevention among Racial/Ethnic Minorities in the United States

Paul D. Juarez *

Department of Family and Community Medicine, Meharry Medical College, Nashville, Tennessee, USA

Introduction

Fatal and non-fatal road traffic injuries are among the leading preventable causes of premature death, disability, and injury worldwide. Each year, it is estimated that over a million persons are killed in road traffic crashes with an additional 50 million persons experiencing a non-fatal injury [1]. The annual, direct economic cost of road traffic crashes internationally has been estimated at over $500 billion. With unprecedented levels of increasing global industrialization and modernization, some are projecting that these numbers could rise by as much as 65% by 2020 without a mobilized effort to manage road safety at a local, national, and international level [2].

A public health framework will be used in this chapter to discuss road traffic crashes and injury prevention among racial/ethnic minorities in the United States. A public health approach suggests that road traffic injuries and death can be studied scientifically, are preventable, and interventions are most effective when there is collaboration across a range of sectors. In this chapter, risk factors and solutions associated with road traffic crashes will be addressed with a focus on modifiable risk factors most pertinent to racial and ethnic minority populations.

For the purpose of this chapter, the ICD-10 Codes for 2007, 10th Revision [3], Chapter XX, Accidents: V01-V89 are used to define road traffic injuries (See Appendix A). Road traffic injuries will be presented in four broad categories: (1) motor vehicles with four or

* Contact Information: Department of Family & Community Medicine, Meharry Medical College, 1005 Dr. D.B. Todd Jr., Blvd., Nashville, TN 37208, Phone: 615 327-5506, Email: pjuarez@mmc.edu.

more wheels autos (V40-V49), pick up trucks and vans (V50-V59), trucks (V60-V69), buses (V70-V79), and other land transport vehicles (V80-V89); (2) two wheel motor cycles (V20-V29) and three wheel motor cycles (V30-V39); (3) pedal cycles (V10-V19); and (4) pedestrians (V01-V09).

The Haddon Matrix [4] will be used both as a model for describing risk factors for road traffic safety and as a guide for suggesting strategies and interventions that can be implemented to mitigate resulting injury and death among racial/ethnic minority groups. The Haddon Matrix describes road traffic injury along two dimensions. The agent-host-environment dimension of the matrix examines injury as being comprised of three components. The *agent*, or road vehicle, is the vector through which energy is channeled that results in the injury; the *host*, or road user, is the recipient of the transmission of energy—the injured party; and the road *environment* in which the injury occurs, including both the physical environment and the social-political-economic context. The second dimension of the Haddon Matrix is time. It looks at an injury along a 3-stage, temporal continuum from pre-event, to event, to post-event and provides a way to consider the stage in time at which an injury might have been prevented or its impact mitigated. The Haddon Matrix provides support for a public health approach that "injuries are not accidents" and that applying a scientific approach to the examination of injuries can provide us with an understanding of modifiable risk factors that can be addressed to prevent and control injury outcomes.

Road Traffic Injuries in the United States

Road traffic injuries are the eighth leading cause of death overall in the United States, the third leading cause of years of person life lost (YPLL) for Americans of all races and ethnicities, and the leading cause of death for persons between 4 and 34 years of age. The mortality rate for all populations in the United States in 2003 from road traffic crashes was 15.2 per 100,000; 21.4 per 100,000 for males 9.3 per 100,000 for females. Motor vehicle traffic fatalities are the most frequent cause of death for young children, children, youth, young adults, and other adults 25–34, and the second most frequent cause of death for toddlers. [5]

Table 1. Age Adjusted Motor Vehicle Related Death Rates per 100,000 by Race and Hispanic Origin and Gender: Total US Population, 2004

Race and Hispanic Origin	Total	Male	Female
Total	15.2	21.4	9.3
White	*	21.8	9.5
Black	*	22.7	8.1
American Indian	*	34.5	17.8
Asian/Pacific Islander	*	9.3	6.3
Hispanic/Latino	*	20.9	7.7

In 2006, there were a total of 42,642 fatal and 2,331,000 non-fatal, injuries resulting from road traffic crashes. Of those, 30,521 fatalities and 1,475,000 non-fatal injuries were passenger vehicle occupants, 1,571 fatalities were passengers in large buses, trucks and other vehicles; 4,810 deaths and 88,000 nonfatal injuries were to motorcycle riders; 773 fatalities and 44,000 nonfatal injuries were among pedalcyclists; and 4,784 fatal and 61,000 nonfatal injuries were among pedestrians. [6]. In recent years, deaths and injuries from road traffic crashes have steadily declined in the United States for all causes of motor vehicle related injuries except those caused by motor cycles and large bus/trucks and other vehicles [7].

Recent reductions in fatal and non-fatal road traffic related injuries have not been experienced equally by all racial/ethnic minority groups, however. Disparities in health outcomes resulting from road traffic injuries are found among males, young drivers, and racial/ethnic minorities. In the remainder of this chapter, an overview of road traffic crash morbidity and mortality among racial/ethnic minorities in the United States will be presented, individual and community risk factors will be reviewed, and a *developmental/ecological model* [8] is proposed as an approach for guiding the development of road traffic injury prevention strategies for racial/ethnic minority populations. This model is offered as a public health approach for conceptualizing comprehensive injury prevention strategies for reducing disparities in risk behaviors, injury, disability, and death resulting from road traffic crashes in racial/ethnic minority communities. While US data are presented, the framework and implications of this chapter can be applied in other countries.

Racial/Ethnic Minorities and Road Traffic Crashes: The Magnitude of the Problem

While road traffic crashes are a leading contributor to premature death, disability, and non-fatal injury in the entire US population, they have a disproportionate negative impact on the health and well-being of members of racial/ethnic minority groups. Causal factors that increase their risk for fatal and nonfatal road traffic deaths and injuries are often described as behavioral, social/cultural, environmental exposure, and lack of access to goods, services, and information.

In the United States, race/ethnicity often is used to characterize people of color. The US Office of Management and Budget (OMB) [9] classify five distinct "races" and persons of Hispanic/Latino origin, who can be of any race (see *Limitations* in this chapter). For instance, *Whites* include all persons of Caucasian ancestry who do not have mixed racial heritage; *Blacks* include persons of African descent, regardless of nationality or mixed heritage; *American Indians and Alaska Natives*, include persons from numerous federally recognized tribes and nations, some of which reside on reservations and others who don't; *Asians* include persons from the far east and southeast Asia; and *Native Hawaiian or Pacific Islanders*. Although 1997 standards modified these classes by separating Pacific Islanders and Hawaiians from Asians, this report uses the earlier classification because of the small numbers in these groups. The US Census considers *Hispanics/Latinos* an ethnic identifier rather than a distinct race, and includes persons of Mexican, Puerto Rican, Cuban, and Central and South American ancestry. For the purpose of this chapter, racial/ethnic groups are limited to a discussion of historically underrepresented minorities in the United States [10]. These include Blacks, American Indians, Asian/Pacific Islanders, and

Latinos/Hispanics. Underrepresented Asians include Asian subpopulations other that Chinese, Filipino, Japanese, Korean, Asian Indian or Thai. While persons of other ethnic groups are recognized, they are not identified by the US federal government as historically underrepresented groups. In this report, race and ethnicity terms are used interchangeably.

Race/Ethnicity, Gender, Age and Motor Vehicle Related Injuries

Motor vehicle related injuries are a leading cause of fatal and non-fatal injuries across all racial/ethnic groups in the United States. In 2002, for Americans of all ages, races and ethnicity, motor vehicle traffic crashes were the eighth leading cause of death in 2002. For all age groups combined, motor vehicle crashes were the third leading cause of death for Native Americans, the fifth leading cause of death for all persons of Hispanic or Latino origin, and the seventh leading cause of death overall for Asians and Pacific Islanders. In contrast to the other groups, motor vehicle traffic crashes did not rank in the top 10 causes for African Americans. [11]

Among racial/ethnic minorities in the United States, American Indian males are at highest risk of dying from a motor vehicle related injury while Asian/Pacific Islanders, of all age groups except for females 65 and over, are at lowest risk (See Table 1). American Indian males ages 20 years and older are twice as likely to die from a motor vehicle crash than American Indian females and nearly four times more likely to die from pedestrian-related injury. [12] The motor vehicle death rate among American Indian and Alaska Native populations is three times the rate for the Asian or Pacific Islander population. The rate for Black non-Hispanics and White non-Hispanic populations, by comparison, is 50-99% higher than that of Asian and Pacific Islanders.

Among males of all ages, the mortality rates vary little among Whites (21.7/100,000), Blacks (22.7/100,000), and Latinos (20.9/100,000); while for American Indian male road traffic mortality rates it is over 50% higher (34.5/100,000) and for Asian males, the rates are less than half the national average for males (9.3/100,000) (see Table 1). For females of all ages, the national fatality rate from road traffic crashes is 9.3. White females (9.5/100,000) have higher rates per 100,000 than Black females (8.1), Hispanic/Latino females (7.7), and Asian/Pacific Islander females (6.3), and are exceeded only by the traffic death rate of American Indian females (17.8).

The age groups with the highest motor vehicle mortality rates in the total US population are 15-24 and 65+ (see Table 2). Black and American Indian/Alaskan Native children have mortality rates that are significantly higher than those of White children for total motor vehicle traffic, motor vehicle occupant, and motor vehicle pedestrians. Compared to Black and White children and youth under 19 years of age, American Indian children and youth have the highest injury death rates for motor vehicle crashes, and pedestrian-related deaths. Although significant declines in total motor vehicle mortality across all racial groups have been experienced in the past two decades, disparities in mortality rates have actually widened for both Black and American Indian/Alaskan Native children compared with White children.

When race/ethnicity, gender, and age are combined to identify those groups at highest risk of motor vehicle related fatalities several trends emerge (see Table 3). Overall, American Indians are at highest risk; they account for 5 of the top 10 rates by race/ethnicity including the top three (see Table 4). Whites and Blacks both account for two of the top 10 categories while Hispanics/Latinos account for the other one. Males are clearly at higher risk across the lifespan than females, accounting for nine of the top 10 race/ethnicity x gender x age categories. Road traffic mortality rates are highest in Black and American Indian/Alaskan Native children, lowest in Asian/Pacific Islander children, and intermediate for Hispanic and White children. Gender differences for motor vehicle related fatality rates increase dramatically after age 15 and are maintained throughout the remainder of the lifespan. Older adults 65 and over account for four of the top race/ethnicity x gender x age categories while youth 15-24 years of age account for three. Of the remaining top ten age categories, adults 25-34 account for two, and persons 45-64 account for one.

Motor Vehicle Occupants

In 2006, more than 6.1 million police-reported motor vehicle crashes occurred in the United States. A total of 42,643 people lost their lives in motor vehicle crashes and another 2,331,000 million people were injured. Sixty-four percent of persons killed or injured in traffic crashes were drivers, 28% were passengers, 3% were motorcycle riders, 2% were pedalcyclists, and 3% were pedestrians. [16]

Table 2. Age Adjusted Motor Vehicle Related Death Rate by Age and Gender: Total US Population: 2004

All Persons	Total	Males	Females
All ages, age-adjusted[4].	15.2	21.4	9.3
All ages, crude.	15.3	21.3	9.5
Under 1 year	3.5	3.8	3.2
1-14 years	4.0	4.5	3.5
1-4 years	4.0	4.2	3.7
5-14 years	4.1	4.7	3.4
15-24 years	26.3	36.4	15.7
15-19 years	25.2	32.5	17.5
20-24 years	27.5	40.4	13.8
25-34 years	17.6	25.8	9.1
35-44 years	15.1	21.9	8.3
45-64 years	14.7	21.1	8.6
45-54 years	15.1	21.9	8.5
55-64 years	14.1	19.8	8.8
65 years and over	20.4	28.2	14.9
65-74 years	16.1	21.3	11.7
75-84 years	24.5	34.7	17.7
85 years and over	26.1	44.2	17.9

Table 3. Motor vehicle-related fatalities, by Race and Hispanic origin, Gender and Age: Total US Population, 2004

2004	All Persons		White, Not Hispanic		Black		American Indian		Asian/Pacific Islander		Hispanic/ Latino	
	Male	Female	Male	Female	Male	Female	Male	Female	Male	Female	Male	Female
All Ages, age adjusted	21.4	9.3	21.7	9.5	22.7	8.1	34.5	17.8	9.3	6.3	20.9	7.7
All Ages, crude	21.3	9.5	22.0	9.8	21.2	7.9	33.7	17.3	8.8	6.0	20.2	7.1
Under 1 year	3.8	3.2	*	3.2	*	*	*	*	*	*	*	*
1-14 years	4.5	3.5	4.5	3.4	4.8	4.0	6.8	7.3	2.6	*	4.7	3.4
15-24 years	36.4	15.7	39.1	16.8	26.4	10.9	47.4	27.0	15.3	9.0	38.3	11.1
25-34 years	25.8	9.1	25.5	9.4	31.8	8.7	46.7	21.6	8.4	4.5	25.4	7.3
35-44 years	21.9	8.3	22.2	8.4	24.7	8.3	37.8	21.4	7.4	5.0	20.8	6.4
45-64 years	21.1	8.6	20.7	8.7	26.9	8.8	38.3	10.4	9.0	6.3	19.6	8.1
65 years +	28.2	14.9	28.5	15.3	28.6	8.6	42.3	30.0	17.0	14.9	26.1	12.3

Table 4. Risk for Motor Vehicle Related Fatalities by Race/Ethnicity, Gender and Age: Total US Population, 2004

Rank	Rate per 100,000	Race/Ethnicity	Gender	Age
1	47.4	American Indian	Male	15-24
2	46.7	American Indian	Male	25-34
3	42.3	American Indian	Male	65+
4	39.1	White	Male	15-24
5	38.3	American Indian	Male	45-64
6	38.3	Hispanic/Latino	Male	15-24
7	31.8	Black	Male	25-34
8	30.0	American Indian	Female	65+
9	28.6	Black	Male	65+
10	28.5	White	Male	65+

(Data for Tables 1-4 abstracted from: Table 44. Death rates for motor vehicle-related injuries, by sex, race, Hispanic origin, and age: United States, selected years 1950-2004, accessed on April 7, 2008 at: www.cdc.gov/nchs/hus.htm). (15)

Fifty-eight percent of fatal crashes involved only one vehicle, compared to 31 percent of injury crashes and 31 percent of property-damage-only crashes. The occupant fatality rate (including motorcycle riders) per 100,000 population declined by 22.7 percent from 1975 to 1992, before leveling off between 1992 to 2005. Fatalities from motor vehicle traffic crashes declined by 868 (2%) from 43,510 in 2005 to 42,642 in 2006 while the occupant injury rate (including motorcycle riders) per 100,000 population declined by 37.2 percent from 1988 to 2005. Compared with other vehicle types, utility vehicles experienced the highest rollover rates in fatal crashes (35.4 percent) while large trucks experienced the highest rollover rate in injury crashes (9.9 percent). [16]

Persons 21 to 24 years of age have the highest fatality rates per 100,000 population while persons 16 to 20 years of age have the highest non-fatal injury rate. Children under 5 years old have both the lowest fatal and nonfatal injury rates per 100,000 population. For every age group, the fatality rate per 100,000 of the population is lower for females than for males. In contrast, the non-fatal injury rate is higher for females than for males in every age group of the population, except for people under 5 years old and those over 65 years old. [16]

Two and Three Wheel Motor Cycles

While travel by motor vehicle has become steadily safer in the United States, motorcycles remain the most dangerous type of motor vehicle to drive. In 2006 there were 4,810 motorcycle fatalities and 88,000 motorcyclists injured [17]. Motorcyclists are involved in fatal crashes at a rate of 35.0 per 100 million miles of travel over 20 times the rate of 1.7 per 100 million miles of travel in cars. Motorcycle rider fatalities increased by 5.1 percent, from 4,576 in 2005 to 4,810 in 2006 and as a proportion of overall traffic fatalities.

The rate of fatal motorcycle crashes among alcohol-impaired drivers was highest among 20-24 year-olds in 1983 and among 40-44 year-olds in 2003.

Pedal Cyclists

Bicycle are a leading cause of serious sports and recreational injury. In the United States, it has been estimated that there are 67 million bicyclists who ride approximately 15 billion hours per year. In 2005, bicycle-related injuries accounted for approximately 900 deaths, 23,000 hospital admissions, 580,000 emergency department visits and more than 1.2 million physician visits per year in the United States, resulting in an estimated annual cost of more than $8 billion. [18] Head injuries account for approximately one-third of emergency department visits for bike injuries, two-thirds of hospital admissions, and three-fourths of deaths. While 90 percent of all deaths involve collisions with motor vehicles, most non-fatal injuries are a result of falls, which often go unreported. The rate of severe injuries in urban areas resulting from riding a bicycle is 37.4 per 100,000 persons in the population. Thirty percent of bicyclist deaths each year occur in the 5-14 year old age group and approximately 20,000 children sustain a non-fatal injury to the head or face while riding. [19] It has been estimated that up to 51 percent of recreational and 85 percent of competitive mountain bikers sustain injuries each year.

Pedestrians

In 2000, 4,739 pedestrians were killed in traffic crashes in the United States, a 27 percent decrease in pedestrian fatalities since 1990 [16]. Sixty-eight percent of the pedestrian deaths in 2000 were males. The pedestrian fatality rate for males was more than double the rate of females (2.4 vs. 1.07 per 100,000 population) while the rate of non-fatal pedestrian injuries for males was 33, as compared to 23 for females. Pedestrian fatalities are far more likely to occur in urban areas (71 percent), at non-intersection locations (78 percent), in normal weather conditions (91 percent), and at night (64 percent). In pedestrian fatalities involving alcohol, pedestrians are more likely than drivers to have been drinking. [20]

African Americans, Latinos, and American Indians all are at much greater risk than Whites for fatal and nonfatal pedestrian injuries[21]. African Americans are at particularly high risk for traffic-related, pedestrian injury and fatality both in urban and rural settings. African American children in the 4–15 age range and Asian and Pacific Islanders older than 64, are at highest risk for pedestrian injuries. Like African Americans, Latinos make more walking and public transit trips than Whites and are more likely than Whites to be killed as pedestrians. The pedestrian fatality rate for American Indians was nearly three times the rate for Whites. [16]

The higher rate of pedestrian injury for African Americans appears to be the result of differences in transportation patterns since African Americans are less likely to own cars and much more likely to use public transit and to walk as compared to Whites. African Americans, American Indians and Latinos are particularly at risk for alcohol-related pedestrian fatalities. Voas and colleagues [22] found the presence of alcohol in about 40% of both African American and Latino pedestrian fatalities and over 70% of American Indian pedestrian fatalities.

Modifiable Risk Factors

Risk factors for road traffic injuries can be separated into four major categories: exposure to risk, risk factors influencing crash involvement, risk factors influencing crash severity, and risk factors influencing severity of post-crash injuries. [1]

Exposure to risk. Exposure to risk includes those factors which are associated with the need to travel such as who, where, why, how, and what time people are traveling. Exposure to risk for road traffic injuries varies based on a host of factors that shape how the need to travel is influenced by the mode of transportation, personal attributes of the traveler, the road environment, and the social/political/ economic context in which they reside and/or travel. The available transportation infrastructure, their socio-economic status, where someone lives and where they are going, the type of work one does and the amount of available leisure time one has all affect the exposure to risk for road traffic injuries. These factors are shaped by the economic wealth of a nation and its government, the expectations of government as a social change agent on behalf of the people, and the knowledge, attitudes, and behaviors of people towards traffic safety create the broader social context of road traffic behavior.

Risk factors influencing crash involvement. Risk factors influencing crash involvement typically are characteristics associated with the mode of travel (the agent), the traveler (the host), and the road environment (the environment) that, if changed, could prevent or minimize the impact of injuries associated with road traffic crashes. Overall, the major risk factors associated with the traveler (host) that influence crash involvement include demographic characteristics (male, 15-24 years of age, and race/ethnicity); excess speed, failure to hold a valid driver's license, failure to use safety features such as seatbelts and child safety seats, alcohol and drug use, age/experience, driver experience, risk taking behavior of the driver, and distractions such as friends in the vehicle and use of cellphones and being a vulnerable road user in urban and residential areas. Social/cultural risk factors include linguistic barriers, immigration status which may affect understanding of motor vehicle laws, larger family sizes, and increased preference of light trucks and vans.

Risk factors influencing injury severity. Other strategies seek to minimize the severity of injuries resulting from a road traffic crash by incorporating protective devices in the safety design and manufacturing of motor vehicles and roads and highways. In the Haddon Matrix activities that attempt to mitigate the severity of injury resulting from a road traffic crash typically target changes of the "agent" or "environment" during the "event." These efforts include adaptation and enforcement of motor vehicle and highway safety design standards and laws, such as front and side airbags, child passenger safety seats, and protective crash helmets by motor and pedal cyclists

Risk Factors influencing post-crash injury outcomes. Risk factors influencing post-crash injury outcomes include improving the response system to enhance the recovery process of crash victims, including improving emergency medical response, trauma, and rehabilitation care.

Interventions influencing post-crash injury outcomes are directly related to the availability and quality of response of the emergency medical service response, transport time, hospital care, and rehabilitation care available to the injured person.

Major Risk Factors for Racial/Ethnic Minorities

The major risk factors most commonly associated with motor traffic injuries include speed, seat belt and safety seat usage, use of alcohol, experience of the driver, distractions valid drivers license, and wearing helmets.

Speed. Speeding is a leading contributing factor to traffic crashes. Speeding reduces a driver's ability to negotiate curves and objects in the roadway, extends the distance necessary to stop, and increases the distance needed for a driver to react to a dangerous situation. Higher crash speeds also reduce the ability of vehicle, restraint system, and roadway hardware such as guardrails, barriers, and impact attenuators to protect vehicle occupants. [23]

Speed is associated with both crash risk and outcomes. The probability of a crash resulting in injury has been identified as proportional to the square of the speed [24]. A meta-analysis of the relationship between motor vehicle speed and risk of crash found a 2% reduction in the number of crashes with every 1 km/h reduction in speed, over 50 km/h [25]. Other studies have found that an increase of 1 km/h of traffic speed results in a 4-5% increase in motor traffic fatalities [26].

Nationally, speed accounts for approximately 34 percent of all fatal crashes. Sixty-three percent of people killed across the nation were killed in speed-related, single-vehicle crashes. Male drivers of all ages are more likely to be involved in speeding-related fatal crashes than female drivers. There is an inverse relationship between speeding related fatalities and driver's age for both males and females. About 41 percent of fatal crashes with drivers that were intoxicated were engaged in speeding (BAC= 0.08+) compared to about 14 percent of sober drivers. Motorcycle operators involved in fatal crashes were twice as likely as drivers of passenger cars, SUVs and pickup trucks to be speeding in 2002. Between 1975 and 2002, speed-related crashes accounted for more than 42 percent (2,501) of all motor vehicle crashes on Indian reservations (5,962). [27]

Seat belts. Ejection from a vehicle is one of the most injurious events that can happen to a person in a crash. In fatal crashes, 75 percent of passenger car occupants who were totally ejected from the vehicle were killed. [16] In 2006, 35 percent of passenger car occupants and 37 percent of light-truck occupants involved in fatal crashes were unrestrained. Research has shown that lap/shoulder seat belts, when used, reduce the risk of fatal injury to front seat occupants (age 5 and older) of passenger cars by 45 percent and the risk of moderate-to-critical injury by 50 percent. [28]

The overall observed seat belt usage rate in the United States in 2006, based on National Occupant Protection Use Survey (NOPUS) findings was 81%; 85% for females and 78% for males. [29] WA DC: National Center for Statistics and Analysis). Seat belt use rates vary widely, however, from state to state, reflecting differences in public attitudes, enforcement practices, legal provisions, and public information and education programs. NHTSA estimates that in 2006, seat belts saved 15,383 lives and that if all passenger vehicle occupants over age 4 wore seat belts, an additional 5,441 could have been saved.

Observed seat belt use rate in 2007 for adults with child passengers was 89% for Whites, 85% for Asians, 81% for Latinos/Hispanics, and 76% for African Americans. Compared to those residing in urban areas, American Indians living in rural areas were 60% more likely than non-Hispanic Whites. [30] Among racial/ethnic minorities, Asians and Pacific Islanders had the highest rate of safety belt use.

Safety Seats. In 2004, nearly 1,200 child passengers died and an estimated 180,000 were treated for motor vehicle injuries in U.S. hospital emergency departments (EDs). The percentage of unrestrained children who were hospitalized was three times that of restrained children. In 2006, it was estimated that 425 children under age 5 were saved as a result of child restraint use. Between 1978 and 2004, annual rates of child fatalities from motor vehicle crashes (MVCs) in the United States declined from 31.8 to 22.3 deaths per million and is attributed largely to the increased use of both child safety seats (for infants and young children) and seatbelts (for older children). [31]

A 2006 study conducted by the CDC found that among children injured in motor vehicle crashes, 45% were either not restrained or inappropriately restrained. Children in trucks were more likely to be inappropriately restrained when compared with children in cars, sports-utility vehicles, and vans (48% versus 40%). Most inappropriate restraint use occurred among children aged 4--8 years who were placed prematurely in seatbelts.

In 2000, less than half of African American, American Indian, and Latino children under 5 years of age in 2000 were restrained in child safety seats as compared to 58 percent of White children. [32] Asian and Pacific Islander children younger than 4 years of age were more likely to be in child safety seats or belted than other racial/ethnic minorities.

Air Bags. Air bags, combined with lap/shoulder seat belts, offer the most effective safety protection available today for motor vehicle occupants. Recent NHTSA analyses found a 14% reduction of motor vehicle fatalities when airbags with no seat belt was used and 11 percent when a seat belt was used in conjunction with air bags. While no studies of racial/ethnic differences were found that examined the role of airbags, Vaca, et al [33] found that Hispanic/Latinos were less knowledgeable about the risk of air bag deployment to young children by restraining them in the front seat.

Alcohol. Overall, thirty-nine percent of traffic crash fatalities and 9% of crashes with non-fatal injuries were alcohol-related. According to NHTSA, alcohol is a contributing factor in 41% of traffic crash fatalities (i.e., those in which a driver or pedestrian had a blood alcohol concentration [BAC] greater than zero) and 35% of crashes involving someone with a BAC of 0.08 percent or higher. Of all alcohol-related crashes in 2002, 4 percent resulted in a death, and 42 percent in an injury. In contrast, in crashes that did not involve alcohol, 0.6 percent resulted in a death, and 31 percent in an injury. Fatal crash risk nearly doubles with each 0.02-percent increase in BAC. Forty-six percent of male traffic deaths are alcohol related compared with 29 percent of female traffic deaths.

Alcohol related traffic deaths are most likely to occur among males, Native Americans and Mexican Americans, and people ages 21 to 45 years of age. American Indians have the highest percentage of alcohol-related traffic fatalities of any ethnic group. Among American Indians, alcohol is involved in 75% of driver fatalities and over 70% of pedestrian fatalities. [22] Alcohol involvement in fatalities related to motor vehicle crashes seems to vary among different Latino ethnic groups. Mexican Americans have a significantly higher rate than Whites, but Puerto Rican Americans, Cuban Americans, and Central and South Americans have the same or lower rates of alcohol related fatalities compared to Whites. [16] Recent research suggests that higher rates of driving after drinking might be because Blacks and Latinos tend to be concentrated in areas associated with community risk factors for drinking (e.g., poverty, billboard advertising, greater numbers of off-premise sales establishments). [34]

Experience. Immaturity and inexperience are primary factors contributing to fatal crashes by young drivers. Characteristics of teens that have been found to be related to motor vehicle morbidity and mortality include race, age, gender, cognition, driving experience, and level of acculturation [34-44] Other risk-factors for motor vehicle crashes among youth include current bio-physiological condition (e.g., motor skills, sleep deprivation, and psychiatric/ neurological status), mental status (e.g., mood, thoughts, feelings) [45], and behavioral dispositions, (e.g., risk taking, impulsivity) that the individual brings to the situation [38, 40, 41-43]. Adolescent drivers also tend to engage in numerous risky behaviors including speeding and other risk-taking behaviors such as following too closely, unsafe accelerations, and rapid lane changes. [44]

Distractions Teen drivers are easily distracted. While cell phones may add to distraction they are not the only distraction or necessarily the worst one. The risk of death increased significantly for drivers transporting passengers irrespective of the time of day or sex of the driver, although male drivers were at greater risk. One additional teen passenger in a car driven by a 16 year-old teen increases crash risk by about 50 percent; three or more teen passengers means the risk of crash is four times greater than driving alone. Driver deaths per 1000 crashes increased for 16- and 17-year-olds transporting male passengers or passengers younger than 30 years [46]. In addition, socio-economic status and family composition may increase risk of motor vehicle crashes by ethnic minority teens by thrusting the burden of family driving responsibilities on them at a young age, such as transporting family members to school, work, and appointments, etc. regardless of their readiness to drive. Increased number of passengers in the vehicle may increase risk by adding potential distractions.

Valid Drivers License. Fatally injured Native American and Hispanic drivers, followed by African American drivers, were less likely to hold valid licenses than White or Asian and Pacific Islander drivers. Native American drivers also were more likely to have had prior driving while intoxicated (DWI) convictions and license suspensions and African American drivers were the most likely to have had convictions for speeding and other moving violations. One out of four motorcycle operators (25%) involved in fatal crashes in 2006 were operating the vehicle with an invalid license at the time of the collision [47].

Helmets. Fatally injured Native American and Latino motorcycle riders were the least likely to wear helmets with a helmet use rate of 47 percent for both groups. Fatally injured White motorcycle riders were helmeted 51 percent of the time, whereas similar Black motorcycle riders wore helmets 58 percent of the time. The highest rate of helmet use by fatally injured motorcycle riders was for Asians and Pacific Islanders, at 67 percent [47].

Physical Environment. Features like left-turn across busy lanes, unprotected turn signals, poorly timed traffic signals, and multilane roads have been demonstrated to increase crash risk. [48-50]

Traffic Safety Promotion Interventions for Racial/Ethnic Minorities

Strategies which have been recommended by the Task Force on Community Preventive Services as effective based on research are presented below in Figure 1 [51]. While these strategies have been demonstrated as effective in reducing the overall fatality and injury rates in the general population, evidence of their effectiveness in reducing rates among racial/ethnic minorities and in reducing disparities in outcomes as compared to the majority population (e.g. non-Hispanic Whites) is not as clear.

In addition to strategies which have been demonstrated to be effective in reducing motor traffic fatalities and injuries in the overall population, increased attention needs to be given to reducing both the rates and disparities of traffic crash outcomes found among racial/ethnic minorities in comparison with non-Hispanic Whites. To accomplish this, targeted interventions that address the unique circumstances and conditions of special populations are needed. In the remainder of this chapter, modifiable risk factors will be reviewed and recommendations provided for adapting general strategies for use with racial/ethnic minority populations.

Exposure to Risk

Planned efforts to reduce exposure to road traffic crashes seek to prevent traffic injuries from occurring in the first place. They fall within the domain of primary prevention strategies and activities. Their aim is to prevent traffic injuries from occurring at all focus by changing the need to travel and are not necessarily limited to the travel itself, but to changing those conditions that create a need to travel. They fall within the range of activities that the Haddon Matrix refers to as "pre-event" and mostly target social, economic, and environmental change. Factors influencing exposure to risk include social/demographic and economic factors, only some of which are modifiable, land use decisions, mixture of road traffic use with vulnerable road users, and road traffic safety policies and engineering and design decisions.

Strategies to reduce exposure to road traffic crashes include a broad range of alternatives including short- and long-term *planning and policy-making* decisions regarding the built environment; promotion of telecommuting or working from home, to enacting mixed use zoning laws that promote co-existence of residential and commercial establishments within neighborhoods, making it possible to walk or cycle to stores, restaurants, and businesses. While these strategies may prove to be effective in reducing overall road traffic crash rate, their impact on reducing disparities between Whites and racial/ethnic minorities is unknown. For instance, successful efforts to decrease the need to travel by providing businesses and/or workers incentives to telecommute may reduce motor vehicle traffic injuries among professionals, but have little or even a negative impact on day laborers, resulting in both increased disparities and rates among low income racial/ethnic minority workers.

For strategies to be effective in reducing traffic fatalities and injury among racial/ethnic minorities through reducing exposure to risk, they must first and foremost target characteristics of the traveler and circumstances associated with the need to travel. Characteristics for consideration include: Is the travel work related and dictated by external constraints? Is the travel to complete personal tasks or for recreational purposes? How much flexibility of travel time is there? Are there options available for the traveler as to mode of travel? Is adaptation of motor vehicle safety limited by socio-economic status? Are there any social/cultural constraints on traveling? Any interventions that do not address the unique circumstances associated with the need to travel by different segments of the community are likely to fall short of their objective. Likewise, the implications of public policies that seek to reduce exposure to risk for the general population should be assessed for impact on different segments of society to ensure social equity.

Risk Factors Influencing Crash Involvement

According to Haddon's Matrix, risk factors influencing crash involvement can be modified to prevent injury to travelers. These activities generally fall within the domain of primary prevention and seek to reduce risk by modifying characteristics of the agent, host, or environment during the pre-injury stage to prevent crashes from occurring.

Pedestrians (V01-V09). Pre-event strategies for reducing pedestrian traffic injuries often target changes in knowledge, attitudes and behaviors of the host through community education and outreach. These include reducing alcohol use by drivers and pedestrians and encouraging pedestrians to make themselves more visible to drivers by wearing bright or reflective clothing, and for cyclists, to use reflectors, head lights, horns, and helmets. Passage, publicity and enforcement of public policies such as "3 foot laws" that seek to separate drivers from cyclists and pedestrians, and public education campaigns to increase pedestrian, cyclist, and motor vehicle driver rights and responsibilities, offer yet another pre-event strategy to reduce risk of crash involvement through education and outreach that targets the host (and driver).

Other pre-event strategies for reducing risk factors for crash involvement have targeted environmental change to separate vulnerable road traffic populations from drivers, vehicle speed management, and road management activities. Environmental strategies to prevent pedestrian road injuries include use of marked crosswalks and pedestrian signals that count down; "stop ahead when flashing" lights and signs; sidewalks; and pedestrian tunnels and bridge crossings. Separation of pedestrians and cyclists from motor vehicles have been achieved by creating separated bike and pedestrian paths and clearly marked and lit and well maintained bike lanes on roads. Efforts to reduce speed of motor vehicles include enhanced enforcement, improved signage, and speed humps. Road management strategies that have been adopted to reduce risk of crash involvement include incorporation of turn lanes, enhanced road visibility, routine road maintenance, barriers to prevent pedestrian access or crossing, traffic signals, and rerouting of traffic away from residential areas and schools.

Pedal cycles (V10-V19). Strategies that have been proposed for preventing pedal cycle injuries target the bike equipment (agent), behavior (host), and environment. Some injury preventive interventions have addressed mechanical concerns associated with the agent (bike) including ensuring correct fit of bicycle, regular safety checks, effective brakes, fenders, spoke guards, child carrier seats, suspension, handlebar padding, and use of reflectors—front, rear, pedal, and wheels. Other primary prevention strategies have targeted the cyclist (host) include *educating* pedal cyclists and motor vehicle drivers about rules, rights, and responsibilities; promoting use of safety helmets; and skills teaching and bike maintenance clinics. They also include getting the cyclist to use protective equipment such as helmets, gloves, eye protection, shoes, reflective and bright clothing, and lights. Environmental interventions to prevent cycling injuries have included improved design and *engineering* of safe and accessible roadways and bicycle facilities; *enforcing* proper behaviors and use of roadway facilities; separated bicycle lands/cycle paths, street lights, and improved connectivity and access to *transit facilities*. Scientific evidence has shown that the single most effective safety equipment available to reduce head injury and death from bicycle crashes is a helmet, which reduces the risk of bicycle-related death and injury. Bicycle helmet education campaigns and improvements in helmet design also have likely made a difference. [52]

Motorcycles. The main risks for motorcycle users arise from failure to wear a crash helmet and low visibility. Therefore, passage and enforcement of public policies and educational strategies to increase the use of helmets and to increase visibility of motorcyclists, by encourage them to operate their lights in the daytime offer the main pre-event opportunities for decreasing risk of serious and fatal crash injuries.

Motor vehicles with four or more wheels. Traffic safety interventions for crash involvement that target the host include better education and training of new drivers, promoting usage of seat belts and child safety seats; reducing alcohol consumption and speeding; and minimizing in-vehicle distractions. Other interventions that target the host include the use of mass media and health education campaigns to promote road traffic safety and the passage and enforcement of laws to minimize risky behaviors.

Passage and enforcement of public policies appear to provide the most effective opportunities for reducing risk of traffic crash injuries. Primary seat belt legislation that authorizes law enforcement officers to pull over a motorist and write a ticket for failure to wear a seat belt and graduated drivers licenses for teen drivers have been demonstrated to be effective in reducing motor traffic fatalities and injuries. The greater decline in alcohol-related traffic deaths among 16- to 20-year-olds is in part attributable to the adoption of age 21 as the legal drinking age, which occurred in all states by 1988. A review of more than 49 studies of changes in the legal drinking age revealed that in the 1980s and 1990s when many states lowered the legal drinking age, alcohol-related traffic crashes involving drivers under 21 increased 10 percent. In contrast, when states increased the legal drinking age to 21, alcohol-related crashes among people under 21 decreased an average of 16 percent [53]. Other policy examples include banning hand-held cell phones, lowering the legal blood alcohol content (BAC) level, sobriety checkpoints, cameras at intersections, and routine vision exams as part of the driver license exams. Other efforts to decrease alcohol use include management-supported intervention training programs for alcohol servers, designated drivers, and free ride programs. The effectiveness of some of these approaches has not yet been demonstrated.

Some strategies to reduce risk of traffic injuries have targeted the vehicle (agent), and include improved motor vehicle manufacturing safety standards, vehicle inspections of commercial vehicles, and adaptation of center mounted brake lights. Efforts to design vehicles that provide better visibility to the driver and to make them more visible to others, maintain safe speeds, and enable the driver to easily change positioning of mirrors, seats, and steering wheel are additional examples of interventions that seek to prevent crashes from occurring through changes of the "agent" or vehicle. Other interventions to increase motor vehicle safety include strategies that have targeted vehicular changes, such as safety belt use monitoring devices, ignition interlock devices, and improvements in comfort and convenience.

Alterations to the physical environment have included changes to the transportation infrastructure through roadway design, roadway hazards, and safety features. Changing roadway design has been used to influence driving behaviors. Traffic safety interventions have included adopting features like turn lanes, four-way stops, speed humps, islands and roundabouts to slow traffic, traffic signals with turn arrows, synchronized signals, and anti-icing systems on roads [54-56]. Efforts to address low lighting conditions and wet or icy roads also have been undertaken to reduce the risk of motor vehicle accidents. Environmental strategies for reducing crash risk also include road width, maintenance, surface quality, speed limit, road lighting, and signage.

Risk Factors Influencing Injury Severity

Strategies to reduce risk of injury severity have focused primarily on efforts to modify the agent and the environment. Risk reduction strategies targeting the agent include use of front and side airbags, collapsible steering column assembly, knee bar structures, and other design features of vehicle interiors to minimize intrusion of the vehicle into the driver or passenger compartments. Research also has shown that the fronts of cars (agent) can be designed to reduce the level of death and injury to pedestrians who are struck by a motor vehicle. Other interventions to reduce risk of injury include modification of the design of motorcycles to incorporate effective leg protection and use of front airbags to protect riders in the case of a head-on collision.

Environmental changes that have been adapted to reduce injury severity resulting from a road traffic crash include enhancing roadside protections such as use of barriers on curves, runaway ramps for trucks on steep road declines, crash cushions, safety barriers, retractable lane delineators, and impact attenuators.

Risk Factors Influencing Post-Crash Injury Outcomes

Environmental risk factors include a lack of access to public transportation and a lack of access to immediate medical care following a motor vehicle crash. Improvements to emergency response systems, including improving emergency medical response, trauma, and rehabilitation care have been demonstrated to be effective measures for enhancing the recovery process of crash victims,

Implications

Over the past twenty years, reductions in injuries resulting from road traffic crashes in the United States have been realized through a broad range of universal activities including better engineering and maintenance of roads and design of vehicles; passage of legislation and increased enforcement to control speed, seat belt use, child passenger restraints, alcohol use, etc; efforts to increase awareness among the general population about motor vehicle safety through health education, community outreach, and the mass media; and improved emergency medical response, trauma care, and rehabilitation services. Efforts to reduce rates of road traffic crashes have yielded significant overall reductions in road traffic mortality and injuries during this period. However, these broad efforts have not had the same impact on all segments of the population. A careful analysis of road traffic fatality and injury rates reveals dramatic differences by characteristics of the agent, host, environment, and the interaction of risk factors.

Injury, disability, and death from motor vehicle crashes among racial/ethnic minorities can be reduced through two broad categories of interventions: 1) those targeting the general population and 2) those that are targeted towards particular racial/ethnic groups. To date, most interventions have relied on strategies that fall into the first category, while few have specifically targeted racial/ethnic minority groups.

Despite a continuing decline in the adverse effects of motor vehicle crashes in the general population, disparities in death, disability, and injury continue to exist for African American, American Indians and Latinos in comparison with non-Hispanic Whites. While it is important to continue efforts to affect changes in behaviors through health education, media and changes at the community level, new efforts also are needed. A model of driving behavior based on ecological theory is presented in Figure 2 that offers a more comprehensive and dynamic approach for increasing traffic safety among racial/ethnic minority populations. For strategies to increase seat belt use in these groups, they also must address the ways in which the physical, social, political, and economic environment of a community, shape individual behaviors. Efforts that employ multiple levels of prevention strategies, culturally and linguistically appropriate messaging, and engage the target population in the development and implementation of targeted strategies are more likely to be effective. Multi-level, multi-faceted interventions hold great promise for not only reducing motor vehicle injury, disability, and death among racial/ethnic minority populations, but also for reducing disparities in these outcomes.

Child safety seat laws	R
Community-wide information and enhanced enforcement	R
Distribution and education campaigns	R
Incentive and education programs	R
Education programs when used alone	IE
Use of Safety Belts	
Safety belt laws	R
Primary enforcement laws	R
Enhanced enforcement	R
Reducing Alcohol- Impaired Driving	
.08 blood alcohol concentration (BAC) laws	R
Lower BAC laws for young or inexperienced drivers	R
Minimum legal drinking age laws	R
Sobriety checkpoints	R
Intervention training programs for servers of alcoholic beverages	R
Mass media campaigns	R
School-based programs	
School-based instructional programs	R
Peer organization programs	IE
Social norming programs	IE
Designated driver programs	
Population-based campaigns	IE
Incentive programs	IE
Multicomponent interventions with community mobilization	R
Ignition Interlocks	R

Accessed on April 7, 2008 at: http://www.thecommunityguide.org/mvoi/default.htm

Figure 1. Community Preventive Services Recommendations to Prevent Motor Vehicle Occupant Injury [71].

Strategies that Target the General Population. Interventions that have been identified as having the greatest impact on increasing motor traffic safety include: changes in public policy, such as primary and secondary enforcement laws; graduated drivers licenses, high-visibility enforcement, and increased sanctions for alcohol use, speeding, and safety belt violations including increased fines and points on the driver's license. A list of interventions that have been demonstrated through research to be effective in preventing motor traffic fatalities and injury is presented in *Figure 1: Community Preventive Services Recommenda-*

tions to Prevent Motor Vehicle Occupant Injury. [71] Many of the strategies that have been demonstrated to be effective in reducing motor traffic injuries in the general population, including racial and ethnic minorities, but they have not reduced the disparities in injury outcomes as compared to non-Hispanic Whites.

Strategies that Target Racial/Ethnic Minority Communities. The conditions, experiences, needs, and resources available to different racial/ethnic minority groups can not be assumed to be the same. Racial/ethnic minorities in the United States have varied needs to travel based on their social/cultural experience, economic condition, and individual circumstance: some live in densely populated urban neighborhoods, others in isolated rural areas; some are engaged in agricultural and seasonal employment while others work from home, connected to the world by their car, telephone, and computer. Still others are dependent on walking, cycling, and public transportation to meet their needs. There is a growing awareness that universal interventions aimed at the general population of a country are received differently and yield different results among subgroups of the population.

In addition to universal interventions and messages, culturally and linguistically appropriate efforts are now needed to reduce the continuing health disparities resulting from road traffic injuries among racial/ethnic minority populations. Furthermore, culturally and linguistically appropriate, targeted efforts to shape messages and interventions must respond to the conditions and circumstances of minority populations if continuing, traffic related, injury disparities are to be reduced among those at greatest risk.

To influence social norms and behaviors in minority communities, strategies will be needed that incorporate multiple levels of interventions such as health education, public media campaigns [91, 92], community messaging, and traffic law enforcement [91, 93]. Community-based strategies that engage the target population in prevention efforts are likely to be the most effective. For instance, focus groups can be conducted with the target population (e.g. African American teens) to help in the development and/or adaptation of developmentally, culturally, linguistically, and environmentally appropriate messages. The most successful media campaigns have employed a social-marketing approach in which multiple themes are directed at specific demographic groups (e.g., Latinos, African Americans, etc.), followed by consumer testing and feedback, and message adjustment based on the feedback. [57-58] Other community messaging strategies could include engaging families, schools, the faith community and other local institutions, organizations, and businesses to reinforce a "buckle up" message that is likely to be more effective than a general media campaign.

Culturally specific campaigns use messengers who come from that community and tailor language, concepts, images, and messages so the target audience can relate, and are responsive to the environmental conditions in which teens and their families live. [59-62] Coordination with local service providers and community leaders can ensure that the messages and visual images developed are both powerful and sensitive to that community. To ensure the strategies, messengers, and message are culturally and linguistically appropriate, consideration should be given to including the target group in the development and/or review of curricula and or health education messaging prior to implementation.

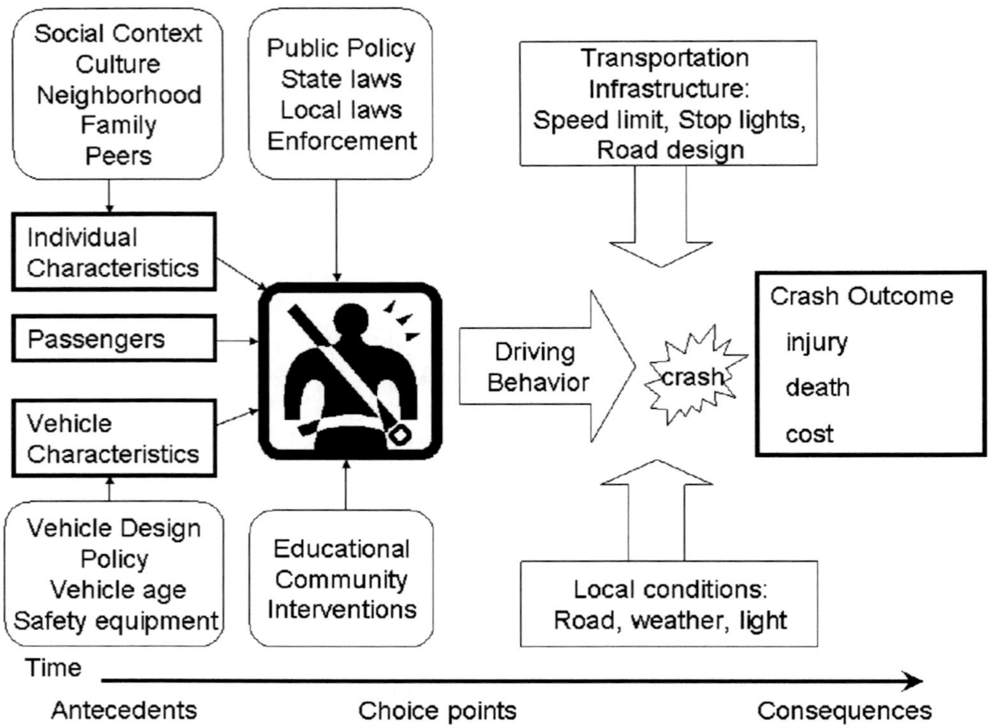

Figure 2. Conceptual Framework: Developmental-Ecological Model.

Inner city and rural communities of high poverty where minority populations are most likely to live, often lack social and economic resources that provide residents with opportunities for healthy growth and development. Interventions that target behavioral change among racial/ethnic minorities must be responsive to their unique physical, social, political, and economic environments. In low income communities of color, strategies that coordinate with and/or are integrated into other public health interventions need to take advantage of existing social capital. Many community organizations already work with racial/ethnic minority groups on issues such as HIV/AIDS prevention, substance abuse prevention, violence prevention, conflict resolution, and sexuality education. Where effective programs exist, advocates should partner with these organizations to add information about seat belt use and other risk factors for motor vehicle crashes.

Even within racial/ethnic minorities, interventions must be responsive to the unique social realities of subgroups within the broader racial/ethnic group. Other differences that shape the way life is experienced and information processed by subgroups include age, gender, ethnicity, rural/urban, and sub-national regions. Safe driving campaigns that target youth, for example, should consider using a range of delivery media such as foreign language radio stations and other nontraditional media outlets to reach the widest audience. At the individual level, health education messages need to be communicated in ways that minority youth will identify. For urban African American youth, this may mean using hip-hop music, advertising, youth websites, and text messaging as potential media [or strategies] for getting the message out. In rural areas, in contrast, strategies might include use of billboards, flyers, and talk radio. In a rural area, influential figures for teens may be more likely to be the faith community, community leaders, and authority figures whereas in an urban environment, the most effective messengers may be entertainers, sports figures, or celebrities.

In addition, concerns of racial/ethnic minority communities must be understood and addressed. Passage of primary seat belt legislation has been resisted by many African Americans, even though it has been demonstrated to be effective in increasing seat belt rates and motor vehicle fatalities. There is a strong level of concern among African Americans and elected officials that increased law enforcement efforts of primary safety belt laws will lead to increased racial profiling of minority drivers. Likewise, even though enhanced, highly visible enforcement and media publicity have been shown to be highly effective in promoting traffic safety, there are significant personnel and financial resource limitations to those approaches in many low income minority communities.

Understanding how racial/ethnic minority populations make decisions regarding driving and risk taking behaviors, and the variables that influence those decisions requires articulation of a dynamic, theoretical framework. The factors that influence the driving behaviors of different minority populations, the likelihood that they will engage in risk taking or health promoting behaviors and activities, and how characteristics of both the motor vehicle and the environment affect them and subsequent outcomes must be incorporated into the framework. [63-65]. In *Figure 2*, a multi-faceted, multi-level model is presented that is based on developmental and ecological theory [66-68] for understanding racial/ethnic minority driving behavior and its consequences. This model views behavior as dynamically interacting with and responsive to a series of expanding spheres of environmental influence. [69-70] This multi-level approach is useful because it allows for the consideration and integration of current and historical, social, cultural, economic and political conditions as potential sources of influence on individual behavior. [8]

According to this model, the same complex systems that create the context for behaviors also mediate and moderate the consequences of these behaviors. Some consequences are immediate, while others are intermediate or long-term. Adverse outcomes of driving behaviors are typically described in terms of personal injury, disability, and death. Yet, outcomes of behavioral choices also have a detrimental effect on others, including family members, peers, neighbors and the community. Some choices having long-term personal physical, emotional, and financial consequences (e.g., serious injury, drunk driving conviction, increases in insurance rates) while others may have incremental effects on social, political, environmental, and economic systems (the activism of Mothers Against Drunk Drivers is an example).

While this model of driving behavior of racial/ethnic minorities is presented as moving through time from left to right, it is in reality, an iterative process, in which new events continually combine with antecedents to influence the choices of the individual in the present. Choices made in the present affect subsequent behavioral decisions creating new situations that influence and constrain future choices. It is in the present, however, that an individual has an opportunity to make choices about driving behaviors that increase or decrease the risk of a crash.

The proposed model is offered as a guide for considering the range and combination of strategies that might be adapted within a community to increase traffic safety outcomes of racial/ethnic minority populations. The model asserts that multi-faceted and multi-level interventions hold the greatest promise for promoting traffic safety and in reducing adverse outcomes among racial/ethnic minority communities. It suggests that interventions that engage communities in their development and implementation are likely to be more effective than solutions imposed by experts or government agencies. While participatory approaches are important in all communities, engaging the community is critically important for racial/ethnic minority populations. Messages must be presented in developmentally, culturally, and linguistically appropriate ways and in a time and place where the message will be heard. The messenger must be someone with whom the targeted audience can readily identify, and the message must be presented through a medium to which the target group is receptive.

Continued efforts that attempt to decrease risky driving behaviors in the general population are an important part of an overall strategy to increase seat belt use among racial/ethnic minority populations. Current efforts need to be reexamined, however, to evaluate their effectiveness in reducing health disparities in motor vehicle injuries found in racial/ethnic minority populations. In areas where disparities in seat belt use and other risky driving behaviors exist, it must be assumed that these efforts are not having their intended impact. In these communities the strategies, messenger, and message need to be examined for their cultural and linguistic appropriateness.

Limitations

The three principal sources of data on road traffic fatalities in the United States are severely limited in the way they report race/ ethnicity. These three data sources include mortality statistics from the National Center for Health Statistics, the *Fatal Analysis Reporting System* (FARS), and NHTSA's National Occupant Protection Use Survey (NOPUS). The difference in classification of race/ethnicity for road traffic fatalities is a major limitation to research conducted on racial/ethnic differences in road traffic outcomes.

The Centers for Disease Control uses vital statistics to identify road traffic fatalities as reported by states to the National Center for Health Statistics (NCHS). The NCHS is dependent on a subjective determination made by a coroner or medical examiner at the city or county level. Medical examiners are typically physicians appointed to office while coroners are generally elected to office without any formal medical training. Differences in personnel and their training introduce sources of variation and inconsistency both in the coding of race/ethnicity as well as in the cause of death.

The *Fatality Analysis Reporting System* (FARS) has only collected data on race/ethnicity since 1999, limiting historical comparisons of road crash fatalities. Prior to 1999, race and Hispanic origin data were obtained by linking FARS data with mortality data from the Centers for Disease Control's National Center for Health Statistics (NCHS). The FARS now reports data on race/ethnicity in accordance with Federal standards set forth by the Office of Management and Budget (OMB) in: "Revisions to the Standards for the Classification of

Federal Data on Race and Ethnicity, Federal Register Notice, Volume 62, Number 210, pages 58781-58790, October 30, 1997," available at www.omb.gov. [9]

Specifically, the following 10 race/ethnicity categories are employed in the survey data collection:

- Not Hispanic or Latino and
  - American Indian or Alaska Native
  - Asian
  - Black or African-American
  - Native Hawaiian or Pacific Islander
  - White

- Hispanic or Latino and
  - American Indian or Alaska Native
  - Asian
  - Black or African-American
  - Native Hawaiian or Pacific Islander
  - White

Likewise the validity of data on race/ethnicity from NHTSA's National Occupant Protection Use Survey (NOPUS), a probability-based annual survey of observed safety belt use in the United States, is limited, relying on observers to subjectively assess race/ethnicity of motor vehicle occupants during random street intersection observations. Observers are asked to judge race as White, Black, or other, and makes no attempt to characterize Hispanic origin.

A second problem with current data used to make comparisons of racial/ethnic differences in road traffic safety, is that data are often presented differently, making comparisons difficult. For instance, a different picture emerges when motor vehicle fatality rates are standardized per 100,000 of a population group than when they are presented per vehicle-miles of travel (VMT).

A third problem associated with using race/ethnicity data to determine the prevalence of injury and death resulting from road traffic crashes is that rates vary dramatically not only across racial/ethnic groups, but within them as well, thus masking intra-racial/ethnic differences. Within any racial/ethnic group the prevalence of road traffic injuries varies by gender, age, social-economic status, educational attainment, urban/rural residence, and level of cultural assimilation. Consequently differences are more likely to be greater within racial groups than between them.

Without more accurate data, it is difficult to sort out the independent effects of race/ethnicity on outcomes of road traffic crashes from other characteristics, such as educational attainment and socio-economic status. Road traffic injuries and deaths for persons living in poor and underserved urban and rural areas may vary, for instance, not due to race/ethnicity, but due to mode of travel, vehicle miles traveled, geographic region of the country in which they reside, or presence of lack thereof of environmental conditions such as crosswalks, traffic signals, and street lighting. Differences in seat belt use also may be due to socio-economic factors such as lack of income to purchase safety equipment such as child passenger safety seats or modern motor vehicles with enhanced safety engineering or to lack of access to culturally and developmentally appropriate messaging promoting road traffic safety. Despite these data gathering limitations, there is sufficient evidence to suggest that there are significant disparities in health outcomes attributable to motor vehicle crashes among racial/ethnic groups and subpopulations of ethnic groups in the United States.

Appendix A International Statistical Classification of Diseases and Related Health Problems 10th Revision, Version for 2007 [3]

Accessed on April 7, 2008 at: http://www.who.int/classifications/apps/icd/icd10online/

This chapter, which in previous revisions of ICD constituted a supplementary classification, permits the classification of environmental events and circumstances as the cause of injury, poisoning and other adverse effects. Where a code from this section is applicable, it is intended that it shall be used in addition to a code from another chapter of the Classification indicating the nature of the condition. Most often, the condition will be classifiable to Chapter XIX, Injury, poisoning and certain other consequences of external causes (S00-T98). Causes of death should preferably be tabulated according to both Chapter XIX and Chapter XX, but if only one code is tabulated then the code from Chapter XX should be used in preference. Other conditions that may be stated to be due to external causes are classified in Chapters I to XVIII. For these conditions, codes from Chapter XX should be used to provide additional information for multiple-condition analysis only.
Categories for sequelae of external causes of morbidity and mortality are included at Y85-Y89.

Chapter XIX: Injury, Poisoning and Certain other Consequences of External Causes (S00-T98)

S00-S09	Injuries to the head
S10-S19	Injuries to the neck
S20-S29	Injuries to the thorax
S30-S39	Injuries to the abdomen, lower back, lumbar spine and pelvis
S40-S49	Injuries to the shoulder and upper arm
S50-S59	Injuries to the elbow and forearm
S60-S69	Injuries to the wrist and hand
S70-S79	Injuries to the hip and thigh
S80-S89	Injuries to the knee and lower leg
S90-S99	Injuries to the ankle and foot
T00-T07	Injuries involving multiple body regions
T08-T14	Injuries to unspecified part of trunk, limb or body region
T15-T19	Effects of foreign body entering through natural orifice

T20-T32	Burns and corrosions
T20-T25	Burns and corrosions of external body surface, specified by site
T26-T28	Burns and corrosions confined to eye and internal organs
T29-T32	Burns and corrosions of multiple and unspecified body regions
T33-T35	Frostbite
T36-T50	Poisoning by drugs, medicaments and biological substances
T51-T65	Toxic effects of substances chiefly nonmedicinal as to source
T66-T78	Other and unspecified effects of external causes
T79	Certain early complications of trauma
T80-T88	Complications of surgical and medical care, not elsewhere classified
T90-T98	Sequelae of injuries, of poisoning and of other consequences of external causes

Chapter XX: Accidents

V01-V99	Transport accidents
V01-V09	Pedestrian injured in transport accident
V10-V19	Pedal cyclist injured in transport accident
V20-V29	Motorcycle rider injured in transport accident
V30-V39	Occupant of three-wheeled motor vehicle injured in transport accident
V40-V49	Car occupant injured in transport accident
V50-V59	Occupant of pick-up truck or van injured in transport accident
V60-V69	Occupant of heavy transport vehicle injured in transport accident
V70-V79	Bus occupant injured in transport accident
V80-V89	Other land transport accidents
V90-V94	Water transport accidents
V95-V97	Air and space transport accidents
V98-V99	Other and unspecified transport accidents

References

[1] Peden M, Scurfield R, Sleet D, Mohan D, Hyder AA, Jarawan E, and Mathers C. 2004. *World report on road traffic injury prevention*. Geneva: World Health Organization

[2] Murray CJL, and Lopez, AD, eds. 1996. The global burden of disease: a comprehensive assessment of mortality and disability from diseases, injuries, and risk factors in 1990 and projected to 2020. Boston, MA: Harvard School of Public Health.

[3] World Health Organization. 2007. ICD-10 Codes for 2007, 10th Revision. Accessed on April 23, 2008 at: http://www.who.int/classifications/apps/icd/icd10online/

[4] Haddon W. On the escape of tigers: an ecologic note. *Am. J. Public Health* 1970;60:2229–34.

[5] Subramanian, R., Motor vehicle traffic crashes as a leading cause of death in the United States, 2000. *Traffic Safety Facts Research Note (DOT HS 809 661).* Traffic Safety Facts Research Note (DOT HS 809 661), 2003.

[6] http://www.nhtsa.dot.gov/portal/site/nhtsa/menuitem

[7] NHTSA, 2008. *Traffic Safety Facts: 2006 Data.* DOT HS 810 809.

[8] Juarez PD, Schlundt DG, Goldzweig I, Stinson Jr. N. A conceptual framework for reducing risky teen driving behaviors among minority youth. *Injury Prevention* 2006; 12(Supplement 1):i49-i55.

[9] Office of Management and Budget (OMB). "Revisions to the Standards for the Classification of Federal Data on Race and Ethnicity, Federal Register Notice, Volume 62, Number 210, pages 58781-58790, October 30, 1997," available at www.omb.gov.

[10] www.hrsa.gov

[11] NHTSA. 2006. Race and Ethnicity Factors in Fatal Motor Vehicle Traffic Crashes 1999 – 2004. WA DC: National Center for Statistics and Analyses.

[12] Wallace LJD, Patel R, Dellinger A. Injury Mortality Among American Indian and Alaska Native Children and Youth --- United States, 1989—1998. *MMWR*. August 1, 2003 / 52(30);697-701.

[13] NHTSA Technical Report. Judith Hilton, Race and ethnicity in fatal motor vehicle traffic crashes: 1999-2004. DOT HS 809 956. May 2006.

[14] Office of Statistics and Programming, National Center for Injury Prevention and Control, CDC. National Estimates of Nonfatal Injuries Treated in Hospital Emergency Departments --- United States, 2000. *MMWR*. May 04, 2001 / 50(17);340-6.

[15] National Center for Health Statistics. Monitoring the nation's health, Health, United States, 2007. Accessed on April 23, 2008 at: http://www.cdc.gov/nchs/products/pubs/pubd/hus/injury.htm#deaths

[16] Fatality Analysis Reporting System (FARS) Encyclopedia. Accessed on April 23, 2008 at: http://www-fars.nhtsa.dot.gov/Main/DidYouKnow.aspx

[17] NHTSA. 2007. *2006 Motorcycles Traffic Safety Fact Sheet (Updated March 2008)* DOT 810806. accessed on April 23, 2008 at: http://www-nrd.nhtsa.dot.gov/CATS/listpublications.aspx?Id=AandShowBy=DocType

[18] Thompson MJ and Rivara FP. Bicycle related injuries. *Am. Fam. Physician* 2001; 63: 2007-14,2017-8.

[19] Rodgers GB, editor. *Bicycle use and hazard patterns in the United States*. U.S. Consumer Product Safety Commission, Washington D.C., 1994.

[20] O'Malley, P.M. and L.D. Johnston, *Unsafe driving by high school seniors: national trends from 1976 to 2001 in tickets and accidents after use of alcohol, marijuana and other illegal drugs. J. Stud. Alcohol*, 2003. 64(3): p. 305-12.

[21] NHTSA. 2003. *Pedestrian Roadway Fatalities*. DOT Technical Report 809456.

[22] Voas RB, Tippetts S, Fisher D, *Ethnicity and Crash Involvement* for National Highway Traffic Safety Administration, Wash., DC, 20590; 17 Feb., 1999; Berkeley: CA Prevention Research Center.

[23] Liu C, Chen CL, Subramanian R, Utter D. 2005. *Analysis of Speeding-Related Fatal Motor Vehicle Traffic Crashes*. NHTSA Technical Report DOT HS 809 839. Springfield, VA: National Technical Information Service.

[24] Nilsson G. 1982. *The effects of speed limits on traffic accidents in Sweden*. Sartryckd: Swedish National Road and Transport Research Institute.

[25] Elvik R. Mysen AB, Vaa T. 1997. *Trafikksikkerhetshandbok tredje utgave [Handbook of traffic safety*, 3rd ed.]. Oslo: Institute of Tranport Economics.

[26] Taylor, MC, Lynam DA, Baruya A. 2000. T*he effects of drivers' speed on the frequency of road accidents.* Crowthorne: Transport Research Laboratory (TRL Report 421).

[27] NHTSA. 2004. *Fatal Motor Vehicle Crashes on Indian Reservations 1975 – 2002.* DOT HS 809 727 WA DC: National Center for Statistics and Analysis.

[28] NHTSA, 2008. *Traffic Safety Facts: 2006 Data.* DOT HS 810 809.

[29] NHTSA, 2007. *Seat Belt Use in 2006 – Demographic Results.* DOT HS 810 766.

[30] Glassbrenne D., Jianqiang Ye T. 2008. *Traffic Safety Facts: 2006 Data.* DOT HS 810 896. WA DC: National Center for Statistics and Analysis.

[31] Insurance Institute for Highway Safety. Fatality facts: 2004. Arlington, VA: Insurance Institute for Highway Safety; 2005. (accessed on April 22, 2008 at: http://www.iihs.org/research/fatality_facts/pdfs/children.pdf

[32] CDC, Nonfatal Injuries and Restraint Use Among Child Passengers --- United States, 2004. *MMWR.* June 9, 2006 / 55(22);624-627.

[33] Vaca F, Anderson CL, Agran P, Winn D and Cheng G. Child Safety Seat Knowledge Among Parents Utilizing Emergency Services in a Level I Trauma Center in Southern California *Pediatrics* 2002;110;e61.

[34] Holubowycz OT and McLean AJ. 1995. Demographic characteristics, drinking patterns and drink-driving behaviour of injured male drivers and motorcycle riders, *Journal of Studies on Alcohol* 56:513–521.

[35] Galovski TE., et al., The psychophsiology of aggressive drivers: comparison to non-aggressive drivers and pre- to post-treatment change following a cognitive-behavioural treatment. *Behav. Res. Ther,* 2003:41(9):055-67.

[36] Deery HA and Fildes BN. Young novice driver subtypes: relationship to high-risk behavior, traffic accident record, and simulator driving performance. *Hum. Factors.* 1999. 41(4)628-43.

[37] Cummings P., et al. Drowsiness, counter-measures to drowsiness, and the risk of a motor vehicle crash. *Inj. Prev,* 2001. 7(3)194-9.

[38] Zuckerman, M. and Kuhlman DM. Personality and risk-taking: common biosocial factors. *J. Pers,* 2000. 68(6)999-1029.

[39] Hoyle, R.H., Personality processes and problem behavior. *J. Pers,* 2000. 68(6): p. 953-66.

[40] Turner C and McClure R. Age and gender differences in risk-taking behaviour as an explanation for high incidence of motor vehicle crashes as a driver in young males. *Inj. Control Saf. Promot,* 2003. 10(3)123-30.

[41] Woodward LJ, Fergusson DM, and Horwood LJ. Driving outcomes of young people with attentional difficulties in adolescence. *J. Am. Acad. Child Adolesc. Psychiatry,* 2000. 39(5)627-34.

[42] Bingham CR Shope JT. Adolescent developmental antecedents of risky driving among young adults. *J. Stud. Alcohol,* 2004. 65(1)84-94.

[43] Anstey KJ et al., Cognitive, sensory and physical factors enabling driving safety in older adults. *Clin. Psychol. Rev,* 2005. 25(1)45-65.

[44] McKnight AJ and McKnight AS. The behavioral contributors to highway crashes of youthful drivers. *Annu. Proc. Assoc. Adv. Automot. Med,* 2000. 44: 321-33.

[45] O'Malley PM and Johnston LD. Unsafe driving by high school seniors: national trends from 1976 to 2001 in tickets and accidents after use of alcohol, marijuana and other illegal drugs. *J. Stud. Alcohol*, 2003. 64(3)305-12.

[46] Carrying Passengers as a Risk Factor for Crashes Fatal to 16- and 17-Year-Old Drivers (Chen L, Baker SP, Braver ER, Li G. *Carrying Passengers as a Risk Factor for Crashes Fatal to 16- and 17-Year-Old Drivers. JAMA.* 2000;283:1578-1582.

[47] NHTSA, 2006 Data. *Motorcycles*. DOT HS 810 806.

[48] Abdel-Aty M and Keller J. Exploring the overall and specific crash severity levels at signalized intersections. *Accid. Anal. Prev*, 2005. 37(3)417-25.

[49] Newton C, et al. Evaluation of an alternative traffic light change anticipation system. *Accid. Anal. Prev*, 1997. 29(2)201-9.

[50] Retting RA, et al., A simple method for identifying and correcting crash problems on urban arterial streets. *Accid. Anal. Prev*, 2001. 33(6)723-34.

[51] Task Force on Community Preventive Services. Recommendations to Reduce Injuries to Motor Vehicle Occupants Increasing Child Safety Seat Use, Increasing Safety Belt Use, and Reducing Alcohol-Impaired Driving. *Am. J. Prev. Med.* 2001;21(4S)16–22.

[52] Wallis AL, Cody BE, Mickalide AD. Report to the Nation: Trends in Unintentional Childhood Injury Mortality, 1987-2000. Washington (DC): National SAFE KIDS Campaign, May 2003.

[53] Shults RA, Sleet DA, Elder RW, Ryan GW and Sehgal M. Association between state level drinking and driving countermeasures and self reported alcohol impaired driving. *Inj. Prev.* 2002;8:106-110.

[54] Bunn F, et al. Area-wide traffic calming for preventing traffic related injuries. *Cochrane Database Syst. Rev,* 2003(1): p. CD003110.

[55] Elvik R. Area-wide urban traffic calming schemes: a meta-analysis of safety effects. *Accid. Anal. Prev,* 2001. 33(3)327-36.

[56] Morrison DS, Petticrew M, Thomson H. What are the most effective ways of improving population health through transport interventions? Evidence from systematic reviews. *J. Epidemiol. Community Health*, 2003. 57(5)327-33.

[57] Lefebvre RC Flora JA. Social marketing and public health intervention. *Health Educ. Q*, 1988. 15(3)299-315.

[58] Maibach E and Holtgrave DR. Advances in public health communication. *Annu Rev Public Health,* 1995. 16:219-38.

[59] Payton JW, et al., Social and emotional learning: a framework for promoting mental health and reducing risk behavior in children and youth. *J. Sch. Health*, 2000. 70 (5)179-85.

[60] Braithwaite RL and Lythcott N. Community empowerment as a strategy for health promotion for black and other minority populations. *JAMA*, 1989. 261(2)282-3.

[61] Chinman M et al., Developing a community science research agenda for building community capacity for effective preventive interventions. *Am. J. Community Psychol,* 2005. 35(3-4)143-57.

[62] Williams DR. and Jackson B. Social sources of racial disparities in health. *Health Aff.* (Millwood), 2005. 24(2): p. 325-34.

[63] Joffe H. Risk: from perception to social representation. *Br. J. Soc. Psychol,* 2003. 42(Pt 1) 55-73.

[64] Neumark-Sztainer D. The social environments of adolescents: associations between socioenvironmental factors and health behaviors during adolescence. *Adolesc. Med,* 1999. 10(1): p. 41-55, v.

[65] Earls F and Carlson M. The social ecology of child health and well-being. *Annu. Rev. Public Health*, 2001. 22:143-66.

[66] Grzywacz, JG Fuqua J. The social ecology of health: leverage points and linkages. *Behav. Med,* 2000. 26(3): p. 101-15.

[67] Green LW, Richard L, and Potvin L. Ecological foundations of health promotion. *Am. J. Health Promot,* 1996. 10(4): p. 270-81.

[68] Kothari AR. and Birch S. Multil*evel health promotion research: conceptual and analytical considerations. Can. J. Nurs Res*, 2004. 36(1)56-75.

[69] Yen IH Syme SL. The social environment and health: a discussion of the epidemiologic literature. *Annu. Rev. Public Health*, 1999. 20:287-308.

[70] McLeroy KR, et al. An ecological perspective on health promotion programs. *Health Educ. Q,* 1988. 15(4)351-77.

[71] Community Preventive Services Recommendations to Prevent Motor Vehicle Occupant Injury. Accessed on April 7, 2008 at: http://www.thecommunityguide.org/mvoi/default.htm

This chapter was supported in part by grants received from: CDC/National Center for Injury Prevention and Control, Grant # U49 CE001022, and NIH/National Center for Minority Health and Health Disparities, Grant # 5P20MD000516

Index

A

abdominal, 36, 40, 41, 65, 70, 72, 96, 97, 107, 108, 191, 192, 196, 200, 201, 203, 204, 206, 210, 226
abnormalities, 70, 75, 87, 88, 99, 100, 108, 118, 122, 123, 179, 181
Aboriginal, 50, 70, 169
abortion, 145, 180, 190, 214, 260, 268, 269, 270
absorption, 202
academic, 60, 92, 284, 297
access, 7, 13, 15, 17, 27, 28, 48, 52, 56, 57, 61, 73, 74, 75, 78, 89, 90, 98, 103, 132, 138, 256, 263, 266, 272, 273, 276, 296, 300, 305, 317, 319, 326
accessibility, 276
accidental, 199, 210, 260
accidents, 189, 268, 292, 304, 327, 328, 329, 330
accountability, 58
accounting, 55, 71, 96, 117, 184, 228, 307
acculturation, 88, 281, 314
accuracy, 7, 36, 183, 266, 299
ACE, 77, 96, 97
achievement, 128, 130, 135, 206, 276, 281, 284
acid, 183, 218, 274
Acquired Immune Deficiency Syndrome (AIDS, 47, 48, 49, 50, 51, 52, 53, 54, 55, 56, 57, 58, 59, 60, 61, 169, 174, 195, 197, 198, 215, 221
acquired immunity, 185, 200, 208
acquired immunodeficiency syndrome, 47, 169, 195
activation, 191
active smokers, 255
activism, 323
acute, 1, 36, 63, 73, 74, 75, 81, 82, 83, 89, 93, 111, 142, 143, 145, 159, 161, 183, 189, 190, 191, 192, 195, 197, 200, 201, 204, 206, 208, 209, 212, 226, 227, 232, 233, 235, 237, 241, 244, 245, 246, 247, 248, 249, 250
acute asthma, 142
acute coronary syndrome, 63, 74, 75, 81, 82
acute infection, 190
acute ischemic stroke, 89
acute myeloid leukemia, 143
ADA, 109
adaptation, 221, 311, 316, 318, 321
adducts, 142
adenine, 10
adenocarcinoma, 5, 20, 146
adenoma, 32, 35, 43
adenomas, 35, 44
adenosine, 24
adenoviruses, 238
adhesion, 185, 216
adiposity, 120
adjustment, 8, 12, 13, 16, 17, 69, 74, 76, 266, 293, 294, 321
administration, 60, 182, 232, 240
administrative, 272, 274
adolescence, 106, 283, 285, 329, 331
adolescent female, 284
adolescents, 2, 47, 101, 107, 111, 152, 155, 205, 279, 280, 281, 282, 283, 284, 331
ADT, 6, 14, 16
adult, 54, 66, 106, 110, 114, 121, 143, 145, 157, 185, 193, 199, 200, 201, 202, 203, 204, 208, 209, 210, 265, 288, 289, 302
adult population, 110, 121, 143, 289
adulthood, 106, 206

adults, 2, 3, 47, 80, 81, 99, 104, 108, 109, 110, 114, 115, 118, 119, 121, 122, 127, 134, 135, 138, 142, 144, 145, 149, 157, 158, 162, 164, 183, 185, 191, 195, 205, 206, 209, 210, 211, 228, 231, 242, 254, 256, 279, 280, 304, 307, 313
advertisement, 150, 153
advertising, 314, 322
advocacy, 78, 161
AEP, 284
aerobic, 8
aerobic exercise, 8
aetiology, 158
Africa, 49, 51, 55, 67, 115, 138, 167, 180, 184, 186, 188, 191, 192, 205, 207, 209, 210, 213, 216, 223, 228, 262, 269
African American, 7, 8, 9, 10, 11, 12, 13, 14, 15, 16, 17, 18, 24, 26, 29, 30, 55, 65, 66, 67, 68, 69, 70, 71, 72, 73, 74, 75, 76, 77, 79, 80, 83, 99, 119, 122, 126, 129, 130, 131, 132, 134, 136, 140, 169, 279, 280, 281, 282, 285, 290, 294, 295, 296, 298, 299, 301, 302, 306, 310, 313, 314, 319, 321, 322, 323
African American women, 55, 68, 72, 296, 302
African continent, 238
agar, 199
ageing, 301
agent, 37, 225, 231, 237, 241, 304, 311, 316, 317, 318, 319
agents, 6, 12, 54, 130, 179, 192, 204, 225, 242, 244
agglutination, 182, 193
agglutination test, 193
aggressiveness, 8, 11, 27
aging, 116
agricultural, 321
aid, 96, 107, 244
AIDS testing, 54
air, 38, 150, 154, 160, 161, 201, 205, 238, 253, 313
air quality, 154, 160
airports, 147
Alaska, 2, 7, 66, 135, 305, 306, 325, 328
Alaska Natives, 2, 7, 135, 305, 306, 307
albumin, 142
alcohol, 48, 65, 72, 87, 88, 166, 290, 310, 311, 312, 313, 314, 316, 317, 319, 320, 328, 330
alcohol abuse, 48
alcohol consumption, 317
alcohol use, 87, 88, 316, 318, 319, 320
alcoholics, 167
alkaline phosphatase, 218
alleles, 9, 11, 77, 106
allergens, 253, 254
allergic, 201, 208, 254, 255, 257
allergic asthma, 257
allergic reaction, 208
allergy, 255, 256, 257
ALS, 302
ALT, 201
alternative, 16, 28, 29, 32, 39, 96, 161, 232, 241, 265, 330
alternative medicine, 16, 28, 29
alternatives, 151, 315
alters, 100
alveoli, 142, 205, 210
Alzheimer, 284
Amazon, 189
amebiasis, 220
amenorrhea, 290
American Cancer Society (ACS), 43, 74, 75
American Heart Association, 97, 108, 133
American Indian, 2, 7, 65, 70, 74, 77, 79, 83, 110, 116, 118, 123, 135, 148, 295, 299, 304, 305, 306, 307, 309, 310, 313, 319, 325, 328
American Indians, 2, 65, 70, 74, 79, 83, 110, 116, 123, 135, 148, 295, 305, 307, 310, 313, 319
amino acid, 232
ammonium, 137
amniocentesis, 183
amniotic, 182, 183, 215
amniotic fluid, 182, 183, 215
amoeboid, 184
amorphous, 198
amputation, 119, 120
anaemia, 177, 179, 181, 185, 186, 187, 188, 191, 200, 203, 205, 212, 217
Anaemia, 216
anastomosis, 39, 41
androgen, 6, 8, 10, 20, 21, 23
androgens, 9, 23
anemia, 36, 186, 268, 269, 270, 271, 273, 274, 278
angina, 75, 82
angiography, 75, 77, 83, 89, 92
angioplasty, 74, 75, 82
animals, 178, 180, 189, 196, 205, 213, 226, 229, 232, 235
annual rate, 313
anorexia, 36, 192, 197, 205

antecedents, 323, 329
anthroposophic, 256
antibiotic, 208
antibiotics, 178, 256
antibodies, 187
antibody, 180, 182, 183, 184, 187, 190, 205, 208, 209, 210, 233, 244
anticonvulsants, 290
antigen, 5, 20, 24, 27, 29, 38, 182, 190, 193, 194, 195, 210, 232
antigenic drift, 235
antihistamines, 208
antimicrobial, 181
antimicrobial therapy, 181
antimony, 194
antioxidant, 12, 143
antiretroviral, 47, 53, 59
antiretrovirals, 53
anti-sense, 240
antisera, 199
antiviral, 240, 250
antiviral therapy, 240
anus, 41
anxiety, 75
APC, 32
apo A-I, 131
apolipoprotein A-I, 127, 131, 136
apolipoprotein A-I (apo A-I), 131
Apolipoprotein E (APOE), 77, 83
apoptosis, 10
appendicitis, 204, 222
appendix, 204
appetite, 177
application, 39, 42, 96, 236, 244, 261
aquatic, 210, 213
Arab countries, 292
Arabs, 87, 88, 292
arachnids, 178
Argentina, 61, 116, 190, 218, 228, 231, 233, 234, 235, 236, 242, 243, 244, 246
argument, 152
armed conflict, 49
aromatase inhibitors, 290
arrest, 56, 199
arrhythmia, 189
arsenic, 137
arterial hypertension, 95, 99, 101, 102, 104, 105
arteries, 41, 210
artery, 39, 63, 77, 80, 81, 87, 88, 129
arthritis, 294, 295, 302
Arthropoda, 178
articulation, 323
AS, 23, 25, 30, 158, 219, 302, 329
asbestos, 275
ascending colon, 39
ASEAN, 120
aseptic, 274
asexual, 184, 196
ash, 328
Asia, 7, 86, 108, 138, 143, 144, 191, 205, 208, 210, 228, 229, 262, 292, 305
Asian, 2, 7, 8, 15, 19, 23, 66, 70, 71, 76, 77, 86, 88, 90, 99, 108, 110, 114, 115, 117, 118, 120, 148, 165, 166, 167, 170, 171, 253, 279, 280, 281, 282, 283, 285, 288, 290, 292, 293, 294, 297, 298, 299, 302, 304, 305, 306, 307, 308, 310, 313, 314, 325
Asian American, 108, 117, 279, 280, 281, 282, 283, 285, 293
Asian Americans, 108, 117, 280, 281, 282, 283, 285, 293
Asian countries, 7, 8, 171, 253
aspirate, 194
assault, 54
assessment, 36, 38, 80, 110, 135, 136, 141, 160, 161, 244, 248, 261, 265, 291, 298, 301, 327
assignment, 18
assimilation, 325
associations, 9, 72, 77, 85, 88, 143, 153, 255, 280, 283, 293, 331
asthma, 138, 140, 142, 145, 146, 156, 157, 158, 206, 208, 253, 254, 255, 256, 257
asymptomatic, 43, 122, 183, 184, 185, 187, 189, 193, 194, 195, 196, 206, 208, 219, 237, 241, 244, 246
atherosclerosis, 70, 77, 79, 80, 81, 83, 89, 92, 109, 134, 147
Atherosclerosis Risk in Communities, 67, 80, 122, 134
atherosclerotic vascular disease, 123
atherothrombAtlas, 157
atopic asthma, 142
atopic eczema, 257
atopy, 254, 257
atrial fibrillation, 87, 88, 89
Atrial fibrillation, 87
atrophy, 197, 209
attachment, 202
attacks, 254, 255

attention, 38, 56, 73, 86, 89, 146, 152, 177, 192, 196, 225, 260, 273, 315
attitudes, 2, 49, 73, 75, 157, 161, 275, 311, 313, 316
attribution, 264
atypical, 6, 218, 231, 243
auditory hallucinations, 179
Aurora, 43
Australia, 7, 31, 50, 58, 108, 191, 210, 237, 238, 246, 253, 297
authority, 323
autonomic, 40, 41
autonomic nerve, 40, 41
autopsy, 5, 8, 20, 22, 266, 271
availability, 57, 119, 228, 272, 274, 285, 312
averaging, 266
avoidance, 40, 152, 161
awareness, 89, 127, 133, 135, 151, 153, 213, 236, 266, 273, 319, 321

B

babies, 106, 179, 190
BAC, 312, 313, 317, 320
back pain, 36
bacteria, 178, 197, 225
bacterial, 141, 142, 200, 226, 231, 233, 238, 241
Badia, 301
Bahrain, 114
Balkans, 213
Bangladesh, 67, 213, 234, 237, 250, 253, 254, 255, 256, 257
Barbados, 86, 91, 116
barium, 33, 38
barium enema, 33, 38
barrier, 27, 73, 272, 276
barriers, 18, 29, 48, 73, 256, 272, 311, 312, 317, 318
B-cell, 191
BDI, 280, 282, 284
beam radiation, 6, 20
behavior, 16, 17, 29, 53, 150, 156, 158, 269, 272, 311, 317, 319, 323, 329, 330
behavioral dispositions, 314
behavioral models, 152
behavioral modification, 150
behavioral problems, 281
Behavioral Risk Factor Surveillance System, 122
beliefs, 14, 75
benchmarks, 132
beneficial effect, 42
benefits, 2, 39, 56
benign, 5, 13, 24, 25, 142
benign prostatic hyperplasia, 24, 25
benign prostatic hypertrophy, 5
benzene, 137
beta cell, 106
beverages, 320
bias, 20, 48, 56, 75, 78, 101, 131, 133, 268
bilateral, 181, 198
binding, 9, 10, 23, 24, 25, 77, 106, 111, 182, 185
binding globulin, 9, 23
bioavailability, 10
biochemical, 22, 28, 131, 152, 232
biologic, 42, 163
biological, 7, 8, 9, 10, 11, 14, 19, 67, 130, 132, 133, 141, 143, 144, 146, 147, 194, 198, 199, 221, 327
biologically, 9, 144
biology, 136, 221, 222, 245
biomarkers, 142
biopsies, 35
biopsy, 5, 13, 37, 182, 194, 195, 199
birds, 180
birth, 52, 65, 66, 67, 70, 80, 106, 140, 141, 156, 164, 168, 170, 180, 181, 183, 185, 186, 187, 190, 194, 195, 196, 217, 235, 263, 265, 267, 272, 276, 281
birth rate, 267
birth weight, 106, 140, 141, 156, 185, 186, 217
births, 180, 188, 262, 263, 264, 267, 274
birthweight, 156
black, 8, 19, 23, 26, 27, 28, 48, 55, 58, 74, 80, 81, 82, 117, 134, 155, 164, 166, 167, 171, 209, 279, 282, 293, 297, 330
black citizens, 164
black women, 74, 293
Blacks, 50, 77, 85, 87, 88, 89, 90, 91, 93, 105, 121, 143, 144, 281, 282, 293, 295, 296, 297, 298, 305, 306, 307, 314
bladder, 6, 212
bladder outlet obstruction, 6
blame, 52
blaming, 49
bleeding, 36, 192, 274
blindness, 181, 209
blood, 3, 39, 63, 64, 65, 70, 72, 80, 99, 104, 108, 117, 118, 121, 134, 136, 141, 149, 160, 178, 182, 183, 184, 186, 187, 188, 189, 192, 194, 202, 204, 205, 207, 208, 212, 215, 216, 217, 233, 270, 273, 313, 317, 320

blood flow, 63, 141
blood glucose, 3, 99, 121
blood group, 233
blood pressure, 64, 70, 72, 80, 99, 104, 118, 134, 149, 160
blood smear, 189
blood supply, 39
blood transfusion, 189, 192, 273
blood transfusions, 192
blood vessels, 63, 117, 212
bloodstream, 184, 189
body fluid, 182, 207
body mass index (BMI), 19, 33, 68, 98, 99, 106, 117, 296
body size, 118
body weight, 101, 293
bone, 5, 6, 169, 193, 287, 288, 289, 290, 294, 295, 296, 297, 299, 300, 301, 302
bone density, 302
bone loss, 289, 294, 299
bone marrow, 193
bone marrow aspiration, 194
bone mass, 287, 290, 294, 301
bone mineral density (BMD), 287, 288, 289, 293, 294, 295, 301
bovine, 196, 241, 250
bowel, 33, 36, 37, 38, 39, 40, 41, 201, 204, 206
bowel obstruction, 36
boys, 49, 283
brachytherapy, 6, 14
brain, 141, 143, 181, 183, 198, 205, 206, 210
brain development, 141
brain injury, 181
brain stem, 198
brain tumor, 143
Brazil, 51, 53, 60, 61, 116, 190, 192, 193, 212, 218, 225, 228, 231, 233, 234, 235, 237, 238, 242, 244, 247, 248, 250
Brazilian, 231, 248
BRCA1, 12, 26
breast, 18, 21, 25, 40, 106, 145, 146, 158, 159, 179, 194, 195, 196, 207, 220, 273, 288
breast cancer, 25, 146, 158, 159
breast feeding, 273
breast milk, 106, 207
brick, 275
bronchial asthma, 257
bronchial hyperresponsiveness, 142
bronchiolitis, 142, 254, 257
bronchitis, 142
bronchospasm, 253
Buenos Aires, 218, 236, 244, 281
buildings, 147, 150
Bureau of the Census, 17
buses, 304, 305

C

CAD, 77
caecum, 203
calcification, 77, 191
calcitonin, 289
calcium, 10, 34, 77, 80, 81, 289, 290, 293, 297, 298
caliber, 36
calorie, 107
CAM, 16
Cambodia, 113, 213
Cameroon, 213
campaigns, 18, 150, 172, 316, 317, 320, 321, 322
cancer, 1, 2, 5, 6, 7, 8, 10, 12, 17, 18, 19, 21, 26, 27, 29, 30, 31, 32, 33, 34, 35, 36, 38, 39, 40, 41, 42, 43, 44, 45, 92, 140, 142, 143, 145, 146, 149, 157, 159, 162
cancer screening, 29, 43
cancers, 5, 7, 21, 32, 33, 38, 39, 143
candidates, 41, 232
CAP, 130, 135
capacity, 57, 58, 61, 142, 143, 177, 330
Cape Town, 115
capital, 54, 172, 274
carbohydrate, 105, 106, 107, 233
carcinoembryonic antigen, 45
carcinogen, 137, 142, 157
carcinogenesis, 8, 9, 32, 146
carcinogenic, 137, 142, 146
carcinoma, 22, 32, 33, 37, 41, 145
carcinomas, 38
cardiac catheterization, 75, 92
cardiac enlargement, 206
cardiac muscle, 63
cardiology, 134, 135
cardiovascular, 31, 64, 65, 66, 67, 68, 69, 73, 74, 76, 77, 78, 79, 80, 81, 82, 83, 86, 89, 92, 95, 96, 97, 99, 100, 103, 107, 108, 109, 110, 125, 130, 132, 133, 134, 136, 138, 160, 268, 269
cardiovascular disease, 31, 79, 80, 81, 82, 83, 86, 89, 92, 95, 96, 97, 103, 107, 108, 109, 110, 125, 134, 138, 268, 269
Cardiovascular disease, 63, 110
cardiovascular function, 160

cardiovascular morbidity, 109
cardiovascular risk, 67, 73, 74, 92, 109, 134, 136
caregiver, 142, 284
caregivers, 279, 281, 282, 283, 284, 285
Caribbean, 50, 61, 66, 70, 71, 80, 86, 90, 91, 116, 117, 121, 210, 281, 284
Caribbean Islands, 210
carotid endarterectomy, 89, 93
carrier, 10, 317
catabolism, 77
Cataracts, 215
categorization, 74
cats, 204
cattle, 211
Caucasian, 7, 26, 29, 66, 70, 96, 119, 126, 129, 130, 132, 167, 280, 282, 290, 294, 295, 296, 297, 302, 305
Caucasian population, 66, 130
Caucasians, 8, 26, 66, 76, 77, 80, 83, 97, 99, 100, 104, 106, 116, 119, 126, 127, 129, 130, 131, 132, 134, 135, 136, 140, 148, 171, 280, 282, 294, 295, 296
causal relationship, 141
causation, 156
cavities, 207
CD, 91, 92, 111, 135, 172, 242, 244, 249
CD4, 183, 189, 191, 197, 201, 216
CD5, 216
CD5+, 216
CD8+, 189
CDC, 47, 50, 57, 58, 59, 60, 61, 79, 122, 313, 328, 329, 331
CDH-1, 11
CEA, 38, 43, 89
cecum, 34, 39, 203
cell, 10, 184, 187, 189, 191, 197, 198, 201, 227, 232, 235, 239, 240, 245, 249, 314, 317
cell culture, 232, 239, 240, 249
cell line, 235, 245
cell lines, 235, 245
cell phones, 314, 317
cellular atypia, 6
cement, 275
Census, 65, 110, 265, 266, 294, 305
Census Bureau, 65, 110, 294
Center for Epidemiologic Studies Depression Scale, 279
Centers for Disease Control, 57, 58, 79, 173, 174, 175, 324
Central America, 180, 189
Central Europe, 291
central nervous system, 183, 190, 209
central obesity, 71, 83, 95, 97, 98, 100, 102, 105, 107, 109, 111
cerebellum, 198
cerebrospinal fluid, 181, 198, 210
cerebrovascular, 71, 85, 88, 89, 93, 103
cerebrovascular disease, 71, 85, 93, 103
CES, 280, 281, 282, 283, 284
Chagas disease, 218, 219
channels, 2
chemical, 12, 152, 199
chemical properties, 152
chemistry, 136
chemoprevention, 12
chemopreventive, 12
chemopreventive agents, 12
chemotherapeutic agent, 40
chemotherapy, 6, 39, 40, 42, 204, 207, 290
chickens, 235
child bearing, 178, 269, 272
child care centers, 237, 247
child welfare, 276
childbearing, 56
childbirth, 262
childhood, 53, 73, 106, 142, 143, 156, 157, 158, 192, 202, 206, 208, 211, 222, 223, 224, 226, 241, 245, 247, 248, 250, 256, 257
Chile, 63, 116, 228, 233, 234, 235, 236, 244
China, 8, 67, 102, 113, 143, 147, 165, 212, 213, 224, 237, 285
Chinese, 8, 66, 70, 74, 86, 92, 102, 106, 110, 113, 120, 159, 170, 171, 281, 282, 283, 285, 294, 301, 306
Chinese women, 159, 294, 301
chlorine, 240
chloroquine, 188, 218
cholecystitis, 192
cholesterol, 64, 68, 69, 70, 72, 77, 83, 87, 89, 99, 101, 102, 105, 106, 108, 109, 126, 127, 128, 129, 131, 132, 133, 134, 135, 136
cholinergic, 141
chorionic villi, 190, 191
chorioretinitis, 181, 182
choroid, 181
chromium, 137
chromosome, 9, 32, 169, 174
chronic, 1, 35, 63, 64, 73, 103, 104, 111, 132, 146, 158, 174, 180, 183, 189, 190, 192, 195,

197, 202, 203, 205, 207, 208, 209, 212, 214, 221, 253, 290, 296
chronic disease, 1, 64, 73, 103, 111, 214
chronic obstructive pulmonary disease, 146, 290
cigarette smoking, 67, 70, 90, 118, 134, 154, 155, 158, 159, 290, 293
cigarettes, 147, 150
circulation, 190, 204, 205, 206, 210
circulatory disease, 31
civil servants, 119
civil society, 53, 54, 57
classes, 305
classical, vii, 191
classification, 36, 108, 232, 243, 305, 324, 326
classified, 5, 6, 73, 179, 235, 236, 264, 268, 326, 327
claudication, 120, 124
cleavages, 236
clients, 51, 54
climatic factors, 242
clinical diagnosis, 20, 118
clinical presentation, 23, 182
clinical symptoms, 188, 196
clinical trial, 1, 2, 18, 19, 20, 29, 30, 39, 45, 48, 126, 133, 136, 240, 298, 300, 302
clinically significant, 5, 9
clinics, 17, 27, 53, 122, 186, 317
cloning, 235
clothing, 203, 316, 317
clustering, 67, 170, 174
clusters, 198, 226, 232
c-Myc, 23
CNS, 181, 197, 198, 209, 210
coal, 145, 158
coastal areas, 208
codes, 10, 226, 326
coding, 10, 235, 324
codon, 169, 171
coenzyme, 129
coercion, 56
co-existence, 315
cognition, 206, 314
cognitive, 177, 202, 280, 296, 298, 329
cognitive function, 177, 202
cognitive impairment, 296
cognitive variables, 280
cohort, 11, 19, 24, 29, 30, 64, 66, 71, 74, 83, 97, 119, 124, 127, 146, 164, 186, 220, 235, 248, 257, 298, 302
colectomy, 33, 39, 42, 44, 45
colic, 39, 201
colitis, 33, 194
collaboration, 61, 277, 303
college students, 280, 281, 282, 283
collisions, 310
Colombia, 116, 236, 247
colon, 31, 33, 34, 35, 36, 38, 39, 40, 43, 44, 45, 189, 203, 222
colon cancer, 31, 35, 36, 38, 39, 40, 44, 45
colonization, 194
colonoscopy, 33, 34, 35, 36, 38, 43, 204
colorectal, 10, 19, 24, 26, 31, 32, 33, 34, 35, 36, 38, 39, 43, 44, 45
colorectal cancer, 10, 19, 24, 31, 32, 33, 34, 35, 36, 39, 43, 44, 45
colostomy, 41
colostrum, 196
combustion, 137
commercial, 268, 315, 318
commodity, 138
common findings, 191
common symptoms, 36
communication, 2, 299, 330
communities, 48, 54, 55, 56, 57, 58, 85, 109, 115, 118, 164, 172, 175, 206, 238, 272, 276, 278, 299, 305, 321, 322, 323, 324
community, 1, 2, 18, 27, 29, 51, 52, 54, 55, 57, 64, 86, 91, 93, 114, 115, 119, 121, 124, 127, 155, 157, 169, 171, 172, 204, 221, 222, 223, 260, 263, 266, 268, 273, 274, 275, 276, 277, 283, 285, 295, 297, 301, 302, 305, 314, 316, 319, 320, 321, 322, 323, 324, 330
community-based, 18, 27, 29, 57, 119, 127, 169
co-morbidities, 295
comorbidity, 75, 292, 297
competency, 48
complement, 201
complementary, 16, 28, 29
complex systems, 323
compliance, 129, 144, 151, 161, 256, 290
complications, 38, 41, 75, 96, 104, 108, 117, 120, 122, 124, 169, 183, 194, 200, 224, 260, 262, 268, 269, 271, 274, 276, 277, 327
components, 95, 97, 98, 99, 101, 104, 105, 107, 149, 304
composition, 131, 268, 293, 314
compounds, 137, 142
computed tomography, 181, 210
concentration, 10, 24, 26, 72, 140, 147, 196, 198, 202, 203, 207, 270, 313, 320

conception, 180, 214
concordance, 48, 102
condoms, 55, 56
conduction, 189
confidence, 67, 212, 266, 267, 293, 297, 299
confidence interval, 67, 212, 266, 293, 297
confidence intervals, 67, 266, 293
confidentiality, 52, 262
conflict, 52, 54, 322
conflict resolution, 322
confounders, 66
confounding variables, 130
congestive heart failure, 83
conjunctivitis, 146, 257
connectivity, 317
consensus, 1, 61, 65, 100, 134, 226, 262, 295, 301
Consensus Development Conference, 300
consent, 29, 56, 150
conspiracy, 48
constitutional, 150, 205
constraints, 316
construction, 147
consultants, 18
consulting, 97
consumption, 49, 65, 105, 106
contaminants, 153
contaminated food, 189
contamination, 201, 203
continuing, 59, 206, 319, 321
continuity, 36, 132
control, 6, 8, 9, 10, 11, 12, 16, 19, 20, 22, 23, 24, 44, 64, 74, 79, 80, 81, 82, 100, 104, 107, 124, 132, 133, 135, 136, 144, 145, 149, 150, 152, 153, 154, 156, 157, 159, 163, 170, 171, 172, 174, 175, 178, 191, 206, 209, 216, 218, 223, 226, 281, 304, 319
control group, 8, 12, 19, 107
controlled, 12, 13, 19, 26, 74, 132, 187, 222, 229, 277, 283
controlled studies, 26
controlled trials, 12
conviction, 323
cooking, 210
COPD, 145, 146
coronary angioplasty, 76, 83
coronary arteries, 63
coronary artery bypass graft, 76, 83
coronary artery disease, 64, 73, 77, 82, 83, 129, 135, 136
coronary heart disease, 64, 66, 75, 79, 81, 82, 83, 103, 110, 118, 123, 126, 134, 136, 159
correlation, 25, 36, 190, 236, 241
correlations, 301
corticosteroids, 208, 290
cortisol, 281, 285
costs, 75, 152, 153, 162, 169, 254, 268, 290
cotinine, 139, 140, 143, 147, 150, 154, 155, 157, 161
cough, 141, 142, 145, 146, 149, 192, 210, 253
counseling, 54, 56, 59
countermeasures, 330
country of origin, 73, 171
couples, 273, 279, 282
coupling, 10
covariate, 170
coverage, 75, 151, 229
covering, 274, 291
cows, 229, 256
CPS, 159
crack, 174
cranial nerve, 210
CRC, 26, 31, 32, 33, 34, 35, 36, 37
C-reactive protein, 72, 76, 83
crime, 72
crops, 26
cross-sectional, 10, 80, 98, 100, 101, 104, 108, 110, 114, 127, 136, 156, 160, 164, 201, 206, 223, 271, 280, 281
cross-sectional study, 10, 110, 127, 136, 160, 164, 223, 271, 281
crustaceans, 178
cryotherapy, 6, 14
cryptosporidium, 197
CS, 21, 24, 28, 79, 81, 91, 285
CSF, 181, 182, 183, 198, 211
CT, 38, 43, 181, 182
CT scan, 38, 43, 182
cultural, 48, 96, 106, 116, 260, 269, 272, 276, 299, 305, 311, 316, 321, 323, 324, 325
cultural beliefs, 106
cultural factors, 96, 269, 272, 276
cultural risk factors, 311
culture, 78, 107, 168, 170, 173, 182, 193, 215, 244, 250, 280, 284
curable, 14, 44
cutaneous larva migrans, 200
cuticle, 199

CVD, 64, 65, 66, 68, 70, 71, 74, 76, 77, 95, 96, 103, 125, 126, 127, 129, 131, 132, 133, 146, 147, 149
cycles, 207, 304, 305, 317
cycling, 317, 321
cyclists, 311, 316, 317
cyst, 180, 198, 224
cysticercus, 211, 224
cysts, 180, 195, 198, 211
cytochrome, 10
cytokine, 186, 191, 221, 222
cytokine response, 191, 221
cytokines, 142, 201
cytomegalovirus, 181
cytoplasm, 198
cytosine, 10, 24
cytotoxicity, 191

D

dairy, 8, 10
dairy products, 8, 10
danger, 54, 273
data collection, 260, 265, 266, 296, 325
data gathering, 326
database, 15, 22, 280, 282, 291, 292, 294, 300, 301
deafness, 181, 184
death rate, 7, 8, 17, 64, 65, 66, 80, 90, 169, 298, 306
deaths, 31, 47, 51, 63, 66, 71, 92, 93, 103, 138, 149, 177, 212, 214, 226, 241, 253, 256, 259, 260, 261, 262, 263, 264, 265, 266, 268, 269, 270, 271, 272, 273, 274, 275, 276, 277, 305, 306, 310, 313, 314, 317, 325, 328
deciliter, 133
decision makers, 300
decision making, 14, 15, 17, 38
decision-making process, 299
decisions, 2, 14, 28, 276, 300, 315, 323
defects, 32, 181
deficiency, 169, 190, 205, 289, 290
deficits, 69, 172, 203
definition, 1, 18, 96, 97, 99, 100, 101, 102, 104, 105, 109, 110, 153, 187, 260, 261
degradation, 10, 216
degree, 32, 33, 35, 36, 38, 71, 77, 97, 123, 178
delays, 78, 272
delivery, 1, 2, 15, 27, 48, 144, 145, 186, 196, 254, 260, 269, 272, 274, 275, 322
delusions, 179
dementia, 281, 282, 285
Democratic Republic of Congo, 242
demographic, 28, 50, 88, 125, 159, 168, 225, 296, 301, 311, 315, 321
demographic characteristics, 311
demographic factors, 88
demographics, 26
denial, 49, 52
density, 68, 72, 77, 134, 169, 186, 207, 209, 287, 288, 294, 295, 296, 297, 300, 301
Department of Defense, 15
Department of Health and Human Services, 154, 284
depressed, 280, 281, 283, 284, 285
depression, 48, 64, 65, 279, 280, 281, 282, 283, 284, 285, 296
depressive disorder, 283
depressive symptomatology, 282, 285
depressive symptoms, 280, 281, 282, 283, 284, 285
deprivation, 6, 73, 81, 106, 160, 167
dermal, 192
dermatitis, 206, 209
dermatologic, 200, 206
dermis, 191
Desert Storm, 178
destruction, 185, 189
detection, 5, 13, 27, 34, 97, 100, 108, 124, 189, 190, 194, 196, 209, 210, 212, 220, 228, 236, 239, 242, 243, 244, 245, 247, 249, 250
detection techniques, 13, 239
detergents, 235
developed countries, 64, 78, 90, 115, 125, 143, 153, 163, 193, 211, 228, 231, 233, 238, 253, 254, 255, 261, 263, 265, 277
developed nations, 195
developing countries, 52, 63, 64, 118, 123, 143, 177, 189, 191, 195, 211, 225, 226, 228, 236, 237, 238, 240, 254, 255, 256, 259, 260, 261, 262, 264, 265, 269, 272, 273, 275, 276
developing nations, 113
DHT, 10
diabetes, 64, 65, 67, 68, 69, 70, 71, 72, 74, 81, 83, 87, 88, 90, 92, 95, 96, 97, 99, 100, 101, 102, 103, 106, 107, 108, 109, 110, 111, 113, 114, 115, 116, 117, 118, 119, 120, 121, 122, 123, 124, 126, 130, 132, 134, 181, 215, 274
diabetes insipidus, 181, 215

diabetes mellitus, 65, 67, 70, 72, 74, 87, 92, 96, 107, 108, 113, 114, 115, 116, 117, 120, 121, 122, 123, 124
diabetic, 66, 99, 100, 103, 105, 106, 117, 122, 123, 124, 132
diabetic patients, 123, 124, 132
diabetic retinopathy, 117, 122
diagnostic, vii, 5, 9, 13, 20, 73, 75, 78, 89, 91, 96, 97, 100, 104, 114, 182, 193, 199, 204, 233, 239, 248, 280, 288, 300
diagnostic criteria, 96, 97, 100, 104, 114
dialysis, 118
diarrhea, 195, 197, 203, 207, 220, 225, 226, 227, 231, 232, 235, 236, 237, 238, 239, 240, 241, 242, 244, 245, 246, 247, 248, 251
diarrhoea, 189, 192, 195, 196, 197, 203, 210, 220, 248, 250
diet, 8, 21, 26, 33, 96, 106, 125, 126, 205
dietary, 12, 16, 32, 33, 105, 106, 169, 297, 300
dietary habits, 106
dietary intake, 34
differentiation, 24, 83, 239
digestion, 202
direct measure, 96
disability, 1, 79, 110, 177, 202, 298, 303, 305, 319, 323, 327
disabled, 288
disclosure, 51, 54
discomfort, 48, 178
discontinuous variation, 201
discrimination, 49, 51, 52, 54, 61, 78
discriminatory, 56
disease-free survival, 15
diseases, iv, vii, 64, 81, 120, 146, 158, 163, 169, 172, 177, 179, 190, 207, 208, 212, 236, 253, 268, 269, 285
disinfection, 240
dislocation, 266
disorder, 104, 208, 269, 270, 271
displacement, 49
disposition, 88
disseminate, 172, 212
distal, 40, 41
distraction, 314
distress, 206
distribution, 2, 18, 21, 26, 68, 71, 72, 88, 90, 104, 109, 121, 152, 153, 184, 197, 208, 222, 227, 230, 237, 238, 243, 247, 292
diversification, 239
diversity, 2, 116, 225, 227, 231, 232, 237, 240, 241, 244, 249
diverticulitis, 204
dizygotic, 180
dizygotic twins, 180
DNA, 26, 32, 143, 146, 183, 194, 197, 248, 249
DNA damage, 143, 146
DNA repair, 26
doctors, 73, 150, 272, 283
dogs, 192, 235
domestic violence, 61, 260, 275
donor, 273
donors, 57, 256
dopamine, 141
DOT, 327, 328, 329, 330
drinking, 205, 271, 310, 314, 317, 320, 329, 330
drinking pattern, 329
drinking patterns, 329
drinking water, 205, 271
drowsiness, 329
drug abuse, 51
drug resistance, 170, 171
drug therapy, 98, 171
drug toxicity, 18
drug treatment, 74, 97, 98, 289
drug use, 2, 49, 165, 167, 169, 173, 174, 268, 311
drug-resistant, 169, 170, 174, 175
drugs, 74, 89, 166, 170, 171, 194, 203, 207, 211, 240, 300, 327
drunk driving, 323
dry, 238, 253
DS-1, 227, 242
dsRNA, 226, 239
DST, 60
duodenal ulcer, 202
duodenum, 201
duration, 33, 36, 66, 80, 117, 122, 150, 184, 194, 196, 203, 232, 233, 240, 260
dust, 178, 201, 203, 253
DWI, 314
DXA, 287, 289, 296, 297
dyslipidemia, 68, 74, 80, 95, 97, 99, 101, 102, 105, 106, 107, 111, 126, 127, 128, 129, 131, 132
dysplasia, 35
dyspnea, 145, 146

E

early retirement, 254
early warning, 90

East Asia, 106, 113, 138, 170, 262
eating, 180, 210
E-cadherin, 11, 25, 26
ECF, 298
ECG, 89, 118
eclampsia, 269, 274
ecological, 164, 173, 305, 319, 323, 331
ecology, 200, 331
economic, 13, 17, 48, 49, 59, 61, 71, 75, 103, 107, 114, 116, 148, 152, 162, 163, 170, 172, 179, 211, 254, 255, 257, 260, 263, 279, 283, 296, 299, 303, 304, 311, 314, 315, 316, 319, 321, 322, 323, 325
economic growth, 103
economic problem, 211
economic resources, 322
economic status, 13, 17, 61, 103, 170, 257, 263, 279, 296, 311, 314, 316, 325
economic systems, 323
economically disadvantaged, 157
ectopic pregnancy, 268, 269
eczema, 255
edema, 189, 191, 224
educated women, 72
education, 8, 16, 17, 19, 20, 29, 49, 58, 59, 66, 67, 71, 72, 78, 138, 139, 144, 150, 153, 167, 172, 255, 273, 274, 275, 280, 281, 295, 313, 316, 317, 320, 322
educational attainment, 134, 325
educational programs, 150
EEG, 211
efficacy, 16, 18, 130, 135, 193, 228, 229, 240, 250
effusion, 143
eggs, 199, 200, 201, 202, 203, 204, 205, 206, 210, 212, 213, 222, 254
Egypt, 114, 115, 121, 212, 213, 238
Egyptian, 115, 248
EIA, 235, 236, 239
elderly, 19, 75, 116, 118, 122, 178, 236, 246, 274, 283, 291, 298, 300, 302
electricity, 271
electrocardiogram, 118, 189
electrocardiographic, 118, 122
electrolyte, 196, 239
electrolytes, 203
electron, 77, 197, 226, 232, 248
electron microscopy, 197, 226, 232, 248
electronic, iv, 19
electrophoresis, 239
elementary school, 157, 282
eligibility criteria, 19, 299
ELISA, 182, 191, 194, 196, 205, 223, 249
embolism, 269
embryos, 199
emergency departments, 313, 328
emergency response, 319
emotional, 280, 323, 330
emotional distress, 280
employees, 138
employers, 138
employment, 51, 73, 321
empowered, 276
empowerment, 152, 330
encapsulated, 205
encephalitis, 183, 198, 209
encoding, 242
encyst, 199, 213
endocrine, 181, 269
endogenous, 187
endoplasm, 198
endoscopic, 37, 38, 41
endothelial dysfunction, 147, 149, 160
endothelium, 185
energy, 147, 197, 203, 287, 289, 304
engagement, 18
engineering, 315, 317, 319, 326
enlargement, 13, 191, 192
enrollment, 2, 18, 19, 299
enrollment rates, 19
enteric, 233, 236, 238, 243, 250
enteritis, 206
entrapment, 200
envelope, 40
environment, 7, 55, 57, 71, 72, 106, 107, 114, 120, 137, 150, 195, 198, 202, 204, 213, 232, 235, 254, 255, 260, 269, 304, 311, 315, 316, 317, 318, 319, 323
environmental, 8, 9, 12, 20, 67, 72, 73, 76, 88, 91, 96, 105, 106, 107, 125, 127, 137, 147, 151, 153, 154, 155, 156, 157, 158, 159, 160, 161, 162, 203, 211, 239, 245, 254, 274, 294, 301, 305, 315, 316, 321, 323, 325, 326
environmental change, 315, 316
environmental conditions, 67, 73, 321, 325
environmental factors, 9, 20, 76, 88, 91, 96, 105, 106, 107, 155, 254, 274, 294
environmental protection, 159
Environmental Protection Agency, 137, 154, 162

environmental tobacco, 154, 155, 156, 157, 158, 159, 160, 161, 162
Environmental tobacco smoke, 137, 155, 156, 159, 160, 161, 162
Environmental tobacco smoke (ETS), 137, 161
enzyme, 10, 12, 193, 235, 239, 244, 246, 249
enzyme immunoassay, 235, 239, 244, 246
enzyme-linked immunosorbent assay, 193, 239
enzymes, 12
EOC, 273, 276
eosinophilia, 181, 201, 203, 204, 208, 209
eosinophils, 202, 208
Epi, 58, 110
epidemic, 48, 49, 50, 51, 53, 55, 57, 58, 59, 60, 61, 101, 103, 161, 169, 172, 185, 231, 233, 246
epidemiologic studies, 126, 131, 159, 287
epidemiological, 9, 19, 50, 64, 85, 97, 99, 114, 122, 124, 127, 131, 156, 159, 171, 191, 192, 219, 236, 239, 240, 250, 254, 257, 261, 292
epidemiology, 7, 20, 21, 22, 26, 48, 79, 108, 115, 124, 125, 134, 135, 136, 158, 162, 167, 170, 171, 172, 173, 174, 175, 222, 225, 226, 228, 236, 242, 243, 244, 245, 246, 247, 248, 293
epigenetic, 32
epilepsy, 211
epithelial cell, 23, 226, 233, 241
epithelial cells, 23, 226, 233, 241
epithelium, 195
equality, 52
equipment, 276, 317, 326
equity, 316
equol, 12, 26
erectile dysfunction, 6
erythrocytes, 184, 185, 186, 187, 188
erythropoietin, 141
Escherichia coli, 199
esophagus, 189
estimating, 6, 143, 267, 268, 291
estrogen, 290, 299
ethical, 262
ethnic background, 2, 49, 68, 85, 170, 279
ethnic diversity, 96, 294
ethnic minority, 12, 16, 18, 47, 48, 57, 59, 65, 72, 75, 90, 93, 103, 164, 167, 170, 173, 279, 284, 285, 299, 303, 304, 305, 314, 315, 316, 319, 321, 322, 323, 324
ethnicity, 2, 12, 14, 17, 20, 28, 49, 50, 54, 58, 65, 67, 76, 77, 79, 80, 81, 85, 87, 89, 92, 93, 95, 96, 97, 98, 99, 100, 101, 105, 109, 118, 122, 125, 126, 127, 128, 139, 143, 148, 152, 158, 167, 170, 173, 174, 281, 291, 292, 293, 294, 295, 296, 298, 299, 301, 305, 306, 307, 311, 322, 324, 325, 328
etiologic agent, 225, 237
etiology, 172, 288
ETS, 137, 138, 139, 140, 141, 142, 143, 144, 145, 146, 147, 148, 149, 150, 151, 152, 153, 154, 155, 156, 158, 160
Euro, 280, 282
Europe, 7, 31, 51, 65, 70, 114, 116, 118, 119, 138, 143, 144, 147, 180, 191, 229, 288, 292, 296, 300
European, 8, 22, 58, 65, 70, 71, 73, 74, 76, 77, 80, 83, 86, 87, 88, 89, 92, 93, 96, 98, 106, 108, 109, 110, 114, 116, 117, 118, 119, 143, 216, 262, 281, 282, 283, 285, 287, 289, 292, 295
European Americans, 83, 281, 283
European Community, 143
Europeans, 70, 71, 73, 75, 76, 77, 86, 88, 89, 110, 114
evidence, 2, 8, 9, 14, 16, 18, 26, 34, 37, 39, 42, 43, 44, 49, 51, 55, 59, 64, 73, 74, 78, 80, 84, 85, 89, 99, 111, 115, 120, 132, 138, 140, 141, 142, 143, 144, 145, 146, 149, 150, 151, 152, 154, 156, 159, 160, 161, 163, 170, 182, 183, 209, 222, 232, 233, 241, 243, 261, 279, 315, 317, 326
evolution, 61, 228
evolutionary, 221, 235
examinations, 35, 43, 207, 211
exchange transfusion, 184
excision, 40, 41, 42, 44
exclusion, 97, 98
excrements, 192
excretion, 196, 204, 212
exercise, 52, 65, 107, 120, 253, 289
expenditures, 288, 300
expert, iv, 131, 134
experts, 76, 184, 324
explosive, 19
exposure, 137, 138, 139, 140, 141, 142, 143, 144, 145, 146, 147, 148, 149, 150, 151, 152, 153, 154, 155, 156, 157, 158, 159, 160, 161, 162, 172, 179, 188, 189, 195, 197, 201, 203, 207, 208, 212, 254, 289, 297, 305, 311, 315, 316
external constraints, 316
external environment, 199, 202, 221
extracranial, 88
eye, 181, 209, 210, 317, 327

eyes, 209, 210

F

faecal, 196, 201, 204, 245
failure, 14, 28, 42, 189, 192, 239, 249, 261, 311, 317
failure to thrive, 189
faith, 321, 323
falciparum malaria, 186, 218
false, 39, 182, 291
familial, 32, 33, 44
family, 17, 32, 33, 35, 36, 49, 51, 54, 71, 142, 174, 226, 231, 235, 254, 255, 266, 271, 273, 274, 280, 283, 284, 285, 290, 311, 314, 323
family history, 32, 35, 290
family income, 71, 254, 255
family members, 17, 49, 142, 271, 314, 323
family planning, 274
family relationships, 285
Far East, 205
fascia, 40
fasting, 70, 71, 97, 99, 101, 102, 104, 105, 115, 121, 122
fasting glucose, 99, 101, 102, 104, 105, 115, 121, 122
fat, 8, 21, 33, 36, 105, 107, 109, 202
fatalities, 260, 304, 307, 308, 309, 310, 311, 312, 313, 314, 315, 316, 317, 320, 323, 324
fatality rates, 90, 91, 307, 309, 325
fatigue, 36, 60
fatty acid, 195
fatty acids, 195
FDA, 287
fear, 49, 51, 52
fears, 49
fecal, 194, 195, 196, 206, 213, 220, 226, 228, 232, 235, 239, 240, 249
fecal smear, 196
feces, 179, 189, 195, 210, 213, 239, 240
federal government, 306
Federal Register, 325, 328
fee, 117
feedback, 321
feeding, 39, 106, 188, 194, 195, 205, 207, 220, 250
feelings, 314
females, 50, 74, 114, 115, 158, 199, 202, 207, 228, 255, 280, 282, 292, 304, 306, 307, 309, 310, 312
femoral neck, 294
femur, 294, 301
fertility, 145, 265, 274
fertilizer, 203, 213
fetal, 73, 141, 142, 180, 182, 183, 185, 186, 187, 190, 215
fetal growth, 73
fetus, 141, 180, 181, 183, 190, 193
fetuses, 181, 183
fever, 188, 191, 192, 196, 205, 209, 210, 212, 226, 257, 274
fiber, 33
fibrillar, 198
fibrillation, 87
fibrinogen, 64, 70, 87
fibrosis, 189, 208
filariasis, 178, 200, 207, 208, 214, 223
financial resources, 56
fines, 320
firearm, 285
firms, 162
first degree relative, 288
fishing, 204, 221, 222
fixation, 36
flatworms, 178, 212
flexibility, 316
flotation, 196
flow, 63, 142, 157
fluid, 182, 183, 194, 195, 196, 197, 207, 210, 215
focus group, 81, 321
focus groups, 321
food, 106, 107, 147, 148, 160, 178, 196, 203, 224, 225, 232, 235, 240, 274
Food and Drug Administration (FDA), 287, 289
food poisoning, 225
foreign language, 322
foreign-born population, 166, 172
foreigners, 51
formaldehyde, 137
fracture, 287, 288, 289, 290, 291, 292, 293, 295, 296, 297, 298, 299, 301, 302
fractures, 287, 288, 289, 290, 291, 292, 293, 295, 296, 297, 299, 300, 301, 302
fragility, 287, 288, 301
Framingham study, 134
freedom, 61, 153
freezing, 235
fresh water, 212, 213
freshwater, 212
fruits, 65, 180
fulminant hepatitis, 235

funding, 56, 57
funds, 19, 273

G

G4, 229, 231
G8, 229, 242
gametocytes, 184
gangrene, 119, 120
gastrectomy, 290
gastroenteritis, 225, 226, 228, 229, 231, 233, 234, 235, 236, 237, 239, 240, 241, 242, 243, 244, 245, 246, 247, 248, 249, 250
gastrointestinal, 195, 202, 205, 212, 222, 232
gastrointestinal bleeding, 202, 222
gastrointestinal tract, 195, 232
gay men, 49, 55
gel, 83, 239
gender, 2, 41, 49, 50, 51, 52, 54, 55, 56, 57, 60, 61, 66, 67, 74, 75, 80, 81, 148, 158, 160, 166, 211, 279, 280, 281, 284, 291, 293, 294, 301, 307, 314, 322, 325, 329
gender differences, 49, 74, 280, 329
gender equality, 56
gender gap, 51
gender identity, 60
gender inequality, 54, 56
gender-sensitive, 56
gene, 10, 11, 23, 24, 25, 26, 32, 77, 106, 111, 169, 174, 220, 221, 227, 231, 239, 242, 243, 249
gene pool, 111
generation, 150, 153, 283
genes, 9, 11, 22, 25, 26, 32, 77, 83, 105, 106, 107, 135, 169, 226, 227, 229, 239, 241, 249
genetic, 7, 8, 9, 10, 11, 12, 17, 22, 23, 25, 26, 32, 33, 76, 83, 88, 90, 96, 105, 106, 107, 113, 116, 125, 133, 157, 169, 170, 171, 172, 181, 221, 226, 227, 231, 232, 242, 243, 246, 247, 249, 288
genetic diversity, 232, 246, 247
genetic factors, 76, 106, 169
genetic linkage, 242
genetic syndromes, 32, 33
genetics, 19, 20, 23, 44, 67, 288
genistein, 12
genome, 9, 226, 227, 233, 235, 239, 243
genome sequencing, 227
genomic, 23, 32, 226, 232, 236, 239, 245
genomic instability, 32
genotype, 11, 77, 136, 227, 228, 231, 235, 236, 237, 240, 241, 243, 244, 247
genotypes, 25, 77, 227, 228, 231, 235, 236, 237, 238, 243, 247
germ line, 25
germline mutations, 32
gestation, 181
gestational age, 217
gestational diabetes, 106
gingival, 192
girls, 49, 54, 55, 56, 158, 205, 283
gloves, 317
glucose, 70, 71, 87, 95, 97, 98, 99, 100, 105, 106, 108, 118, 120, 121, 135
glucose metabolism, 95, 100, 106
glucose tolerance, 98, 100, 118, 135
glutathione, 12
glutathione peroxidase, 12
glycemia, 98
glycoprotein, 226
glycosylated, 72
glycosylated hemoglobin, 72
goal attainment, 135
goals, 19, 56, 78, 125, 129, 135, 259, 263, 276, 299
government, iv, 53, 54, 56, 57, 120, 272, 273, 311, 324
government policy, 272
grades, 13
grading, 6, 20
gram-negative bacteria, 199
grants, 331
granulomas, 200, 204, 211
gravitation, 51
growth, 8, 10, 24, 25, 125, 140, 177, 179, 181, 192, 199, 200, 202, 203, 212, 322
growth factor, 10, 24, 25
growth hormone, 181
Guam, 206, 222
Guatemala, 234, 250
guidelines, 43, 78, 85, 99, 129, 131, 136, 265
Guillain-Barré syndrome, 192
gut, 201, 202, 205, 233
gynecologist, 271

H

Haiti, 197
half-life, 208
handling, 189
hands, 203

haplotypes, 11, 25
harbour, 202
harm, 169, 199
hazards, 318
HDL, 68, 70, 72, 98, 99, 101, 102, 104, 105, 106, 126, 127, 129, 130, 131, 134
head, 310, 316, 317, 318, 326
head injury, 317
headache, 210
Health and Human Services, 154, 284
health care, 2, 7, 8, 18, 27, 29, 48, 51, 52, 57, 67, 73, 75, 76, 78, 82, 84, 89, 103, 132, 133, 150, 172, 256, 260, 261, 263, 266, 269, 272, 273, 276, 279, 288, 300
health care professionals, 48, 260, 273
health care sector, 51
health care system, 48, 73, 76, 133, 263, 273, 276
health education, 273, 317, 319, 321, 322
health effects, 137, 138, 144, 149, 152, 156, 160, 162
health insurance, 51, 53, 75, 90, 291, 292, 298, 300
health services, 19, 74, 150, 272, 296
health status, 52, 67, 103, 169, 263, 273, 299
healthcare, 1, 2, 15, 16, 17, 73, 74, 78, 290, 302
heart, 63, 64, 65, 66, 67, 75, 79, 80, 81, 82, 83, 97, 102, 103, 104, 105, 108, 109, 110, 111, 118, 123, 134, 135, 141, 145, 149, 159, 160, 189, 274, 279
heart disease, 63, 66, 79, 103, 109, 111, 123, 135, 145, 159, 160, 274, 279
heart rate, 141, 149, 160
heating, 145, 158
height, 295
helmets, 311, 312, 314, 316, 317
hematemesis, 202
hematologic, 216
hematoxylin-eosin, 191
hemoglobin, 43, 142, 187, 270
hemorrhage, 90, 268, 269, 270, 271
hemorrhagic stroke, 118
hemostasis, 40
hepatitis, 169, 173, 174, 192, 205, 246, 268, 269
hepatitis a, 268
hepatitis B, 169, 173, 174
hepatitis C, 169, 173
hepatomegaly, 191, 205
hepatosplenomegaly, 181, 189
herbal, 16
heroin, 185
heroin addicts, 185
heterogeneity, 116
heterogeneous, 103, 116, 125
heterosexuals, 47
high blood cholesterol, 108
high blood pressure, 90, 103, 104
high density lipoprotein, 70, 134
high fat, 8
high risk, 26, 34, 35, 39, 40, 42, 47, 75, 78, 129, 130, 184, 187, 274, 295, 310
high school, 71, 72, 166, 280, 295, 328, 330
high-density lipoprotein, 68, 87, 126, 136
high-fat, 8
highlands, 237
high-risk, 13, 82, 132, 134, 169, 171, 172, 173, 175, 236, 329
high-risk populations, 173, 175
highways, 311
hip, 96, 98, 287, 288, 292, 293, 294, 295, 297, 298, 299, 300, 302, 322, 326
hip fracture, 288, 292, 297, 298, 300, 302
hip fractures, 292, 297, 298, 302
Hispanic origin, 281, 308, 309, 324, 325
Hispanic population, 48, 80, 96, 110, 130, 174, 292, 306
Hispanics, 2, 15, 16, 65, 66, 74, 75, 76, 77, 79, 83, 85, 87, 88, 90, 91, 99, 100, 103, 105, 106, 107, 110, 111, 116, 117, 122, 125, 127, 130, 131, 133, 134, 135, 140, 143, 148, 164, 174, 280, 284, 293, 295, 296, 298, 299, 300, 305, 306, 307, 313
histologic type, 38
histological, 6, 20, 191, 198, 199, 204
histology, 35
HIV, 47, 48, 49, 50, 51, 52, 53, 54, 55, 56, 57, 58, 59, 60, 61, 72, 165, 166, 168, 169, 170, 173, 174, 177, 179, 180, 183, 190, 192, 194, 197, 198, 207, 214, 219, 254, 269, 322
HIV infection, 47, 48, 49, 50, 51, 53, 54, 55, 56, 57, 58, 60, 168, 169, 190, 197
HIV test, 57
HIV/AIDS, 47, 49, 50, 51, 52, 53, 54, 55, 56, 57, 58, 59, 60, 61, 169, 173, 177, 254, 269, 322
homeless, 163, 167, 171, 175
homelessness, 48, 166, 170
homes, 107, 138, 152, 155, 236, 274
homocysteine, 70, 87
homogeneous, 64, 76
hookworm, 177, 200, 205, 206, 221, 222
hormone, 6, 8, 9, 10, 23, 289, 295, 299

hormones, 10
hospital, 73, 75, 82, 89, 91, 119, 120, 146, 151, 161, 173, 237, 256, 261, 272, 273, 274, 291, 292, 296, 297, 300, 302, 310, 312, 313
hospital care, 261, 312
hospital death, 89
hospitalization, 75, 194, 225, 229, 240, 257
hospitalizations, 226, 229, 235, 240
hospitalized, 103, 196, 219, 233, 236, 237, 238, 244, 246, 247, 248, 249, 250, 313
hospitals, 75, 89, 147, 150, 190, 203, 232, 272, 298
host, 73, 114, 171, 178, 179, 181, 190, 191, 196, 199, 201, 202, 203, 205, 206, 208, 209, 211, 212, 213, 233, 304, 311, 316, 317, 319
host population, 114
hostility, 49
household, 139, 143, 145, 146, 151, 152, 155, 178, 195, 201, 204, 240, 255, 257, 265, 266, 268
households, 137, 138, 143, 150, 254, 268, 274, 275, 279, 282
housing, 72
human, 8, 18, 22, 23, 26, 47, 50, 52, 56, 57, 61, 76, 111, 134, 173, 178, 179, 180, 184, 191, 197, 199, 201, 207, 208, 209, 212, 213, 216, 218, 219, 220, 221, 222, 223, 227, 228, 229, 230, 231, 235, 236, 237, 238, 241, 242, 243, 245, 246, 247, 248, 249, 250, 276
human genome, 22
human immunodeficiency virus, 47, 50, 173, 180, 207, 219
human milk, 220
human rights, 52, 56, 57, 61
humans, 12, 137, 178, 184, 195, 197, 199, 201, 202, 204, 205, 206, 208, 210, 211, 212, 213, 221, 222, 226, 227, 228, 229, 231, 232, 233, 235, 240, 243, 245
humerus, 287, 291, 292
humidity, 227, 238
humoral immunity, 187, 195
husband, 145, 146
hybridization, 23, 227, 242, 249
hydatid, 224
hydatid disease, 224
hydatidosis, 211
hydramnios, 215
hydration, 196
hydrocele, 208
hydrocephalus, 181
hydrogen, 137
hydrogen cyanide, 137
hydrops, 180, 181
hygiene, 177, 211, 226, 255, 257, 269
hygienic, 213
hyperactivity, 145
hyperbilirubinemia, 189
hypercholesterolemia, 72, 87, 88, 126, 127, 135
hypergammaglobulinemia, 191
hyperglycemia, 70, 109, 123
hyperinsulinaemia, 70
hyperlipidemia, 126, 127, 133
hypermethylation, 32
hyperparathyroidism, 290
hyperreactivity, 142
hypersensitivity, 201, 209, 212
hypertension, 65, 67, 69, 71, 72, 74, 75, 81, 87, 88, 92, 99, 105, 108, 109, 123, 126, 134, 269, 270
hypertensive, 63, 76, 80, 99, 104, 268, 271
hyperthyroidism, 290
hypertriglyceridemia, 72, 101, 104, 105
hypogammaglobulinemia, 181
hypogonadism, 290
hypomethylation, 32
hypoplasia, 142
hypothesis, 73, 95, 97, 100, 141, 146, 255, 257
hypothyroidism, 181
hypovitaminosis D, 297
hypoxia, 141, 142

I

IBD, 33
ICD, 67, 260, 303, 326, 327
icosahedral, 226, 236
identification, 18, 38, 39, 100, 198, 204, 221, 247, 266, 296, 299
identity, 2, 60
idiopathic, 215
IDU, 169
IFA, 182
IgE, 142, 201, 204, 208, 255
IGF, 10, 11, 23, 24, 25
IGF-1, 10, 11, 24
IGF-I, 23, 24, 25
IgG, 182, 183, 188, 190, 208
IHD, 63, 64, 65, 66, 67, 70, 71, 76, 77, 78
IL-2, 189
IL-4, 189, 201
illegal drugs, 328, 330

illusion, 131
images, 321
imaging, 5, 74
immigrants, 21, 66, 67, 71, 73, 86, 104, 163, 171, 206, 294, 301
immigration, 168, 171, 173, 178, 311
immune response, 189, 191, 199, 200, 205, 212, 213, 233, 243
immune system, 179, 185, 239
immunity, 169, 179, 185, 187, 188, 201, 208, 216, 217, 219, 221, 226, 228, 231, 233, 235, 240
immunization, 242
immunocompetence, 191
immunocompromised, 178, 180, 190, 195, 196, 197, 198, 236
immunodeficiency, 168, 220, 245
immunofluorescence, 182, 191, 193, 196, 209
immunoglobulin, 181, 257
immunohistochemistry, 190
immunological, 190, 223
immunosuppression, 206
immunosuppressive, 178, 207
immunosuppressive agent, 207
immunosuppressive drugs, 178
impaired glucose tolerance, 98, 121, 122, 123
impairments, 184, 202, 296
implementation, 2, 74, 78, 82, 147, 150, 151, 160, 161, 163, 243, 319, 321, 324
impulsivity, 314
in situ, 37
in utero, 106, 157
in vitro, 218, 220
inactivation, 32
inactive, 211, 290
incarceration, 166
incentives, 316
inclusion, 1, 29, 52, 53, 96, 151, 261, 262
income, 8, 17, 19, 71, 79, 107, 118, 138, 139, 144, 166, 167, 238, 255, 263, 272, 281, 299, 316, 322, 323, 326
incubation, 180, 192, 199, 226, 232
incubation period, 180, 192, 226, 232
independence, 21
India, 38, 55, 58, 59, 60, 67, 110, 114, 120, 165, 177, 188, 192, 193, 204, 205, 210, 211, 213, 214, 217, 218, 219, 223, 224, 234, 235, 237, 244, 248, 253, 259, 260, 262, 263, 265, 267, 268, 270, 271, 272, 273, 274, 276, 277, 278
Indian, 66, 70, 80, 83, 86, 89, 102, 110, 111, 113, 114, 120, 121, 158, 167, 168, 192, 194, 203, 220, 221, 222, 224, 257, 259, 265, 270, 271, 276, 277, 278, 306, 307, 308, 311, 312, 329
Indians, 65, 66, 106, 113, 114, 117, 120, 121, 167, 237, 247, 295, 305, 310, 314
indication, 38, 55, 263
indicators, 67, 126, 133, 151, 167
indices, 70, 143, 181, 262
indigenous, 51, 58, 115, 178, 193
indirect bilirubin, 189
indolent, 5
Indonesia, 113, 188, 203, 208, 213, 234, 250
inductor, 142
industrialization, 303
industrialized countries, 171, 195
industry, 151, 161, 162
inequality, 55, 85
inequity, 89
inertia, 129
infancy, 106, 156, 157, 179, 206, 216, 217, 220, 222, 254, 255, 256
infant mortality, 51, 185, 186, 216
infants, 56, 111, 141, 155, 156, 157, 158, 178, 179, 180, 181, 182, 183, 184, 185, 186, 187, 188, 189, 190, 192, 194, 195, 196, 202, 206, 207, 214, 215, 216, 217, 219, 220, 221, 222, 225, 226, 229, 237, 240, 243, 244, 272, 313
infarction, 103
infections, 50, 51, 53, 57, 73, 156, 169, 177, 178, 179, 181, 184, 185, 187, 188, 194, 195, 197, 198, 199, 200, 201, 202, 203, 204, 205, 206, 207, 208, 209, 212, 217, 220, 221, 222, 223, 226, 227, 228, 231, 236, 237, 238, 240, 242, 244, 246, 248, 251, 254, 255, 256, 268, 269
infectious, 64, 103, 142, 169, 174, 177, 179, 195, 214, 219, 248, 255
infectious disease, 64, 103, 169, 174, 179, 214, 219, 255
infectious diseases, 64, 103, 169, 174, 179, 214, 219, 255
infestations, 202
inflammation, 13, 147, 181, 203, 208, 209
inflammatory, 32, 35, 185, 189, 191, 208, 209, 223, 294
inflammatory bowel disease, 32, 35
inflammatory response, 185
inflammatory responses, 185
informed consent, 16, 299
infrastructure, 19, 171, 267, 311, 318

ingest, 180
ingestion, 180, 194, 195, 199, 200, 201, 202, 203, 204, 206, 210, 212, 213
inhalation, 178, 201
inheritance, 55
inherited, 17
inhibitor, 70
inhibitors, 129
inhibitory, 11
initiation, 11, 34, 55, 152
injection, 166, 169, 173, 174
injections, 194
injuries, 110, 262, 303, 304, 305, 306, 309, 310, 311, 312, 313, 315, 316, 317, 318, 319, 321, 324, 325, 327, 328, 330
injury, iv, 6, 177, 296, 303, 304, 305, 306, 309, 310, 311, 312, 313, 315, 316, 317, 318, 319, 320, 321, 323, 325, 326, 327, 328
innate immunity, 208
inner ear, 181
innovation, 1
inoculation, 182
insects, 178
insight, 96
inspections, 318
instability, 32
institutionalization, 302
institutions, 57, 204, 273, 321
instruments, 52, 298
insulin, 10, 23, 24, 25, 66, 70, 71, 74, 83, 95, 96, 97, 98, 99, 102, 104, 106, 108, 109, 111, 120, 122, 123, 124, 147
insulin dependent diabetes, 106, 120
insulin resistance, 71, 83, 95, 96, 97, 98, 102, 104, 106, 108, 109, 111, 147
insulin sensitivity, 106, 109
insulin-like growth factor, 24, 25
insulin-like growth factor I, 24
insurance, 8, 48, 73, 75, 132, 292, 298, 323
insurance companies, 132
Insurance Institute for Highway Safety, 329
integration, 323
integrity, 56, 185
intensity, 28, 57, 74, 142, 146, 147, 159, 179, 200, 201, 203, 205, 216
interaction, 25, 77, 218, 233, 280, 319
interleukin, 189, 191, 201
interleukin-2, 189
international, 2, 21, 52, 60, 73, 109, 157, 170, 171, 259, 263, 284, 303
International Agency for Research on Cancer, 21, 22
International Classification of Diseases, 74
International Covenant on Economic, Social and Cultural Rights, 52
interpretation, 104, 193, 289
intervention, 8, 19, 52, 57, 73, 75, 76, 108, 149, 150, 151, 154, 222, 255, 266, 294, 302, 318, 330
intervention strategies, 108
interview, 162, 284, 296
interviews, 254, 280
intestinal tract, 179
intestine, 204, 206, 220, 232
intracranial, 88, 181, 211
intraperitoneal, 182
intrauterine growth retardation, 186, 217
intravenous, 92, 167, 173, 188, 194, 240
intrinsic, 172
intussusception, 229, 240, 250
invasive, 14, 34, 41, 77, 83, 90, 194
invasive cancer, 34
involuntary smoke, 153
iodine, 202
ionic, 198
iridocyclitis, 181
iron, 177, 200, 203, 205
iron deficiency, 177, 200, 205
irradiation, 6
irritability, 188
irritation, 145, 208
ischaemic heart disease, 93, 159
ischemia, 118
ischemic, 63, 64, 67, 78, 86, 87, 88, 89, 90, 92, 118, 122
ischemic heart disease, 63, 64, 67, 122
ischemic heart disease (IHD), 63
ischemic stroke, 86, 88, 89, 90, 92
Islam, 220
Islamic, 211, 213
island, 86
isoflavones, 12, 26
isoforms, 77
isolation, 49, 140, 182, 196, 209, 214, 215, 235, 239, 245, 275
isoniazid, 166, 170, 171

J

Jamaica, 116

Japanese, 7, 8, 10, 11, 12, 20, 21, 22, 23, 25, 26, 27, 66, 68, 69, 83, 116, 118, 119, 123, 146, 156, 158, 281, 282, 283, 296, 306
jaundice, 181, 188, 192, 270, 271, 274
jejunum, 232
jobs, 148
judge, 325
Jun, 79, 80, 82, 134, 136, 154
Jung, 243
justice, 153, 162, 179

K

Kaiser Family Foundation, 53, 55, 59
Kenya, 49, 59, 186, 203, 217
kidneys, 117, 204

L

labeling, 49
labor, 143, 268, 270, 274
labour, 188, 214, 269
lactating, 195
lactose, 202
lakes, 197
lamina, 37
land, 304, 315, 327
land use, 315
language, 52, 54, 57, 96, 321
Laos, 113
laparoscopic, 6, 39, 42, 44, 45
laparoscopy, 42
laparotomy, 39
large intestine, 200, 202
large-scale, 14
larva, 200, 204, 207, 222
larvae, 199, 200, 201, 202, 203, 204, 205, 206, 208, 209, 210
larval, 199, 200, 201, 204, 205, 211, 212, 223
later life, 254
late-stage, 28
Latin America, 31, 61, 69, 103, 104, 107, 111, 116, 121, 122, 139, 143, 144, 147, 154, 189, 229, 236, 237, 240, 242, 243, 279, 281, 284
Latin American countries, 116, 240
Latino, 66, 68, 69, 107, 279, 281, 282, 284, 304, 305, 306, 308, 309, 311, 313, 314, 325
Latino women, 69
Latinos, 2, 55, 69, 281, 282, 305, 306, 307, 310, 313, 314, 319, 321
law, 151, 161, 317, 321, 323
law enforcement, 317, 321, 323
laws, 311, 315, 316, 317, 320, 323
lawyers, 162
LDL, 68, 70, 71, 77, 89, 126, 127, 128, 129, 130, 131, 132, 133
lead, 20, 53, 56, 57, 77, 117, 131, 147, 153, 180, 185, 190, 207, 227, 262, 269, 289, 295, 298, 323
leakage, 41
learning, 330
legislation, 52, 150, 153, 161, 317, 319, 323
leishmaniasis, 178, 191, 192, 193, 219
leisure, 311
leisure time, 311
lens, 198
leptin, 23, 109
Lesbian, 59, 60
lesions, 35, 41, 76, 77, 189, 192, 198, 207, 209, 211, 232
leukemia, 143, 157
liberation, 142
licenses, 314, 317, 320
life course, 281
life cycle, 195, 198, 199, 204, 208, 210, 211
life expectancy, 5, 6, 16, 65, 71, 79, 80, 116, 126
life quality, 152
life style, 67
life-cycle, 202
lifespan, 307
lifestyle, 8, 21, 23, 24, 31, 32, 57, 73, 76, 81, 113, 116, 125, 127, 133, 256, 290
lifestyle changes, 21, 116
life-threatening, 193, 211, 271
lifetime, 33, 146, 152, 253, 263, 288, 290
ligand, 10, 233
light trucks, 311
likelihood, 14, 16, 143, 146, 148, 149, 178, 268, 289, 294, 296, 323
limitation, 16, 324
limitations, vii, 39, 75, 141, 178, 323, 326
linear, 95, 190
linguistic, 1, 311, 324
linguistically, 319, 321, 324
linkage, 9, 49, 106, 169, 207
links, 61, 142, 276
lipid, 63, 71, 74, 76, 78, 89, 97, 98, 101, 104, 106, 126, 127, 130, 131, 133, 135, 136
lipid metabolism, 106
lipid profile, 71, 78, 101, 130, 135
lipids, 65, 109, 132, 134

lipoprotein, 68, 70, 83, 87, 92, 126, 127, 134, 136
Lipoprotein, 131, 134, 136
lipoproteins, 77, 83, 134
literacy, 260
literature, 19, 96, 113, 116, 198, 221, 271, 279, 288, 291, 296, 331
lithium, 290
litigation, 272
liver, 38, 43, 184, 189, 190, 194, 201, 204, 206, 212, 290
liver abscess, 194
liver disease, 290
liver function tests, 43
localization, 168
location, 36, 40, 67, 93, 117, 148, 191, 194, 200, 233, 296
locus, 22, 25
longitudinal study, 23, 158, 283
long-term, 27, 42, 55, 82, 123, 149, 183, 233, 315, 323
losses, 141, 202
low risk, 55, 73
low-density, 77, 87, 126, 135, 136
low-density lipoprotein, 77, 87, 126, 135, 136
lower respiratory tract infection, 156
low-income, 151, 299
lumbar, 294, 326
lumbar spine, 294, 326
lumen, 202
lung, 2, 19, 26, 138, 140, 142, 145, 146, 149, 157, 158, 160, 204, 208, 212, 224
lung cancer, 2, 138, 142, 146, 149, 157, 158
lung function, 138, 140, 142, 145, 149, 157, 160
lungs, 198, 199, 201, 204, 205, 206, 211
lymph, 6, 14, 39, 41, 45, 168, 181, 189, 191, 192
lymph node, 6, 14, 39, 41, 45, 168, 191, 192
lymphadenopathy, 181, 189
lymphatic, 38, 189, 200, 207, 208, 214, 223
lymphatic system, 189
lymphocytes, 214
lymphoid, 201
lymphoid tissue, 201
lymphoma, 143
lysosomes, 218

M

M1, 37
machinery, 54
macrophages, 191, 222
magnetic resonance, 210
magnetic resonance imaging, 210
MAI, 57
maintenance, 239, 317, 318, 319
major depression, 283
majority group, 125, 126
malabsorption, 177, 195, 200, 207
malabsorptive, 290
malaise, 210
malaria, 177, 178, 179, 184, 185, 186, 187, 188, 189, 216, 217, 218, 268, 269, 274
Malaysia, 113, 203, 213
males, 22, 23, 24, 50, 66, 68, 74, 101, 114, 115, 228, 289, 292, 294, 304, 305, 306, 309, 310, 312, 313, 329
malignancy, 204, 290
malignant, 7, 13, 18
malnutrition, 177, 195, 196, 203, 206, 222
mammalian cell, 179
mammals, 180, 195, 197, 199
management, 1, 9, 14, 15, 16, 28, 38, 48, 75, 76, 78, 82, 83, 85, 89, 90, 93, 108, 129, 134, 136, 215, 224, 233, 253, 256, 260, 274, 316, 318
manganese, 26
manganese superoxide, 26
manganese superoxide dismutase, 26
manipulation, 151, 153, 162
manners, 13
manual workers, 71
manufacturer, 295
manufacturing, 311, 318
mapping, 22, 39, 45
margin of error, 267
marijuana, 328, 330
market, 143, 152, 240
marketing, 152, 321, 330
markets, 106, 138
marriage, 274
marriages, 146
marrow, 193
masking, 325
mass media, 18, 19, 317, 319
mastoid, 181
maternal, 139, 141, 143, 180, 182, 183, 185, 186, 187, 188, 189, 190, 202, 214, 217, 231, 254, 255, 259, 260, 261, 262, 263, 264, 265, 266, 268, 269, 270, 271, 272, 273, 274, 275, 276, 277, 278
maternal care, 261, 262
maternal smoking, 141, 143
matrix, 304

maturation, 142, 199, 205
maxillary sinus, 159
MDR, 169, 170
measles, 177
measurement, 19, 89, 131, 265, 277, 283, 284, 288, 289, 293, 296
measures, 1, 17, 20, 54, 78, 90, 99, 149, 150, 172, 259, 260, 264, 273, 274, 277, 283, 319, 329
meat, 8, 180
mechanical, iv, 38, 317
mechanics, 147
media, 19, 56, 143, 152, 153, 172, 199, 319, 320, 321, 322, 323
median, 51, 68, 147, 192, 233, 292
mediation, 285
mediators, 201
medical care, 15, 27, 73, 78, 90, 271, 319, 327
Medicare, 17, 21, 28, 117, 136, 297, 298
medication, 52, 118, 130, 145
medications, 289, 296
medicine, 134, 135, 136, 214, 216
Mediterranean, 114, 138, 192, 205
Melanesian, 118
meninges, 181
meningitis, 210, 223
meningoencephalitis, 189, 197, 198, 210, 221
menopause, 290
menstrual, 290
mental health, 285, 330
mental retardation, 184
merozoites, 184, 195
mesentery, 40, 41
messages, 321, 322
messengers, 321, 323
meta-analysis, 44, 77, 83, 153, 156, 157, 159, 284, 312, 330
metabolic, 70, 95, 96, 97, 98, 99, 100, 101, 102, 103, 104, 105, 106, 107, 108, 109, 110, 111, 140, 269
metabolic syndrome, 70, 95, 96, 97, 98, 99, 100, 101, 102, 103, 104, 105, 106, 107, 108, 109, 110, 111
metabolism, 77, 100, 147, 155
metastases, 23, 36, 37, 38, 40, 42
metastasis, 5, 6, 13, 37, 192
metastatic, 5, 6, 11, 12, 25, 31, 38, 40, 44
metastatic disease, 5, 6, 12, 31, 38, 40
meteorological, 228
Mexican, 66, 68, 72, 74, 79, 86, 91, 99, 101, 103, 104, 105, 106, 107, 110, 111, 118, 123, 125, 126, 134, 144, 162, 220, 235, 246, 280, 284, 292, 293, 296, 305, 313
Mexican Americans, 66, 68, 72, 86, 91, 103, 104, 110, 134, 284, 313
Mexican-Americans, 68, 101, 125, 126, 296
Mexico, 1, 31, 32, 36, 43, 44, 65, 74, 95, 100, 103, 104, 105, 106, 107, 111, 116, 165, 189, 195, 237, 244, 280
mice, 182, 191, 235
microarray, 249
microbes, 223, 257
microfilariae, 207, 208, 209
micronesian, 118
microscopy, 193, 197, 198
microsurgery, 41
microvascular, 124
microvasculature, 185
Middle East, 114, 115, 295, 301
middle-aged, 24, 119, 134, 158
migrant, 70, 114, 115
migrants, 66, 70, 71, 80, 103, 114
migration, 28, 49, 67, 113, 201, 202, 204, 205, 226, 239, 266
military, 13, 232, 236, 246
milk, 254, 256
Millennium Development Goals, 53, 54, 259
minks, 235
minorities, vii, 1, 2, 18, 19, 48, 49, 50, 51, 53, 55, 56, 57, 60, 64, 65, 66, 67, 69, 70, 71, 72, 73, 74, 75, 76, 77, 78, 81, 84, 85, 87, 89, 90, 126, 131, 138, 151, 152, 153, 163, 164, 165, 167, 168, 169, 170, 171, 172, 175, 279, 288, 291, 292, 297, 298, 299, 300,□303, 305, 306, 313, 315, 316, 319, 321, 322, 323
minority groups, 1, 85, 86, 125, 126, 131, 132, 133, 167, 168, 169, 295
minority students, 280
miracidium, 213
mitochondria, 197
mobility, 36, 226
modalities, 6, 14, 16
modality, 14, 34, 38
models, 12, 152, 201, 293
modernization, 303
molar ratio, 10
molecules, 9, 199
mollusks, 210
money, 153, 201

monkeys, 202
monoclonal, 196, 210, 236, 239, 245
monoclonal antibodies, 196, 210, 236, 245
monozygotic twins, 180
mood, 280, 281, 283, 284, 285, 314
morbidity, 6, 15, 20, 39, 41, 42, 57, 65, 66, 125, 126, 133, 152, 169, 173, 174, 179, 188, 189, 203, 212, 223, 225, 253, 255, 261, 276, 277, 287, 305, 314, 326
morning, 145, 149, 204
morphological, 198, 199, 235
morphology, 36
mortality rate, 7, 8, 13, 14, 15, 29, 31, 32, 64, 65, 66, 67, 69, 70, 71, 90, 103, 125, 184, 193, 212, 259, 263, 264, 273, 298, 304, 306, 307
mortality risk, 146
mosquitoes, 178, 184, 187
mother tongue, 96
motherhood, 259, 263
mothers, 141, 142, 180, 185, 186, 187, 190, 194, 195, 202, 220, 269
motion, 87, 88
motivation, 1, 75
motor skills, 314
motor vehicle accident, 318
motor vehicle crashes, 306, 307, 312, 313, 314, 319, 322, 326, 329
motorcycles, 309, 318
mouse, 8, 201
mouse model, 201
mouth, 192, 202
movement, 153
MPA, 59
MRI, 38, 43
MSI, 32
MTHFR, 77
mucosa, 32, 37, 38, 189, 191, 197, 202, 203, 205, 210, 226, 241
mucous membrane, 192
mucous membranes, 192
multidisciplinary, 129
multi-ethnic, 81, 301
multilateral, 57
multiple factors, 299
multiple myeloma, 290
Multi-Society Task Force, 43
multivariate, 15, 76
murmur, 192
muscle, 6, 189, 203, 212
muscle strength, 6
muscles, 40
music, 322
mutation rate, 32
mutations, 23, 32
myalgia, 196
Myanmar, 113
Mycobacterium, 169, 171, 174, 175
myocardial infarction, 63, 79, 81, 82, 83, 103, 110, 111, 130, 132, 133, 135, 151, 161
myocarditis, 181, 189

N

nation, 57, 91, 231, 311, 312, 328
national, 19, 50, 52, 58, 59, 66, 70, 74, 85, 89, 92, 101, 103, 109, 115, 117, 119, 123, 125, 135, 136, 155, 161, 162, 164, 168, 175, 259, 263, 264, 266, 283, 292, 303, 306, 322, 328, 330
National Health Interview Survey, 71
National Highway Traffic Safety Administration, 328
national income, 263
National Institutes of Health, 1, 18, 29, 225, 284
nationality, 305
Native American, 102, 106, 116, 129, 280, 282, 293, 306, 313, 314
Native Americans, 129, 280, 282, 293, 306, 313
Native Hawaiian, 66, 68, 69, 282, 283, 305, 325
native population, 188
natural, 34, 65, 73, 86, 142, 148, 150, 163, 185, 211, 228, 260, 281, 284, 326
natural killer, 142, 284
natural killer cell, 142, 284
nausea, 36, 210
neck, 210, 326
necrosis, 191, 223
needles, 184
negative consequences, 2
negative experiences, 14
negotiation, 151, 152
nematode, 199, 200, 201, 203, 206, 221, 223
nematodes, 199, 200, 205
neonatal, 183, 185, 186, 273, 276, 278
neonate, 196
neonates, 194, 197
neoplasia, 6, 20, 24
neoplasm, 7
neoplasms, 159
Nepal, 55, 59, 197
nephritic syndrome, 181

nephropathy, 117, 122
nerves, 41
nervous system, 168, 181, 190, 197
nested PCR, 249
neural tissue, 40
neuroendocrine, 106
neurologic disorders, 91
neurologic symptom, 184
Neuropeptide Y, 284
neutralization, 232
New World, 192, 205
NGO, 52
NHTSA, 313, 324, 325, 327, 328, 329, 330
Nicaragua, 175, 231, 243
nicotine, 137, 139, 141, 142, 144, 147, 148, 150, 161
Nicotine, 141, 142, 154, 155, 158, 161, 162
Nigeria, 7, 213, 214, 216, 262
NIH, 29, 131, 331
Nile, 212
nitric oxide, 201
nodes, 36, 37, 38
nodules, 209
non diabetic, 98, 104
non-biological, 14, 15
nongovernmental, 54
nongovernmental organization, 54
nongovernmental organization (NGO), 54
non-Hodgkin's lymphoma, 143
non-insulin dependent diabetes, 123
nonsense mutation, 77
nonsmokers, 158, 159, 160, 162
non-smokers, 141, 146, 149, 153
non-smokers, 159
non-smokers, 255
nonwhite, 288, 293, 294
normal, 6, 27, 32, 33, 35, 39, 43, 99, 106, 109, 118, 123, 135, 189, 196, 267, 289, 294, 310
norms, 49, 56, 273
North Africa, 115, 295, 301
North America, 8, 31, 65, 114, 118, 119, 161, 289, 292, 295
North Carolina, 29, 164, 172
Northeast, 238
nuclear, 141, 182
nucleotide sequence, 236
nucleotide sequencing, 246
nucleotides, 239
nucleus, 181, 198
nursing, 207, 232
nursing home, 232
nutrient, 177, 199
nutrients, 10, 24, 178, 272
nutrition, 73, 107, 120, 155, 177, 202, 284, 300
nutritional deficiencies, 272
nutritional transition, 111

O

obese, 71, 100, 109, 134
obesity, 8, 21, 22, 65, 67, 69, 70, 71, 72, 88, 90, 95, 96, 97, 98, 99, 101, 103, 105, 106, 107, 108, 110, 111, 113, 116, 120, 126
obligate, 179
observations, 64, 65, 70, 74, 100, 132, 153, 231, 325
obstetricians, 272
obstruction, 201, 269
obstructive lung disease, 158, 253
occupational, 20, 147
odds ratio, 9, 141, 143, 145, 297
oedema, 192
Office of Management and Budget, 305, 324, 328
OFS, 115
old age, 167, 310
older adults, 118, 284, 302, 329
older people, 76, 301
olfactory, 197
OMB, 305, 324, 328
onchocerciasis, 200, 207, 223
oncogene, 32
oncology, 18, 44
online, 19, 60
opposition, 151, 153
optic nerve, 181
oral, 118, 178, 194, 195, 205, 226, 228, 232, 239
orchitis, 208
organ, 22, 189, 192, 211, 261, 262
organic, 12, 190, 235
organic solvent, 235
organic solvents, 235
organism, 178, 179, 181, 182, 195, 197
organization, 54, 55, 84, 245, 320
organizations, 57, 58, 59, 61, 96, 321, 322
orientation, 60
orthopaedic, 291
osteopenia, 288, 293, 295, 301
osteoporosis, 6, 287, 288, 289, 290, 292, 293, 294, 295, 296, 297, 298, 299, 300, 301, 302
osteoporotic fractures, 287, 288, 300, 301
otitis media, 143

out-of-hospital, 65
outpatient, 17, 82, 292
outpatients, 129, 234, 236
ovarian, 26, 33, 288
ovarian cancer, 26, 288
oversight, 132
overweight, 70, 99, 106, 111
oxidative, 10, 143, 147, 157, 160
oxidative stress, 143, 147, 157, 160
oxygen, 63, 141, 201

P

P. falciparum, 184, 186, 187, 188
Pacific, 2, 7, 66, 86, 88, 90, 108, 138, 210, 299, 304, 305, 306, 307, 308, 310, 313, 314, 325
Pacific Islander, 2, 7, 66, 90, 299, 304, 305, 306, 307, 310, 313, 314, 325
Pacific Islanders, 2, 90, 305, 306, 310, 313, 314
PAI-1, 77, 87
pain, 6, 42, 73, 74, 82, 120, 152, 196, 203, 207, 210, 226
Pakistan, 67, 114, 115, 234, 253
Pakistani, 70, 166, 251
Palestine, 193
palliative, 6
pallor, 189, 192
pancreatic, 196
pandemic, 53, 54, 56, 166
Papua New Guinea, 186, 187, 207, 217
paradox, 65, 80, 110
Paraguay, 225, 228, 231, 242, 243
paralysis, 181
paralytic ileus, 206
parameter, 99, 106
parasitaemia, 180, 185, 186, 187, 188, 190
parasite, 178, 179, 182, 184, 185, 186, 187, 189, 191, 192, 194, 195, 199, 200, 202, 204, 206, 208, 211, 212, 213, 214
parasites, 178, 179, 184, 185, 186, 187, 188, 189, 190, 191, 200, 201, 205, 207, 208, 209, 210, 212, 216, 219, 221, 225, 257
parasitic infection, 177, 178, 179, 192, 203, 205, 213, 238
parasitic infestation, 224
parathormone, 297
parathyroid, 289
parathyroid hormone, 289
parenchymal, 184, 198, 211
parenchymal cell, 184
parent-adolescent relationships, 283
parental smoking, 139, 156, 157
parents, 139, 141, 150, 152, 155, 156, 161, 255
particles, 131, 226, 232, 235, 239, 241, 244
partnerships, 53
passenger, 305, 311, 312, 313, 314, 318, 319, 326
passive, 153, 155, 156, 157, 158, 159, 160, 162, 217
passive smoke, 157, 158
passive smokers, 158
paternal, 139, 142, 143, 254, 255
pathogenesis, 204, 224
pathogenic, 179, 198, 220
pathogens, 214, 248, 250
pathology, 197, 221
pathophysiology, 81, 100, 185, 216
pathways, 131, 141, 143
PCR, 183, 186, 194, 196, 236, 237, 239, 243, 245, 248, 249, 250
pedal, 304, 311, 317
pedestrian, 306, 310, 313, 314, 316
pedestrian traffic, 316
pedestrians, 304, 305, 306, 307, 310, 316, 318
pediatric, 164, 172, 208, 211, 245, 248
pediatric patients, 248
peers, 55, 323
PEF, 149
pelvic, 41, 204, 287
pelvis, 326
penalties, 150
penetrance, 13
per capita, 263
percentile, 98
perception, 75, 155, 260, 331
perceptions, 58, 60
perfectionism, 280
perforated bowel, 204
perforation, 36
performance, 13, 43, 183, 329
perinatal, 57, 180, 181, 216
perineum, 204
periodic, 207, 265, 273
peripheral blood, 182, 184, 185, 187, 193, 207, 209
peripheral vascular disease, 124, 130
peritoneal, 41, 204
peritoneal cavity, 204
peritoneum, 37, 204
peritonitis, 202, 204
permit, 266
peroxide, 143

personal, 35, 50, 78, 177, 240, 311, 316, 323
personal history, 35
personal hygiene, 240
personality, 179
person-to-person contact, 232
Peru, 105, 190, 197, 213, 218
PET, 43
PET scan, 43
petechiae, 192
pets, 178, 204
pH, 232, 235
phagocyte, 191
phagocytic, 142, 189
pharmacological, 179, 199
phenotype, 83, 109, 244
phenotypes, 76
Philippines, 113, 165, 213
phlegm, 141, 145, 146, 149
phone, 19
phylogenetic, 232
physical abuse, 53
physical activity, 33, 302
physical environment, 304, 318
physical exercise, 64, 107, 253
physical factors, 329
physical fitness, 177, 221
physical health, 284
physicians, 14, 17, 75, 76, 89, 92, 129, 132, 299, 324
physiological, 24, 85, 88, 111, 260, 314
physiology, 95
pigs, 202, 229
pilot study, 30, 248
placebo, 12, 130
placenta, 181, 182, 183, 185, 188, 190, 191, 216, 271, 272, 277
placental, 141, 180, 181, 185, 186, 188, 191, 216, 217, 218
planning, 263, 315
plaque, 77
plaques, 63
plasma, 9, 10, 11, 23, 24, 25, 76, 77, 83, 96, 97, 99, 121, 131, 136, 143
plasma levels, 10, 11, 24, 76, 77
plasma proteins, 83
plasminogen, 70, 92
plasmodium falciparum, 216, 217
plasmodium malariae, 216, 217
plasmodium vivax, 184, 217, 218
platelet, 147, 184
platelet aggregation, 147
Platyhelminthes, 178
plausibility, 146
play, 8, 11, 32, 88, 178, 233, 272, 288, 289, 300
plexus, 181
pneumonia, 189, 254, 255, 256
pneumonitis, 181, 201
point mutation, 227, 239
poisoning, 326, 327
police, 54, 55, 56, 307
policy makers, 89, 273
policymakers, 260
political, 31, 50, 55, 276, 304, 311, 319, 322, 323
pollen, 253
pollutants, 137, 138
pollution, 153, 178
polonium, 137
polyacrylamide, 239
polymerase, 183, 194, 215, 221, 236, 246
polymerase chain reaction, 183, 194, 215, 221, 236, 246
polymorphism, 10, 11, 23, 25, 26, 77, 83, 106, 169, 175, 243
polymorphisms, 10, 11, 25, 26, 77, 169, 171, 174
Polynesian, 118
polyp, 34
polypectomy, 34
polyps, 32, 33, 34, 35
PON1, 77
pools, 197
poor, 6, 16, 38, 39, 48, 57, 73, 74, 75, 132, 153, 163, 164, 177, 182, 187, 189, 190, 195, 202, 205, 240, 254, 256, 259, 260, 263, 264, 266, 268, 269, 271, 272, 273, 274, 276, 278, 283, 290, 296, 325
poor health, 283
population group, 2, 66, 67, 68, 73, 153, 203, 296, 325
population growth, 115
pores, 198, 199
positive correlation, 9
postmenopausal, 146, 289, 293, 297, 302
postmenopausal women, 146, 289, 293, 302
postmortem, 182
postnatal exposure, 141, 142
postoperative, 38, 41, 42, 43
postpartum, 269, 271
posttraumatic stress disorder, 48
poverty, 48, 49, 50, 54, 107, 148, 159, 163, 164, 167, 172, 173, 314, 322

poverty line, 148
powder, 229
power, 12, 49, 100, 138, 152, 153, 293
preclinical, 134
precocious puberty, 181
prediction, 6, 136, 293
predictors, 12, 24, 44, 135, 139, 295
prednisone, 21
pre-existing, 14, 49
preference, 311, 326
pregnancy, 141, 143, 156, 158, 180, 182, 183, 185, 186, 188, 190, 193, 214, 215, 216, 217, 219, 260, 262, 263, 266, 268, 269, 271, 274, 276, 277
pregnant, 51, 54, 156, 158, 181, 183, 184, 185, 186, 190, 193, 205, 214, 217, 260, 261, 269, 271
pregnant women, 51, 156, 183, 184, 185, 186, 190, 193, 214, 217, 269, 271
prehospital, 81
prejudice, 78
premature death, 303, 305
premature infant, 216
prematurity, 186, 190, 216, 217
premenopausal, 146, 294
premenopausal women, 146, 294
preoperative, 38, 40, 41, 42
preparation, iv
preschool, 155, 200, 202
preschool children, 155
pressure, 160
preterm delivery, 144
prevention, 11, 19, 29, 44, 48, 53, 54, 55, 56, 57, 58, 59, 60, 61, 78, 79, 82, 90, 96, 110, 126, 132, 138, 163, 170, 172, 175, 217, 240, 261, 289, 303, 305, 315, 316, 317, 319, 321, 322, 327
preventive, vii, 1, 78, 85, 88, 172, 173, 179, 259, 260, 273, 298, 317, 330
primary care, 100, 298
primary school, 203
primary tumor, 37
primates, 207
primigravidae, 186
printing, 110
prisoners, 163
privacy, 56
private, 18, 53, 54, 78, 150
pro-atherogenic, 131
probability, 169, 268, 279, 312, 325
probable cause, 266
probe, 248
problem behavior, 284, 329
problem behaviors, 284
procedures, 16, 42, 57, 75, 78, 85, 89, 90, 93, 194, 269, 272
process indicators, 272
proctoscopy, 43, 203
producers, 12, 26
production, 18, 142, 201, 222
productivity, 152, 162
profession, 18
prognosis, 6, 11, 20, 39, 41, 42, 67, 76, 78, 81, 142, 181, 190
prognostic marker, 215
program, 7, 13, 14, 15, 29, 32, 57, 60, 75, 76, 83, 109, 129, 150, 265, 273, 274
programming, 56
progressive, 64, 100, 191
proliferation, 10, 201
promote, 2, 14, 17, 19, 272, 275, 315, 317
promoter, 11, 25, 32
promoter region, 11, 32
propagation, 240, 244, 245
prophylactic, 33
prophylaxis, 183, 197, 220
prostate, 5, 6, 7, 8, 9, 12, 13, 19, 20, 21, 22, 23, 24, 25, 26, 27, 28, 29, 30
prostate cancer, 6, 7, 8, 12, 20, 21, 22, 23, 24, 25, 26, 27, 28, 29, 30
prostate carcinoma, 23, 27, 29
prostate gland, 5, 6
prostate specific antigen, 27
prostatectomy, 6, 20, 21, 22, 27, 28
prostitution, 55
protection, 2, 34, 52, 138, 160, 185, 188, 195, 200, 240, 313, 317, 318
protective factors, 65, 280
protein, 10, 24, 25, 32, 64, 72, 202, 203, 207, 226, 232, 240, 243, 254
proteins, 9, 117, 226, 228, 232, 235, 236, 239, 242
proteinuria, 117
proteolysis, 202
protocol, 194
protocols, 89
proto-oncogene, 9, 32
protozoa, 179
proximal, 41, 232, 287, 291, 294, 301
proxy, 12

PRP, 6
pruritus, 205, 206
PSA, 5, 6, 7, 8, 12, 13, 14, 15, 17, 20, 28
pseudopodia, 198
PSG, 216
psychiatric disorder, 53, 57
psychiatric disorders, 53, 57
psychological, 279, 284, 289
psychological distress, 279
psychological health, 284
psychology, 284, 285
psychosis, 179
psychosocial, 28, 58, 64, 65
psychosocial factors, 65
public, 2, 9, 17, 20, 31, 52, 57, 78, 99, 107, 125, 127, 138, 144, 147, 150, 151, 152, 153, 154, 159, 160, 162, 167, 170, 171, 172, 177, 211, 213, 240, 254, 263, 272, 280, 287, 294, 303, 304, 305, 310, 313, 316, 317, 319, 320, 321, 322, 330
public affairs, 2
public awareness, 78, 172
public education, 316
public health, 9, 17, 20, 31, 52, 57, 99, 107, 150, 159, 160, 162, 171, 177, 211, 213, 240, 263, 272, 287, 294, 303, 304, 305, 322, 330
public opinion, 153, 162
public policy, 320
public relations, 162
public transit, 310
Puerto Rican, 155, 305, 314
pulmonary arteries, 210
punishment, 56

Q

Qatar, 85, 87
QOL, 6, 16
quality improvement, 78
quality of life, 1, 6, 16, 28, 146, 279, 295, 298, 299
quality of service, 272
quality research, 299
questionnaire, 17, 78, 114, 255, 266
questionnaires, 265, 297, 299
quinine, 188

R

race, 2, 7, 8, 12, 13, 14, 15, 17, 20, 21, 22, 24, 28, 29, 48, 49, 50, 52, 60, 67, 72, 79, 82, 85, 88, 89, 90, 92, 93, 96, 105, 108, 109, 118, 122, 125, 126, 127, 128, 129, 132, 136, 139, 148, 152, 167, 173, 281, 285, 289, 291, 292, 293, 294, 297, 305, 307, 309, 311, 314, 324, 325
racial categories, 50
racial differences, 10, 11, 80, 82, 155
racial groups, 49, 51, 85, 306, 325
racial minorities, 2, 51
racism, 51, 52, 61
radiation, 40, 42
radiation damage, 40
radiation therapy, 42
radical, 6, 20, 21, 22, 27, 28, 41
radio, 18, 322
radio station, 322
radiotherapy, 6, 8, 15, 16, 40, 42
rainfall, 200
random, 117, 280, 296, 325
range, 19, 51, 100, 102, 115, 148, 152, 198, 228, 231, 233, 237, 240, 289, 295, 303, 310, 315, 319, 322, 324
rape, 49, 54, 55
ras, 32
rash, 181, 189, 205, 206, 209, 210, 212
ratings, 291
rats, 210
reactivity, 157, 236
reading, 231, 235
reagents, 228
reality, 49, 323
real-time, 239, 243, 248, 249
receptors, 10
recognition, 34, 78, 177, 260
recombination, 227
recovery, 42, 93, 198, 210, 311, 319
recreational, 310, 316
recruiting, 18, 19, 29
rectal examination, 5, 27
rectal prolapse, 203
rectum, 36, 40, 41, 43, 45, 202, 203
recurrence, 15, 22, 28, 39, 40, 42, 43, 88, 92, 191
red blood cells, 141, 187
red meat, 34
reduction, 40, 65, 66, 70, 78, 101, 107, 129, 130, 142, 143, 150, 153, 169, 171, 248, 259, 261, 263, 270, 272, 273, 288, 312, 313, 318

reflection, 41, 79, 90, 140, 152
refractory, 6, 10, 21, 233
refugees, 163
regional, 6, 7, 14, 27, 28, 29, 37, 53, 59, 189, 259
registries, 7, 19, 291
regression, 6, 21, 281, 297
regression analysis, 281
regular, 107, 275, 317
regulation, 141, 150, 161
regulations, 148, 150, 151, 152, 153
regulators, 25
rehabilitation, 75, 82, 289, 312, 319
rehabilitation program, 75
rehydration, 34, 239
relapse, 6, 150, 194
relapses, 196
relationship, 12, 16, 48, 49, 64, 65, 68, 77, 96, 106, 199, 213, 222, 223, 241, 254, 296, 312, 329
relationships, 108, 138, 159, 232, 283
relatives, 8, 33, 35, 55, 266
relevance, 261, 288, 294
reliability, 298
religion, 96
renal, 75, 117, 122, 290
renal disease, 122, 290
renal failure, 75, 117, 118
renal replacement therapy, 117
renin, 76
repair, 32, 292
reperfusion, 75, 82
replication, 196, 232, 241
repolarization, 75
reproduction, 152
reproductive age, 264, 275
research, 1, 2, 8, 18, 19, 29, 48, 52, 60, 78, 90, 96, 99, 147, 149, 150, 151, 152, 153, 160, 202, 256, 268, 284, 296, 299, 300, 302, 314, 315, 320, 324, 329, 330, 331
researchers, vii, 9, 49, 271
resection, 38, 39, 41, 42, 43, 44, 45
reservoir, 191, 192, 208
reservoirs, 192, 209
residential, 311, 315, 317
resistance, 8, 71, 95, 96, 97, 98, 166, 169, 170, 171, 175, 194, 201, 218, 232, 233, 235, 243
resolution, 54, 177, 205, 233
resources, 19, 49, 57, 74, 138, 153, 261, 272, 273, 276, 321
respiratory, 138, 140, 141, 142, 145, 146, 149, 151, 152, 156, 157, 158, 160, 161, 163, 168, 205, 250, 253, 254, 255, 256, 257, 269, 270, 271
respiratory disorders, 271
respiratory problems, 142, 149
respiratory syncytial virus, 257
responsibilities, 314, 316, 317
responsiveness, 149, 158, 208
restaurants, 144, 147, 148, 149, 150, 152, 160, 161, 315
restitution, 298
retardation, 205
retention, 271, 302
retina, 205
retinitis, 181
retinochoroiditis, 205
retinol, 23, 25
retinopathy, 117, 122
retrovirus, 245
revascularization, 75, 132, 133
reverse transcriptase, 245, 246
rheumatoid arthritis, 287, 290, 301
rheumatoid factor, 182
ribosomal, 194, 245
ribosomal RNA, 194
rings, 184
Rio de Janeiro, 218, 219, 221, 225, 233, 244, 247
risk assessment, 9
risk behaviors, 48, 58, 60, 305
risk factor profiles, 85, 86, 87
risk factors, 12, 34, 64, 65, 67, 68, 69, 70, 71, 73, 74, 76, 77, 78, 79, 80, 81, 85, 87, 88, 90, 92, 95, 110, 111, 116, 118, 120, 121, 122, 123, 124, 125, 126, 134, 135, 140, 165, 166, 170, 171, 175, 215, 218, 244, 254, 262, 274, 279, 284, 288, 289, 293, 295, 297, 299, 300, 301, 303, 304, 305, 311, 312, 314, 315, 316, 319, 322, 327
risk profile, 71, 81, 105
risks, 2, 9, 32, 40, 50, 55, 64, 69, 71, 123, 138, 151, 152, 153, 158, 263, 302, 317
risk-taking, 314, 329
risky driving, 324, 329
rivers, 197, 314
RNA, 53, 226, 227, 231, 232, 235, 242, 245
road safety, 303
robustness, 106
rodents, 185, 192
rolling, 268

room temperature, 229, 232
rotavirus, 226, 227, 228, 229, 230, 231, 237, 238, 239, 240, 241, 242, 243, 247, 248, 249, 250
roundworms, 178, 202, 204
RRP, 6
RSV infection, 254
runaway, 318
rural, 2, 113, 114, 115, 116, 120, 121, 159, 175, 193, 203, 208, 211, 214, 217, 237, 253, 254, 255, 257, 269, 271, 272, 273, 274, 275, 310, 313, 321, 322, 325
rural areas, 2, 114, 193, 208, 254, 269, 272, 273, 274, 275, 313, 321, 323, 325
rural communities, 115, 322
rural population, 114, 121, 211

S

safeguard, 106
safety, 43, 135, 304, 311, 312, 313, 315, 316, 317, 318, 319, 320, 323, 324, 325, 326, 328, 329, 330
salt, 76
salts, 206
sample, 18, 92, 114, 115, 117, 123, 144, 196, 204, 232, 264, 265, 267, 268, 279, 281, 283, 285, 295, 296
sampling, 193, 266, 267, 268
sampling error, 266
sanctions, 320
sand, 204
sanitation, 177, 180, 195, 238, 248
satellite, 40
satisfaction, 48
saturated fat, 10
Saudi Arabia, 114, 121, 212
scaling, 57
scanning electron microscopy, 199
schistosomiasis, 177, 212, 223, 224
school, 51, 55, 71, 72, 147, 150, 156, 165, 166, 178, 201, 202, 204, 232, 236, 254, 255, 257, 314, 317, 321
school performance, 203
schooling, 17, 51
science, 26, 153, 162, 330
scientific, vii, 1, 65, 108, 131, 138, 304
scolex, 224
scores, 6, 13, 130, 281, 282, 293, 294
screening programs, 18, 295
SES, 125, 126, 167
severity, 2, 75, 76, 77, 83, 85, 91, 180, 183, 208, 226, 231, 236, 243, 253, 260, 311, 318, 330
severity levels, 330
sex, 9, 23, 29, 49, 51, 52, 53, 55, 56, 58, 60, 72, 80, 92, 120, 122, 125, 178, 268, 280, 288, 289, 298, 309, 314
sex differences, 80
sex hormones, 23
sexual assault, 49
sexual contact, 53, 178
sexual intercourse, 192
sexual orientation, 49
sexual reproduction, 196
sexual violence, 54
sexuality, 49, 54, 322
sexually transmitted infections (STIs), 51, 53, 54
shape, 198, 235, 311, 319, 321, 322
sharing, 96
sheep, 211
shelter, 54, 199
shortness of breath, 146, 253
short-term, 42, 147, 162, 233
Short-term, 44, 160, 233
shoulder, 312, 313, 326
sickle cell, 187
side effects, 207, SIDS, 141
sigmoid, 39, 203
sigmoid colon, 203
sigmoidoscopy, 33, 34, 35
sign, 106
signals, 9, 185, 315, 316, 318, 325
signs, 13, 74, 81, 90, 181, 182, 183, 193, 196, 209, 253, 266, 273, 316
similarity, 88
single nucleotide polymorphism, 11, 77
sinus, 145, 146
sites, 6, 19, 189, 202, 204, 212, 287, 296
skeletal muscle, 180
skills, 317
skin, 178, 189, 192, 198, 199, 200, 204, 205, 206, 208, 209, 210, 212
slavery, 223
sleep, 141, 314
sleep deprivation, 314
sleeping sickness, 189
sludge, 249
slums, 203, 269, 271, 272, 274, 277
small intestine, 200, 201, 206, 222, 232

smoke, 70, 141, 145, 146, 147, 150, 151, 152, 153, 154, 155, 156, 157, 158, 159, 160, 161, 162, 254
smoke exposure, 154, 155, 156, 161, 162, 254
smokers, 69, 138, 139, 140, 141, 144, 145, 150, 152, 153, 155, 159, 162
smoking, 64, 65, 67, 69, 70, 87, 88, 137, 138, 139, 141, 142, 143, 144, 145, 146, 147, 148, 149, 150, 151, 152, 153, 154, 155, 156, 157, 158, 159, 160, 161, 162
SNPs, 11, 77
sobriety, 317
social, 48, 49, 50, 52, 54, 57, 59, 67, 71, 72, 73, 127, 152, 153, 154, 158, 163, 170, 172, 179, 204, 263, 266, 269, 272, 276, 281, 284, 304, 305, 311, 315, 316, 319, 321, 322, 323, 325, 331
social capital, 322
social change, 311
social class, 71, 204
social context, 152, 311
social environment, 331
social exclusion, 49, 52
social factors, 54, 67, 127
social inequalities, 49, 50
social movements, 57
social norms, 321
social participation, 72
social roles, 153
social sciences, 284
social services, 59
social support, 73
socially, 151, 163, 169
society, 2, 49, 51, 138, 152, 153, 163, 170, 178, 275, 299, 316
socioeconomic, 1, 2, 7, 14, 15, 16, 17, 18, 19, 20, 29, 65, 67, 71, 73, 76, 82, 88, 90, 91, 93, 107, 125, 133, 134, 144, 152, 154, 157, 167, 173, 297, 299, 301, 302
socioeconomic background, 17
socioeconomic status, 1, 2, 14, 15, 17, 18, 20, 29, 65, 67, 76, 82, 88, 90, 93, 107, 125, 144, 152, 154, 167, 173, 299
sodium, 194
sodomy, 55
soft drinks, 107
soil, 12, 177, 178, 180, 200, 202, 206, 213
solutions, 153, 303, 324
Somali, 299
Somalia, 170
South Africa, 53, 55, 61, 114, 115, 121, 139, 212, 238, 246, 248
South America, 7, 171, 189, 191, 192, 205, 209, 213, 228, 231, 233, 237, 243, 269, 305, 314
South Asia, 66, 70, 71, 73, 74, 76, 77, 80, 81, 82, 86, 87, 88, 89, 91, 92, 93, 99, 102, 106, 110, 114, 167, 262, 269
Southeast Asia, 208, 292
soybean, 26
Spaniards, 96
spasticity, 184
specialists, 74
speciation, 197
species, 131, 178, 184, 188, 191, 192, 194, 195, 197, 198, 199, 200, 206, 207, 209, 210, 212, 213
specificity, 5, 99, 182, 193, 223, 239
spectrum, 108, 200, 224, 272, 294
speed, 296, 311, 312, 316, 318, 319, 328, 329
speed limit, 318, 328
sperm, 143
spheres, 54, 323
sphincter, 40, 41, 42
spinal cord, 209, 212
spine, 198, 288, 293, 294, 295, 299
spine fractures, 299
spleen, 190, 194, 204
splenomegaly, 188, 192
sporadic, 32, 180, 192, 231, 233, 234, 235, 237, 244, 247
spore, 197
sports, 310, 313, 323
spouse, 75, 283
sprue, 206
sputum, 207
squamous cell, 159
Sri Lanka, 188, 217, 257
SRS, 265, 270
stable angina, 63
stages, 13, 36, 38, 73, 198, 199
stakeholders, 58
standard deviation, 289, 294
standard error, 263, 265
standardization, 260
standardized mortality ratio, 71
standards, 52, 56, 305, 311, 318, 324
statin, 129, 130, 132, 135
statins, 129, 130, 131
statistics, 21, 51, 54, 71, 122, 133, 212, 324
status of children, 200

STD, 50, 58, 59, 60, 174
stenotic lesions, 87, 88
stereotypes, 2, 49, 56, 76
stereotyping, 2
stigma, 49, 50, 51, 52, 54, 61
stigmatized, 49
stillbirth, 180, 181, 260, 277
stoma, 39
stomach, 33
strabismus, 181
strain, 170, 174, 187, 190, 227, 229, 231, 232, 233, 243, 247
strains, 166, 169, 170, 227, 228, 229, 231, 232, 233, 239, 240, 241, 242, 243, 244, 247, 249
strategies, 18, 19, 30, 48, 57, 58, 59, 78, 79, 85, 88, 107, 110, 144, 161, 163, 169, 172, 239, 273, 302, 304, 305, 311, 315, 316, 317, 318, 319, 321, 322, 324
stratification, 82
streams, 209
strength, 65, 67, 98, 293
stress, 64, 65, 75, 142, 143, 160, 284, 285
stressful events, 283
stressors, 72
stroke, 63, 70, 73, 85, 86, 87, 88, 89, 90, 91, 92, 93, 118, 119, 123, 133, 146, 147, 159, 297
strokes, 85, 86, 93, 118, 119
stroma, 198
strontium, 289
structural changes, 142
structural gene, 175
structural protein, 226, 232
students, 138, 139, 154, 246, 280
subacute, 198
subarachnoid hemorrhage, 90
subcutaneous tissue, 209
subgroups, 70, 82, 105, 129, 226, 241, 288, 321, 322
subjective, 324
submucosa, 37, 38
sub-Saharan Africa, 53, 54, 55, 115, 168, 184, 186, 187, 212, 216, 262
Sub-Saharan Africa, 217, 262
substance abuse, 48, 322
substance use, 2
substances, 63, 327
suburban, 282, 283, 297
Sudan, 115, 121, 193, 213
sudden infant death syndrome, 137, 156
Sudden Infant Death Syndrome (SIDS), 141
suffering, 152, 178
sugar, 196
suicidal, 284
suicidal behavior, 284
suicide, 268, 270, 271, 281, 285
sulfate, 185, 216
sulfur, 12
summer, 204, 297
supplemental, 206
supplements, 26, 44, 297, 300
supply, 130, 177, 226
suppression, 20
suppressor, 32, 209
Surgeon General, 140, 145, 154
surgery, 6, 16, 31, 38, 39, 40, 42, 43, 44, 76, 83, 163, 210, 273
surgical, 6, 15, 22, 32, 38, 39, 40, 78, 327
surgical resection, 39
surrogates, 232
surveillance, 8, 15, 35, 43, 166, 170, 172, 179, 228, 236, 237, 238, 239, 240, 242, 261, 265
survival, 6, 8, 13, 15, 16, 17, 21, 24, 25, 27, 28, 29, 39, 40, 42, 43, 101, 106, 159, 174, 186, 203, 261, 265
survival rate, 6, 15, 39, 42, 43
susceptibility, 8, 11, 22, 70, 72, 76, 90, 106, 146, 169, 171, 174, 181, 185, 191, 233, 243, 287
suspensions, 314
sustainability, 273
swelling, 209
symbiotic, 199
symptom, 211
symptoms, 6, 13, 36, 74, 82, 138, 140, 141, 142, 145, 146, 149, 151, 156, 158, 179, 182, 185, 186, 195, 196, 197, 200, 205, 207, 208, 210, 212, 226, 233, 240, 243, 253, 255, 256, 257, 266, 279, 280, 281, 282, 283, 284, 289
synchronous, 35, 38, 43, 207
syncytium, 185
syndrome, 35, 44, 70, 74, 95, 96, 97, 99, 100, 101, 102, 104, 105, 106, 107, 108, 109, 110, 140, 192, 203, 207, 208, 216
synthesis, 187, 240, 245
synthetic, 199
syphilis, 181
systematic, 14, 29, 44, 84, 131, 134, 150, 296, 330
systematic review, 29, 44, 84, 134, 150, 330
systems, 15, 57, 78, 148, 160, 228, 240, 260, 261, 265, 318, 319

T

T cells, 191, 201
T lymphocyte, 183
T regulatory cells, 185
tachycardia, 192
Tanzania, 115, 121, 216, 223, 269
tapeworm, 178, 211
target behavior, 322
target population, 299, 319, 321
targets, 51, 54, 151, 228, 239, 279, 316
task force, 278
taxation, 150, 153
taxonomy, 245
teachers, 246, 282
teaching, 173, 296, 317
Technology Assessment, 287
teen driving, 328
teenage girls, 49
teens, 314, 321, 323
Tehran, 113
telephone, 117, 281, 296, 321
television, 60, 107, 172
TEM, 41
temperate zone, 228
temperature, 200, 227, 232
temporal, 304
testosterone, 9, 10, 23, 290
testosterone levels, 9, 23, 290
text messaging, 322
textile, 147
Thai, 113, 120, 210, 306
Thailand, 113, 114, 120, 186, 188, 210, 213, 217, 218, 223, 233, 234, 237, 244
thawing, 235
theoretical, 151, 227, 323
theory, 88, 272, 319, 323
therapeutic, 6, 38, 48, 129
therapeutic relationship, 48
therapy, 6, 14, 15, 20, 38, 39, 40, 41, 43, 47, 53, 59, 74, 75, 78, 118, 127, 129, 130, 131, 135, 171, 173, 175, 182, 183, 191, 196, 224, 289, 290, 295, 296, 299, 302
third party, 151
thoracic, 168
thorax, 326
threat, 56
threatened, 261
threshold, 99, 102, 149
thresholds, 97, 98, 99, 101, 104, 105, 107, 294
throat, 140, 149, 192
thrombocytopenia, 181, 192, 193
thrombosis, 136
time, 8, 13, 14, 15, 18, 21, 27, 34, 35, 39, 40, 42, 48, 55, 57, 63, 70, 74, 75, 89, 97, 109, 117, 130, 132, 140, 142, 144, 146, 171, 178, 180, 186, 191, 196, 213, 250, 255, 261, 264, 266, 268, 279, 283, 291, 298, 304, 311, 312, 314, 323, 324
time constraints, 48
time consuming, 266
time periods, 255
timing, 186
tissue, 38, 92, 180, 182, 183, 189, 191, 193, 198, 200, 201, 205, 208, 244, 287
TMP, 197
tobacco, 137, 149, 151, 152, 153, 154, 155, 156, 157, 158, 159, 160, 161, 162, 254
tobacco smoke, 153, 154, 155, 156, 158, 159, 160
toddlers, 304
Togo, 115
tolerance, 118, 181, 216
toluene, 137
total cholesterol, 68, 89, 105, 126, 127, 129, 134, 135
toxemia, 270
toxic, 137, 142
toxicity, 150, 208
toxins, 141
Toxocara canis, 204
toxoplasmosis, 179, 180, 181, 182, 183, 184, 214, 215
traffic, 72, 268, 292, 303, 304, 305, 306, 307, 309, 310, 311, 312, 313, 315, 316, 317, 318, 319, 320, 321, 323, 324, 325, 327, 328, 329, 330
training, 48, 49, 273, 275, 317, 318, 320, 324
trans, 55
transcription, 10, 236, 246, 249
transcriptional, 10
transfer, 185, 188
transfusion, 184
transient ischemic attack, 89, 92
translation, 78, 236, 240
transmission, 48, 49, 50, 53, 54, 56, 57, 164, 166, 169, 170, 172, 173, 179, 180, 183, 184, 185, 186, 187, 188, 190, 193, 195, 196, 199, 200, 201, 203, 205, 207, 208, 214, 216, 217, 218, 219, 220, 223, 224, 229, 232, 245, 304

transplant, 207
transplantation, 118, 189
transport, 266, 269, 272, 273, 274, 275, 276, 304, 312, 327, 330
transportation, 90, 144, 150, 170, 299, 310, 311, 318, 319, 321
transurethral prostatectomy, 5
transurethral resection, 6
transverse colon, 39
trauma, 57, 72, 119, 202, 312, 319, 327
travel, 51, 178, 309, 311, 315, 316, 321, 325
travel time, 316
treatable, 126, 195
trend, 12, 50, 70, 76, 114, 250, 253, 261, 279, 295
trial, 1, 19, 29, 30, 39, 40, 42, 44, 130, 135, 222, 229, 248, 299
tribes, 305
trichuriasis, 200, 203, 222
triglycerides, 70, 71, 77, 83, 87, 103, 105, 126, 127, 129
tropical areas, 184, 192
trucks, 304, 305, 309, 312, 313, 318
trypanosomiasis, 218
trypsin, 244
tuberculosis, 163, 164, 166, 167, 169, 171, 172, 173, 174, 175, 177, 268, 269, 271, 274
tubular, 35
tumor, 5, 6, 11, 13, 14, 19, 27, 32, 36, 37, 38, 39, 40, 41, 42
tumor growth, 6
tumor progression, 32
tumorigenesis, 12
tumors, 6, 8, 9, 36, 38, 39, 41, 42, 143, 146
Tunisia, 114, 115, 121, 193, 213
turkeys, 235
turnover, 297
twins, 180, 214
type 1 diabetes, 116
type 2 diabetes, 80, 81, 95, 96, 97, 98, 100, 106, 107, 111, 116, 117, 120, 122
type 2 diabetes mellitus, 95, 106, 120, 122

U

ubiquitous, 179, 185, 236
UDP-glucuronosyltransferase, 26
Uganda, 7, 8, 21, 51, 59
ulcer, 120
ulceration, 124, 208
ulcerative colitis, 33
ultrasonography, 5, 38, 70, 181, 183
ultrasound, 43
ultra-thin, 197
umbilical cord, 141, 182, 217
umbilical cord blood, 182, 217
UN General Assembly, 52
uncertainty, 107
unclassified, 88
unemployment, 167
UNESCO, 60
UNFPA, 276
UNICEF, 276
uninsured, 75
United Nations (UN), 1, 52, , 53, 54, 55, 217, 259
United States, vi, 7, 8, 23, 27, 28, 29, 32, 47, 50, 55, 57, 58, 59, 60, 65, 73, 79, 80, 81, 85, 90, 91, 93, 96, 101, 103, 116, 117, 118, 119, 122, 125, 133, 155, 164, 172, 173, 174, 180, 215, 218, 233, 244, 249, 253, 279, 284, 292, 293, 294, 300, 301, 303, 304, 305, 306, 307, 309, 310, 312, 313, 319, 321, 324, 325, 326, 327, 328, 329
universities, 19, 147, 280
unstable angina, 63, 75
urban, 102, 110, 113, 114, 115, 116, 120, 121, 157, 159, 168, 175, 193, 203, 208, 211, 248, 254, 255, 274, 275, 281, 284, 296, 297, 300, 310, 311, 313, 321, 322, 325, 330
urban areas, 115, 116, 274, 310, 313
urban population, 114, 115, 120, 274, 281
urbanization, 103, 106, 115, 116, 253
urinary, 6, 13, 33, 41, 139, 140, 155, 212
urinary bladder, 212
urinary dysfunction, 6
urinary tract, 13, 33
urine, 113, 142, 155, 157, 183, 212
URL, 79, 174
Uruguay, 116, 211, 224, 231
US Department of Health and Human Services, 154
users, 273, 315, 317
uterus, 141, 268

V

vaccination, 228, 229, 240, 250
vaccine, 177, 219, 226, 228, 229, 232, 240, 241, 243, 248, 250
vaccines, 228, 229, 240, 241, 242
vacuole, 198

vagina, 204
vaginal, 53, 272
validation, 109
validity, 298, 299, 325
values, 13, 27, 49, 68, 76, 97, 99, 100, 105, 106, 126, 127, 131, 188, 267, 293, 294
variability, 77, 85, 99, 149, 157, 160, 183, 236, 300
variable, 72, 100, 208, 211
variables, 21, 22, 74, 100, 126, 133, 225, 280, 293, 296, 323
variance, 9, 280, 282, 283
variation, 10, 11, 12, 14, 24, 25, 26, 77, 83, 88, 109, 148, 159, 169, 174, 189, 223, 243, 249, 257, 285, 324
vascular, 38, 131, 136, 149
vascular disease, 131
vasoconstriction, 141
vector, 177, 178, 190, 191, 200, 304
vegetables, 65, 180, 201
vegetarianism, 169
vehicles, 152, 303, 305, 309, 310, 311, 313, 316, 317, 318, 319, 326
vehicular, 242, 245, 318
velocity, 107
Venezuela, 105, 111, 212, 237, 242, 247
ventilation, 141, 142, 148, 151, 160, 161
ventricular, 87, 88
venue, 2
very low density lipoprotein, 71
vessels, 77, 198, 204
veterans, 74, 81, 178
victims, 312, 319
Vietnam, 113, 165, 178, 203, 213
Vietnamese, 66
village, 114, 268
violence, 49, 54, 55, 56, 61, 284, 322
violent, 55
viral, 53, 225, 226, 231, 232, 233, 239, 240, 242, 244, 245, 246, 248, 255, 256, 269
viral gastroenteritis, 240, 246, 248
viral hepatitis, 269
viral infection, 255
virology, 241
virulence, 181, 191, 231
virus, 168, 169, 174, 225, 226, 228, 229, 231, 232, 233, 236, 238, 239, 240, 243, 244, 250, 254, 257
virus infection, 174, 236, 238, 243
viruses, 178, 215, 225, 227, 231, 232, 233, 235, 236, 238, 239, 240, 243, 244, 246, 250, 257
viscera, 189, 204, 206
visible, 316, 318, 323
vision, 278, 318
visual, 181, 184, 296, 321
visual acuity, 181, 296
visual images, 321
visualization, 34, 203
vitamin A, 202
vitamin C, 34, 143, 157
vitamin D, 11, 25, 169, 174, 289, 290, 297, 300, 302
Vitamin D, 169, 289, 290, 297
vitamin D deficiency, 174, 290
vitamin D receptor (VDR), 11, 25, 169, 174
vitamin E, 26
VLDL, 77
volvulus, 209
vomiting, 36, 192, 207, 210, 226, 240
voters, 153
vulnerability, 55
vulva, 204

W

walking, 296, 310, 321
war, 56, 178, 266
war on terror, 56
warfarin, 89
warrants, 48
water, 177, 178, 179, 195, 197, 203, 212, 226, 232, 243
weakness, 98
wealth, 114, 311
wear, 314, 317
weight loss, 36, 141, 191, 192, 196, 207
well-being, 2, 305, 331
West Africa, 66, 115, 121, 169, 174, 217
West Bank, 193, 219
West Indies, 86, 92
western countries, 86, 89
wheeze, 141, 142, 145, 146, 158, 253, 254, 255, 257
wheezing, 142, 201, 205, 255, 256, 257
white blood cell count, 202
white blood cell differential, 203, 204
white women, 117, 281, 282, 285, 288, 297, 300, 302
winter, 238, 297
work environment, 148

workers, 49, 53, 55, 56, 138, 147, 148, 149, 152, 160, 161, 268, 273, 281, 282, 316
working conditions, 73
working population, 138, 149, 151
working women, 138
workplace, 138, 143, 144, 146, 147, 148, 149, 150, 151, 154, 160
World Bank, 277
World Development Report, 277
World Health Organization (WHO), 49, 50, 51, 55, 60, 61, 95, 96, 97, 99, 102, 103, 104, 108, 115, 121, 139, 151, 153, 154, 161, 212, 214, 216, 217, 259, 260, 262, 263, 265, 266, 272, 276, 278, 287, 288, 289, 293
World War, 178
World War I, 178
World War II, 178
worm, 177, 199, 200, 202, 203, 204, 205, 206, 208, 209, 212
worms, 179, 199, 200, 201, 202, 203, 204, 206, 207, 209, 210, 222

X

xenograft, 8, 21
x-ray, 38, 43, 189, 287
X-ray, 289

Y

Yemen, 209
yield, 19, 36, 43, 149, 182, 294, 321
young adults, 91, 106, 109, 111, 160, 192, 197, 289, 294, 304, 329
young men, 49, 60, 208
young women, 49, 53, 54
younger children, 139, 142

Z

Zimbabwe, 8, 51
zoning, 315
zoonosis, 224
zoonotic infections, 210